The Underactive Bladder

Michael B. Chancellor • Ananias C. Diokno
Editors

The Underactive Bladder

Springer

Editors
Michael B. Chancellor
Department of Urology
Oakland University William Beaumont
School of Medicine
Royal Oak, MI
USA

Ananias C. Diokno
Department of Urology
Oakland University William Beaumont
School of Medicine
Royal Oak, MI
USA

ISBN 978-3-319-23686-5 ISBN 978-3-319-23687-2 (eBook)
DOI 10.1007/978-3-319-23687-2

Library of Congress Control Number: 2015956541

Springer Cham Heidelberg New York Dordrecht London

Printed on acid-free paper

Springer International Publishing AG Switzerland is part of Springer Science+Business Media (www.springer.com)

Foreword

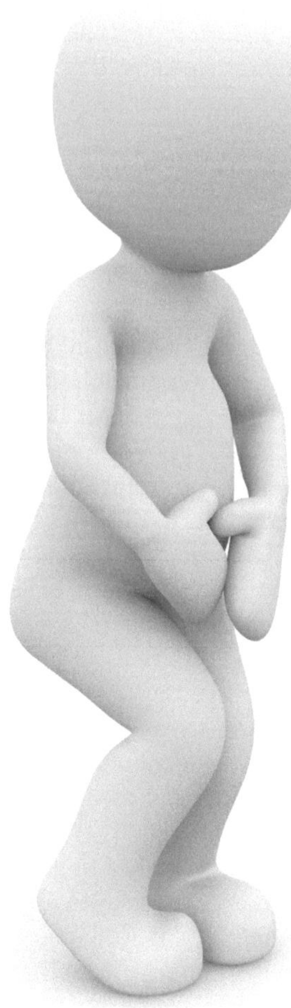

While most practitioners are familiar with overactive bladder (OAB), the converse condition of underactive bladder has generally remained far below the radar. Yet if you have known anyone struggling with underactive bladder (UAB), you are keenly aware of the suffering they and their family endure. Underactive bladder is a life-altering condition that dramatically effects a patient's and his or her family's lives.

UAB is a name given to a group of troubling symptoms including hesitancy, weak and or interrupted urine stream, straining, incomplete bladder emptying, and frequent urination or leakage due to overflow incontinence. The symptoms and severity of UAB vary between patients, and the course of the disease is often unpredictable. UAB is a multifactorial condition that can be caused by myogenic and neurogenic conditions as well as aging and medication side effects.

UAB is closely related to detrusor underactivity, which is a clinical and specific urodynamic definition. Detrusor underactivity due to impaired detrusor contractility is the most classic pathology of the underactive bladder. Diseases such as diabetes and heart disease or conditions that cause peripheral nerve damage are culprits of UAB also. And although many others are known, the scientific community has of yet been unable to create a working pathogenesis, let alone a standardized clinical definition.

A recent study highlighted the levels of prevalence and lack of awareness of underactive bladder in the general population. The survey revealed that 23 % of men and women reported having a problem emptying the bladder completely, yet only 11 % had ever heard of UAB (Chap. 1).

The most common method to manage UAB is to treat the urine retention mechanically with intermittent self-catheterization and indwelling catheter as there is no currently available treatment to restore normal voiding function. Intermittent self-catheterization and indwelling catheterization. This "solution" results in high expenses, infections, and pain. The complications of catheterization can lead to emergency room visits and hospitalization; embarrassment and even admission into nursing homes; and a severe reduction in quality of life (Chap. 5). Catheters are associated with blockage, dislodgement, bleeding, strictures, leakages, and excess healthcare costs, and complications affect quality of life. Recurrent infections and antibiotic use have been associated with drug-resistant superbug catheter-associated epidemic.

The problem of UAB is big and getting bigger with the aging population and rapidly increasing rate of diabetes that may result in diabetic bladder dysfunction. Lacking effective therapy for UAB, general urologists have hardly noticed the elephant in the room. A quick search on PubMed noted 40-fold less publication in UAB versus OAB (Chancellor and Diokno 2014). It is our hope that this first book on the underactive bladder will be the catalyst to generating interest in this condition that can lead to rapid advancement in education, research, and, ultimately, a cure for this life-altering condition.

The book is written in a concise, uniform, and clinically relevant style edited by two leading pioneers in the field, Drs. Michael Chancellor and Ananias Diokno, who organized the First International Congress on Underactive Bladder in 2014.

The landmark meeting, CURE-UAB, was organized by Drs. Chancellor and Diokno from Beaumont Health System and Oakland University William Beaumont School of Medicine in Michigan in conjunction with the National Institute of Aging and the Underactive Bladder Foundation (www.underactivebladder.org). The Second International Congress on CURE-UAB will be held in Denver in December 2015.

The first book devoted to underactive bladder is designed to be of practical assistance to all doctors and nurses wishing to help improve the lives of UAB patients. This book discusses in detail the pathophysiology and research being conducted toward a cure. Practical evaluation and management with reviews of the latest clinical series are highlighted. *The Underactive Bladder* will be of interest to all clinicians who take care of patients with bladder emptying problems.

Sincerely,

Michael B. Chancellor, MD
Ananias C. Diokno, MD

Reference

Chancellor MB, Diokno AC (2014) Frontier in urology; the underactive bladder. Int Urol Nephrol 46(Suppl 1):S1–S46

Preface

The condition of the underactive bladder is important and a major unmet need in medicine. Although the term underactive bladder (UAB) seems new, looking back, we realize that we have been researching this topic most of our career. One of us (AD) has been performing National Institute of Health research on the aging bladder since the 1980s, and the other (MC) has been researching stem cell and regenerative medicine to restore bladder function for urinary retention and stress incontinence since the 1990s.

It is only over the past 2 years that the term underactive bladder has become widely accepted and momentum is building for UAB to become a top priority in urology research over the next decade. We believe the First International Congress for Underactive Bladder (CURE-UAB), sponsored by the Aikens Center for Neurourology Research at Beaumont Health System, the Underactive Bladder Foundation, and the National Institute of Aging, was the catalyst that captured the global scientific community's interest in UAB. The First International CURE-UAB was held in February 2014 in Washington, DC. The second international meeting is to be held in December 2015 in Denver, CO.

As a result of the first meeting in Washington, DC, a special issue of *International Urology and Nephrology*, Volume 46, Supplement 1, pages 1–46, was published discussing disease definition, clinical guidelines, therapeutic directions, and suitable animal models to allow accurate testing of potential therapeutic candidates for UAB. Additional professional material and videos remain available online (www. nderactivebladder.org). Another major outcome of the international meeting is the Program Announcement by the National Institutes of Health in December 2014 requesting new grant applications that focus on UAB (PA-15-049 Underactive Bladder in Aging) by the National Institute on Aging (http://www.nia.nih.gov) and National Institute of Diabetes and Digestive and Kidney Diseases (http://www.niddk.nih.gov). We are delighted and proud of the accomplishments of CURE-UAB.

The need for education was also identified at CURE-UAB and is why we have written this book. There are researchers, physicians, nurses, and many other healthcare professionals in the world dedicated to finding answers to both the cause and effective treatments for those who experience symptoms of underactive bladder. It was our goal to bring together these thought leaders and write this book to educate the medical community and to ultimately help improve the lives of patients living with UAB

Royal Oak, MI, USA

Michael B. Chancellor, MD
Ananias C. Diokno, MD

Acknowledgment

As we have traveled this path to bring much-needed attention to the international medical community about the underactive bladder (UAB) condition, we have been helped and supported by a long list of friends and colleagues. We may not be able to acknowledge you individually here, but please know your conversation, email, or encouragement has been invaluable.

First of all, we would like to thank all of the authors who have contributed to this important book. We would also like to thank the incredible people who participated in the successful First International Congress for Underactive Bladder (CURE-UAB) in Washington, DC, in 2014 and those who will be joining us for the Second International CURE-UAB in Denver, CO, in December 2015.

On the national and international stage, we are much appreciative of the work and support from the Underactive Bladder Foundation, the National Institutes of Health and the Urology Care Foundation.

Both of us are physicians and researchers at Beaumont Health System in Michigan, and it is with the support of Beaumont that we were able to vanguard the global initiative on CURE-UAB. We would like to recognize Bob and Ann Aikens for their generous support and the formation of the Aikens Neurourology Research Center at Beaumont Health System and Oakland University William Beaumont School of Medicine. Some of the members of the Aikens Center and those who contribute daily to its success include Margaret Casey, Bill Dow, Laura Lamb, Peter Levanovich, Andrew Vereecke, and Bernadette Zwaans. We would like to show our appreciation for our department faculty and staff for their support including Kenneth Peters, Debbie Hasenau, Kim Killinger, Shelly Lajiness, Ann Robinson, Jason Gilleran, Melissa Fischer, Sarah Bartolone and Jennifer Bowlus. We like to thank Janet Okonski and Margie O'Leary for their editorial assistance and Ryan Pruchnic, Ron Jankowski, Jaclyn Mycka and members of Cook Myosite for their research support. We like to especially recognize Ronald and Maureen Hirsch for their friendship and help. Finally, we like to thank the member of the faculty of the Oakland University William Beaumont School of Medicine and Beaumont Health.

We would finally like to thank our family for allowing us to take time out to write this book on an important topic for which we are very passionate.

Thank you.

Michael B. Chancellor, MD
Ananias C. Diokno, MD

Contents

Contributors

Editors

Michael B. Chancellor, MD Department of Urology, Aikens Research Center, Oakland University William Beaumont School of Medicine, Rochester, MI, USA

Neurourology Program, Beaumont Health System, Royal Oak, MI, USA

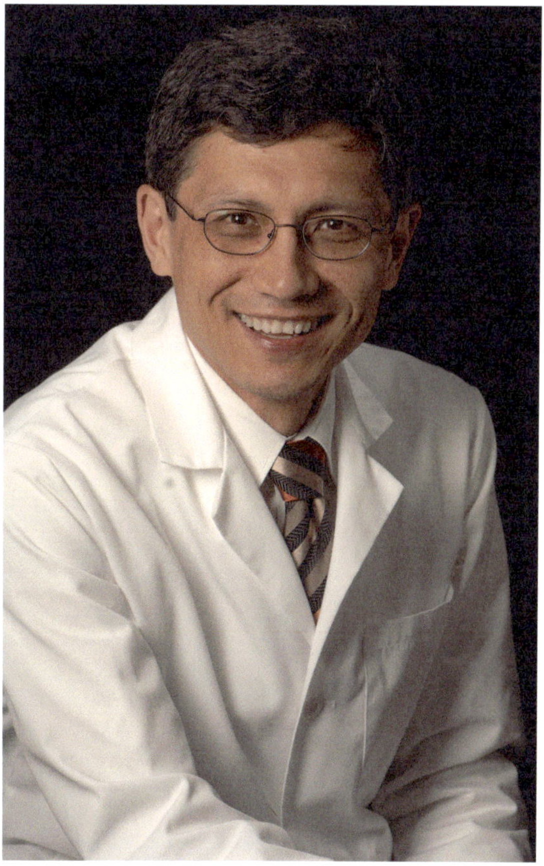

Ananias C. Diokno, MD Department of Urology, Oakland University William Beaumont School of Medicine, Rochester, MI, USA

Beaumont Health System, Royal Oak, MI, USA

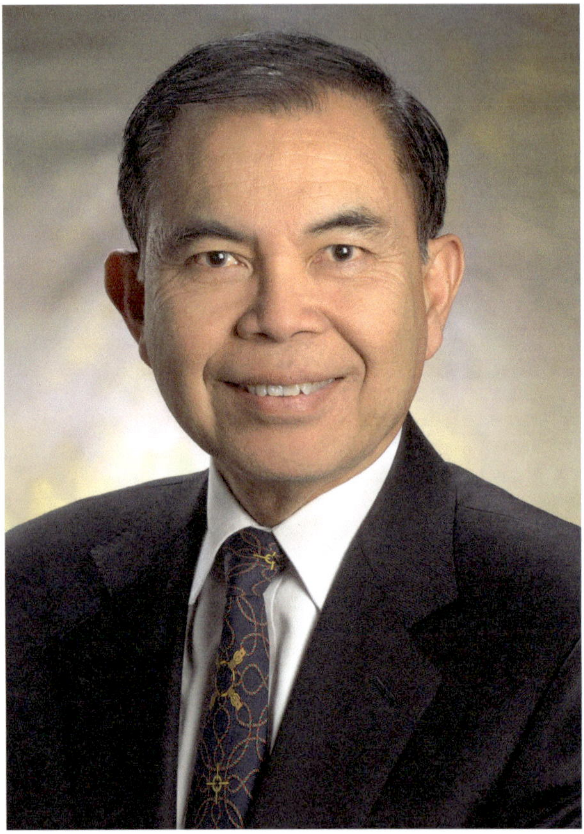

Authors

Marcus A. Austenfeld, MD Department of Urology, School of Medicine, The University of Kansas, Kansas City, KS, USA

David D. Chancellor, BS Executive Director, The Underactive Bladder Foundation, Pittsburgh, PA, USA

Yao-Chi Chuang, MD Department of Urology, Kaohsiung Chang Gung Memorial Hospital, Chang Gung University College of Medicine, Kaohsiung, Taiwan

Tomas L. Griebling, MD, MPH Department of Urology, School of Medicine, The Landon Center on Aging, The University of Kansas, Kansas City, KS, USA

Israel Franco, MD Section of Pediatric Urology, New York Medical College, International Children's Continence Society, Maria Fareri Children's Hospital, Valhalla, NY, USA

Mahendra Pratap Kashyap, PhD Department of Urology, University of Pittsburgh School of Medicine, Pittsburgh, PA, USA

Michelle J. Lajiness, FNP-BC Department of Urology, Aiken Neurourology Research Center, Urology Associates, Beaumont Health, Royal Oak, MI, USA

En Meng, MD, D Phil Division of Urology, Department of Surgery, Tri-Service General Hospital, Taipei, Taiwan

National Defense Medical Center, Taipei, Taiwan

Janet Okonski, BS Department of Urology, University of Pittsburgh School of Medicine, Pittsburgh, PA, USA

Margie O'Leary, RN, MSN, MSCN Department of Neurology, UPMC Multiple Sclerosis Clinic, University of Pittsburgh School of Medicine, Pittsburgh, PA, USA

Hikaru Tomoe, MD, PhD Department of Urology and Pelvic Reconstructive Surgery, Tokyo Women's Medical University, Tokyo, Japan

Pradeep Tyagi, PhD Department of Urology, University of Pittsburgh School of Medicine, Pittsburgh, PA, USA

Naoki Yoshimura, MD, PhD Departments of Urology and Pharmacology & Chemical Biology, University of Pittsburgh School of Medicine, Pittsburgh, PA, USA

Chapter 1
Epidemiology and Demographics of Underactive Bladder

Michael B. Chancellor

Introduction

Underactive bladder (UAB) is a term clinically under recognized due to a lack of consensus on terminology and insufficient standardization of diagnostic criteria. Yet, despite its limited clinical recognition, the breadth of the effect of UAB should not be underestimated. Lower urinary tract dysfunction is especially prevalent among the elderly population, and as the population continues to grow older in all the developed countries, the number of people affected by underactive bladder and the associated costs will dramatically escalate over the next decade (Chancellor and Diokno 2014; Chancellor and Kaufman 2008; van Koeveringe et al. 2011; Miyazato et al. 2013).

While a variety of descriptors, symptom constellations, and related terms have been used regarding bladder emptying problems; the only formal definition for the underactive bladder is provided by the International Continence Society (ICS). Detrusor underactivity (DU) is defined by the ICS as "a contraction of reduced strength and/or duration, resulting in prolonged bladder emptying and/or a failure to achieve complete bladder emptying within a normal time span (Abrams et al. 2002)."

Solid epidemiology is dependent on accurate and precise definition of disease of entity studied. The ICS definition serves as an excellent starting point. Unclear or inaccurate definitions lead to over- or underestimation of incidence and prevalence of medical disease. Moreover, the astute clinician should always keep in mind the clinically relevant question: "Does incidence and prevalence equate to significance."

M.B. Chancellor, MD
Department of Urology, Aikens Research Center, Oakland University William Beaumont School of Medicine, Rochester, MI, USA

Neurourology Program, Beaumont Health System, Royal Oak, MI, USA
e-mail: Michael.Chancellor@beaumont.edu

M.B. Chancellor, A.C. Diokno (eds.), *The Underactive Bladder*,
DOI 10.1007/978-3-319-23687-2_1

A number of conditions complicate the picture of UAB and DU. Research indicates that age-related changes and bladder outlet obstruction are common but difficult to distinguish from underactive bladder. The symptoms of UAB range from physically bothersome to socially restrictive and include straining, incontinence, and loss of bladder sensation. Nuotio et al. (2003) reported that incontinence is an important predictor of institutionalization in the elderly. Diagnosis of UAB and DU based upon clinical symptoms is complex (Taylor et al. 2006). A recently published paper by Osman et al. reviewed the current understanding of UAB and concluded that attempts at redefinition must address the limitations of the ICS definition as well as the inability to distinguish DU from other LUTS on the basis of symptoms alone (Osman et al. 2014).

There is a wide range of prevalence values across clinical studies and patient populations. Diokno et al. (1986) found that 22 % of men and 11 % of women over 60 years age had difficulties with bladder emptying. Taylor et al. (2006) found detrusor underactivity (often secondary to impaired contractility) in two-thirds of incontinent institutionalized patients. Abarbanel and Marcus (2007) reported 48 % of men aged >70 years ($n=82$) and 12 % of women aged >70 years ($n=99$) had UAB. Jeong et al. (2012) reported 40 % of men aged >65 years ($n=632$) and 13 % of women aged >65 years ($n=547$) had UAB. UAB and increased post-void residual volume (PVR) have been reported to be associated with aging (DuBeau 2006; Malone-Lee and Wahedna 1993).

Defining Urinary Retention, Detrusor Underactivity, and Underactive Bladder

National Library of Medicine: *Urinary Retention* as:

- Inability to empty the urinary bladder with voiding (urination)
- Incomplete emptying of the bladder

International Continence Society: Detrusor Underactivity (Abrams et al. 2002) as:

- A contraction of reduced strength and/or duration, resulting in prolonged bladder emptying and/or a failure to achieve complete bladder emptying within a normal time span

European Urology 2015 Underactive Bladder (Chapple et al. 2015) working definition as:

The underactive bladder is a symptom complex suggestive of detrusor underactivity and is usually characterized by prolonged urination time with or without a sensation of incomplete bladder emptying, usually with hesitancy, reduced sensation on filling, and a slow stream.

ICD-10-CM (United States), diagnosis code R33.9 *Retention of Urine* as:

- A disorder characterized by accumulation of urine within the bladder because of the inability to urinate

The Underactive Bladder Foundation (www.underactivebladder.org) working terminology: *Underactive Bladder Syndrome* as:

- Urinary symptoms including hesitancy, straining, and incomplete bladder emptying in the absence of anatomic obstruction

Lower Urinary Tract Overactive and Underactive Bladder Symptoms

We need to apply to UAB research what we learned from OAB research when the known prevalence of symptoms based on well-designed clinical trials is high (Irwin et al. 2006). Most clinicians know from years of clinical care that the majority of OAB patients, even with symptoms, do not seek medical intervention. As reported, the prevalence of OAB is 30 million versus less than 5 million with treatment seeking behavior. Therefore, as we advance in UAB, we need to distinguish between clearly defined syndrome and true significance.

Lower urinary tract symptoms (LUTS) including OAB and UAB exert both an economic and emotional toll. Studies have found that urinary incontinence is a significant prognostic indicator of institutionalization among older adults (Nuotio et al. 2003). The symptoms of UAB and DU, including straining, urinary incontinence, and loss of bladder sensation, range from physically bothersome to socially restrictive (Fry et al. 2011). The clinical features of UAB and DU are sometimes indistinguishable from other lower urinary tract diseases. Urinary flow rate is used as a screening test for bladder outlet obstruction (BOO), but a slow flow rate and increased residual urine volume are common to both BOO and UAB/DU (see Chap. 3).

Urinary Retention: Acute and Chronic

Urinary retention is an important term that has significant insurance value. And yet urinary retention is, if carefully considered, a nonspecific term that can be either restricted to complete inability to urinate or encompass inadequate bladder emptying with large post-void residual volume.

Acute urinary retention such as immediately after a surgical procedure with anesthesia and narcotics that resolves after a few hours and a single catheterization is not within the scope of UAB or DU. Chronic urinary retention is more consistent with the definition of UAB. Chronic urinary retention has been defined by the ICS as a post-void residual (PVR) >300 mL or rather committing to an absolute volume, stating that it is a non-painful bladder, which remains palpable after the patient has passed urine (Abrams et al. 2002).

Epidemiology Based on Symptoms Perspectives

Valente et al. (2014) reported a large epidemiology survey in the United States regarding urinary symptoms with UAB. Men and women aged 60 and above received the self-administered questionnaire via mail. The mailing list was randomly generated by an independent third party, and "difficulty completely emptying" the bladder was used as an indication for UAB.

A total of 633 subjects (13 %) returned the survey, and respondents ranged from 33 to 92 years old, though 97 % were aged 60 and above, with a mean of 74.3 years and a median age of 74. Distributions were similar between the two sexes (54 % men, 46 % women). Nearly one-quarter (23 %, $n=137$) of respondents reported difficulty emptying his/her bladder (DESx), yet only 11 % ($n=70$) had ever heard of UAB. There was no significant association between DESx and gender ($p=0.079$) or age ($p=0.075$) (Fig. 1.1). While 52 % of all respondents reported never having to strain to empty their bladder, the other 48 % recounted needing to push, bear down, or strain to empty, at least rarely to very often.

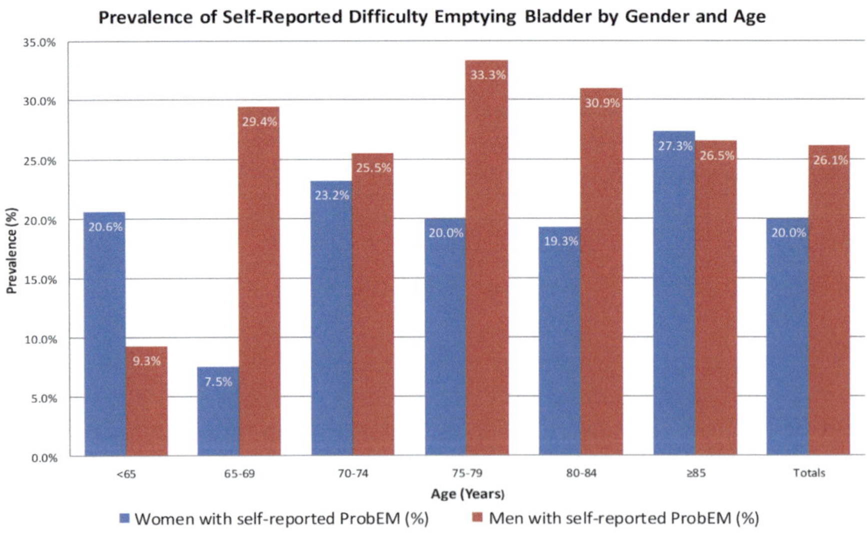

Fig. 1.1 Prevalence of self-reported difficulty emptying bladder by gender and age (Permission obtained Valente et al. 2014)

Table 1.1 Self-reported coexisting conditions related to underactive bladder

Characteristic/question	UAB question positive[a]	UAB question negative	N
Q3: Do you have any of the following problems? *(check all that apply)*	*N (%)*		
Diabetes[b]	39 (34.5)	74	113
Stroke[b]	8 (40.0)	12	20
Cancer[b]	14 (29.8)	33	47
Parkinson's	0 (0.0)	5	5
Heart disease	27 (25.5)	79	106
Multiple sclerosis	2 (28.6)	5	7
None	40 (16.1)	208	248
Others[b]	47 (27.8)	122	169

Permission obtained Valente et al. (2014)
[a]Answers yes to question, "Do you ever have difficulty emptying your bladder?"
[b]$p < 0.05$

A number of coexisting conditions have been implicated in UAB development and progression. The DESx group was more likely to report diabetes, stroke, and recurrent bladder infections ≥3 per year (Table 1.1). Additionally, women with a history of hysterectomy or prolapse/incontinence surgery were significantly more likely to have difficulty with bladder emptying. UAB was more common in men with prior prostate surgery.

Persons reporting UAB symptoms were twice as likely to describe their health as "poor" or "fair" compared to those without the complaint (26 % vs 12 %, $p < 0.001$). Those with difficulty emptying their bladder were 70 % more likely to describe their health as "poor" or "fair" than expected (Valente et al. 2014). According to an epidemiologic survey on LUTS in Japan (Homma et al. 2006) of 10,096 men and women 40 years old or older and the analysis of responses from 4,570 subjects (effective collection rate 45 %), prevalence rates for slow stream more than once a week were 37 % in men, 18 % in women, and 27.0 % in the overall population. Prevalence rates for slow stream more than once a day were 28 % in men, 13 % in women, and 20 % in the overall population. Similarly, the prevalence rates for feeling of incomplete emptying more than once a week were 26 % in men, 10 % in women, and 18 % in the overall population.

Epidemiology Based on Urodynamic Perspectives

Abarbanel and Marcus (2007) reported a study of 181 community-dwelling elderly with LUTS identified impaired detrusor contractility (IDC) in urodynamic studies in 48 % of men and 12 % of women. Of the men in this study, 40 % were found to have concomitant bladder outlet obstruction (BOO); 10 % of those with IDC had BOO. 16 % were found to have IDC in the absence of involuntary contractions or obstruction of the bladder outlet

A recent study by Jeong et al. (2012) examined the prevalence of DU in 1,179 elderly men and women aged over 65 years with nonneurogenic voiding dysfunction presenting with LUTS and found that upwards of 40 % of men and 13.3 % of women met urodynamic parameters for DU, and the numbers increased with age in both groups.

Studies based on urodynamic parameters suggest the prevalence of DU is higher among men than women. In addition, the presence of bladder outlet obstruction, diabetes, neurologic diseases, and retention complicates the picture and appears to be positively associated with UAB. These studies imply that DU is common and morbid, yet the true prevalence remains largely unknown.

Bladder Outlet Obstruction and UAB

The relationship between BOO and UAB/DU is poorly understood and complex. Not all men with BOO develop UAB/DU and similarly not all men with UAB/DU have BOO (Thomas et al. 2005). Detrusor contractility is commonly and irreversibly impaired due to chronic BOO and may persist even after the obstruction is relieved. Following 69 men for over a decade diagnosed with DU (Qmax <15 ml/s, Pdet@Qmax <40 cmH_2O) and initially managed with watchful waiting, Thomas et al. (2005) found no significant deterioration in symptomatic or urodynamic parameters over time. Only eleven patients (16 %) failed the initial watchful waiting approach and underwent prostate surgery, 8 (12 %) due to worsening symptoms and 3 (4 %) due to acute retention. The authors concluded that DU is not progressive in the majority of men and an initial conservative approach may be justified.

BOO as the primary cause of UAB in women is uncommon, occurring in 3 % of those referred for urodynamic studies from a general population (Massey and Abrams 1988). Cases of BOO in women are probably associated with pelvic floor dysfunction/spasticity and cause such as Fowler's syndrome (Fowler et al. 1988). Anatomical BOO in women may be iatrogenic after pelvic prolapse and anti-incontinence surgery or pelvic organ prolapse, urethral stricture, and urethral diverticula.

Association Between OAB and UAB (Fig. 1.2)

- Both OAB and UAB are common in older patients.
- Both are syndromes with shared symptoms including frequency and nocturia.
- Both can occur together – detrusor hyperreflexia impaired contractility (DHIC).
- Both are associated with common underlying etiologies – bladder outlet obstruction, neurological diseases, e.g., diabetes mellitus.

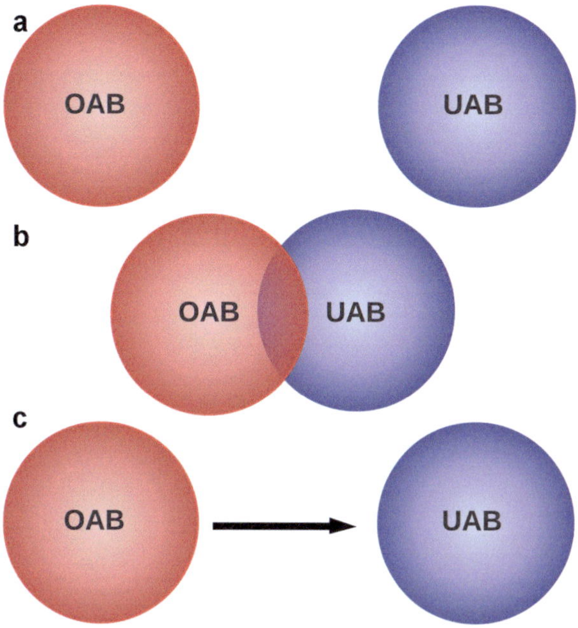

Fig. 1.2 Several ways to consider the relationship between the overactive bladder (*OAB*) and underactive bladder (*UAB*). (**a**) OAB and UAB as separate conditions; (**b**) OAB and UAB as overlapping syndromes; (**c**) OAB may progress to UAB (Permission obtained Chancellor 2014)

Skeletal muscle sarcopenia increases with aging, and impaired bladder emptying is also associated with increasing age in both men and women (Cucchi et al. 2008; Madersbacher et al. 1998; Malone-Lee and Wahedna 1993). It has also been established that impaired bladder emptying is often associated with detrusor overactivity with or without bladder outflow obstruction (Resnick and Yalla 1987; Elbadawi et al. 1993). Detrusor hyperreflexia impaired contractility (DHIC) is a common and important finding based on urodynamic studies in both healthy and symptomatic elderly (Ameda et al. 1999) (Fig. 1.3). Griffiths et al. (2007) noted the coincidental occurrence and overlap of OAB and UAB with different etiological factors. Histological studies including electron microscopic analysis detected age-related change in the bladder associated with both detrusor overactivity and underactivity in DHIC patients (Elbadawi et al. 1993).

Chronic untreated or treatment refractory OAB – be it due to neurological diseases such as diabetes, bladder outlet obstruction, or aging sarcopenia and frailty – may progress to DHIC and finally UAB. The progression of OAB to UAB hypothesis suggests that early education, behavioral modification, and medical treatment may alter and prevent the progression to UAB (Fig. 1.4) (Chancellor 2014).

Mechanisms of UAB; that may apply to OAB include:

- Aging: slow decline in neural and non-neural functions due to degeneration of cells or random cellular damage and genetic aging programs

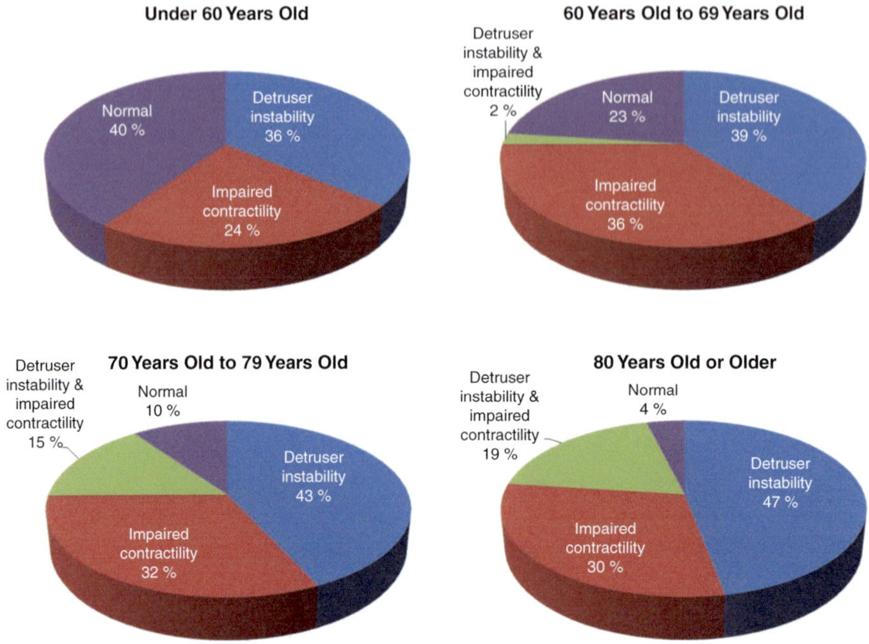

Fig. 1.3 Distribution of urodynamic diagnoses relative to age (Adapted from Ameda et al. 1999). Incidence of detrusor instability with impaired contractility increases, while proportion of patients without urodynamic abnormalities decreases in men older than 70 years (Permission obtained Chancellor 2014)

- Neural: injuries or diseases affecting the central or peripheral nervous system
- Non-neural: diseases affecting bladder smooth muscle, urothelium, interstitial cells, or connective tissue

How does the transfiguration of OAB to UAB happen? Chronic muscular overactivity in OAB may lead to muscle fatigue, or progressive ischemia, inflammation, and oxidative damage caused by factors of OAB can lead to hypocontractility (Chancellor 2014). Studies have demonstrated that the bladder wall thickens with increased mass with OAB (Ukimura et al. 2003) and that urine nerve growth factor levels escalate (Kim and Park 2006).

Decreased bladder sensations may also be a more common cause of UAB than previously reported. Efferent nerve activity stimulates and maintains the detrusor contraction depending on sensory input (Smith 2010; Griffiths et al. 2007). Urethral afferent neurons may also be important for sensory feedback during voiding to maintain micturition and efficient bladder emptying (Shafik et al. 2003). Abnormalities of the urothelium, interstitial cells, ganglia, and smooth muscle cells which form a sensor-transducer system that activates afferent nerve fibers may be a more common cause than previously suspected (Collas and Malone-Lee 1996; Smith 2010).

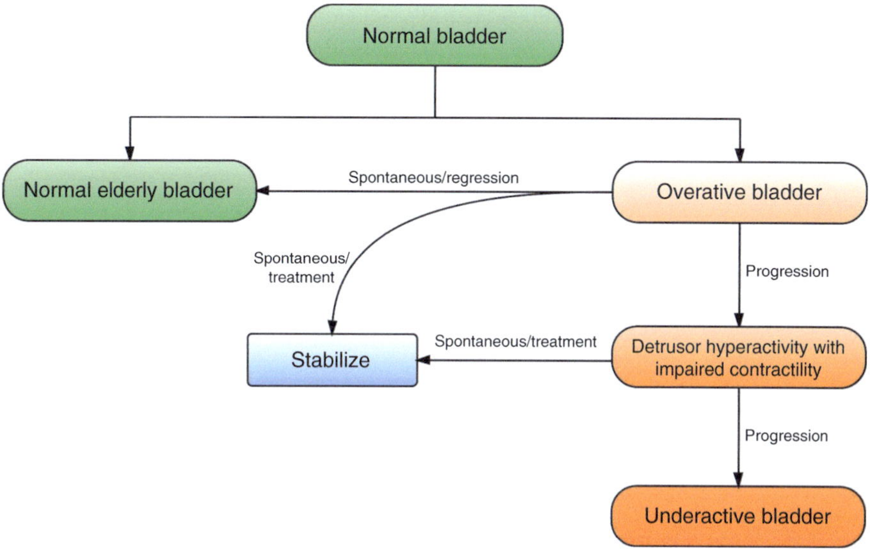

Fig. 1.4 The OAB to UAB hypothesis: patients with chronic untreated or treatment refractory overactive bladder have a significant risk of progression to underactive bladder (Permission obtained Chancellor 2014)

Underactive Bladder Nursing Perspective

There are excellent epidemiology studies of catheter treatment-associated complications that would be beneficial for those interested in the UAB. The use of intermittent or indwelling catheters in patients with UAB contributes to catheter-associated urinary tract infection, encrustation, urethral stricture, dislodgment, and leakage of urine (Subcommittee WSCPC 2009). Catheter-related complications also contribute to excess health-care costs and compromise quality of life (Wilde et al. 2013a). In a study, 202 long-term indwelling catheter users reported having experienced the following problems: 31 % infection, 24 % blockage, 12 % dislodgement, 43 % leakage, and 23 % catheter-associated pain

Catheter-associated infection contributed to excess health-care expenditures with additional nursing home care visits (19 %), clinic visits (25 %), emergency department visits (35 %), and hospitalizations (27 %). Overall, 70 % required a catheter change for blockage, and 19 % were treated at the emergency department for it. Outside of usually scheduled changes, additional catheter changes took place in 37 % of the sample, and one-third of these took place in the emergency department (Wilde et al. 2013b).

Intermittent catheterization is better than indwelling catheter, but patients have reported difficulties staying dry between catheterizations. Being able to find a discreet location and time for catheterization outside the home is widely reported (Wilde et al. 2011). Not performing catheterizations frequently enough can cause bladder overdistention and UTI. Sometimes patients and their family give up on intermittent catheterization and resort to an indwelling catheter.

Conclusions

Recent studies suggest that nearly one quarter of the population has difficulty emptying their bladder and yet only 11 % had ever heard of UAB. The pathogenesis, epidemiology, clinical management, and treatment options for the condition of the underactive bladder remain largely unknown because of a large gap in awareness and understanding of the underactive bladder. We lack longitudinal population studies in patients with lower urinary tract symptoms including OAB and UAB. Challenges remain to determine the true epidemiology for the potential different patient populations and effective treatment guidance.

References

Abarbanel J, Marcus EL (2007) Impaired detrusor contractility in community-dwelling elderly presenting with lower urinary tract symptoms. Urology 69:436–440

Abrams P, Cardozo L, Fall M et al (2002) The standardization of terminology of lower urinary tract function: report from the Standardisation Subcommittee of the International Continence Society. Neurourol Urodyn 22:167–178

Ameda K, Sullivan MP, Bae RJ, Yalla SV (1999) Urodynamic characterization of nonobstructive voiding dysfunction in symptomatic elderly men. J Urol 162:142–146

Chancellor MB (2014) The overactive bladder progression to underactive bladder hypothesis. Int Urol Nephrol 46(Suppl 1):S23–S27

Chancellor MB, Diokno A (2014) CURE-UAB: shedding light on the underactive bladder syndrome. Int Urol Nephrol 46(Suppl 1):S1–S46

Chancellor MB, Kaufman J (2008) Case for pharmacotherapy development for underactive bladder. Urology 72:966–967

Chapple CR, Osman NI, Birder L et al (2015) The underactive bladder: a new clinical concept. Eur Urol 68:351–353. http://dx.doi.org/10.1016/j.eurouro.2015.02.030

Collas DM, Malone-Lee JG (1996) Age-associated changes in detrusor sensory function in women with lower urinary tract symptoms. Int Urogynecol J Pelvic Floor Dysfunct 7:24–29

Cucchi A, Quaglini S, Rovereto B (2008) Development of idiopathic detrusor underactivity in women: from isolated decrease in contraction velocity to obvious impairment of voiding function. Urology 71:844–848

Diokno AC, Brock BM, Brown MB, Herzog AR (1986) Prevalence of urinary incontinence and other urological symptoms in the noninstitutionalized elderly. J Urol 136:1022–1025

DuBeau CE (2006) The aging lower urinary tract. J Urol 175:S11–S15

Elbadawi AE, Yalla SV, Resnick NM (1993) Structural basis of geriatric voiding dysfunction. II. Aging detrusor: normal versus impaired contractility. J Urol 150:1657–1667

Fowler CJ, Christmas TJ, Chapple CR, Parkhouse HF, Kirby RS, Jacobs HS (1988) Abnormal electromyographic activity of the urethral sphincter, voiding dysfunction, and polycystic ovaries: a new syndrome? BMJ 297:1436–1438

Fry CH, Bayliss M, Young JS, Hussain M (2011) Influence of age and bladder dysfunction on the contractile properties of isolated human detrusor smooth muscle. BJU Int 108(2 Pt 2):E91–E96

Griffiths D, Tadic SD, Schaefer W, Resnick NM (2007) Cerebral control of the bladder in normal and urge-incontinent women. Neuroimage 37:1–7

Guideline for prevention of catherassociated urinary tract infections (2009) (www.cdc.gov/…/pdf/CAUTI/CAUTIguideline2009final.pdf) The underactive bladder foundation. www.underactivebladder.org

Homma Y, Yamaguchi O, Hayashi K, Neurogenic Bladder Society (2006) Epidemiologic survey of lower urinary tract symptoms in Japan. Urology 68:560–564

Irwin DE, Milsom I, Hunskaar S et al (2006) Population-based survey of urinary incontinence, overactive bladder, and other lower urinary tract symptoms in five countries: results of the EPIC study. Eur Urol 50:1306–1315

Jeong SJ, Kim HJ, Lee YJ et al (2012) Prevalence and clinical features of detrusor underactivity among elderly with lower urinary tract symptoms: a comparison between men and women. Korean J Urol 53:342–348

Kim JC, Park EY (2006) Nerve growth factor and prostaglandin E in the urine of female patients with overactive bladder. J Urol 175:1773–1776

Madersbacher S, Pycha A, Schatzl G, Mian C, Klingler CH, Marberger M (1998) The aging lower urinary tract: a comparative urodynamic study of men and women. Urology 51:206–212

Malone-Lee J, Wahedna I (1993) Characterisation of detrusor contractile function in relation to old age. Br J Urol 72:873–880

Massey JA, Abrams PH (1988) Obstructed voiding in the female. Br J Urol 61:36–39

Miyazato M, Yoshimura N, Chancellor MB (2013) The other bladder syndrome: underactive bladder. Rev Urol 15:11–22

Nuotio M, Tammela TL, Luukkaala T, Jylha M (2003) Predictors of institutionalization in an older population during a 13-year period: the effect of urge incontinence. J Gerontol 58:756–762

Osman NI, Chapple CR, Abrams P, Dmochowski R, Haab F, Nitti V et al (2014) Detrusor underactivity and the underactive bladder: a new clinical entity? A review of current terminology, definitions, epidemiology, aetiology, and diagnosis. Eur Urol 65:389–398

Resnick NM, Yalla SV (1987) Detrusor hyperactivity with impaired contractile function. An unrecognized but common cause of incontinence in elderly patients. JAMA 257:3076–3081

Shafik A, Shafik AA, El-Sibai O, Ahmed I (2003) Role of positive urethrovesical feedback in vesical evacuation. The concept of a second micturition reflex: the urethrovesical reflex. World J Urol 21:167–170

Smith PP (2010) Aging and the underactive detrusor: a failure of activity or activation? Neurourol Urodyn 29:408–412

Taylor JA, Kuchel GA (2006) Detrusor underactivity: clinical features and pathogenesis of an underdiagnosed geriatric condition. J Am Geriatr Soc 54:1920–1932

Thomas AW, Cannon A, Bartlett E, Ellis-Jones J, Abrams P (2005) The natural history of lower urinary tract dysfunction in men: minimum 10-year urodynamic follow-up of untreated detrusor underactivity. BJU Int 96:1295–1300

Ukimura O, Kojima M, Iwata T et al (2003) Ultrasonic measurement of bladder weight as a novel urodynamic modality. Ad Exp Med Biol 539:311–315

Valente S, DuBeau C, Chancellor D et al (2014) Epidemiology and demographics of the underactive bladder: a cross-sectional survey. Int Urol Nephrol 46(Suppl 1):S7–S10

van Koeveringe GA, Vahabi B, Andersson KE, Kirschner-Herrmans R, Oelke M (2011) Detrusor underactivity: a plea for new approaches to a common bladder dysfunction. Neurourol Urodyn 30:723–728

Wilde MH, Brasch J, Zhang Y (2011) A qualitative descriptive study of self-management issues in people with long-term intermittent urinary catheters. J Adv Nurs 67:1254–1263

Wilde MH, McDonald MV, Brasch J, McMahon JM, Fairbanks E, Shah S, Tang W, Scheid E (2013a) Long-term urinary catheter users self-care practices and problems. J Clin Nurs 22:356–367

Wilde MH, Zhang F, Fairbanks E, Shah S, McDonald MV, Brasch J (2013b) Perceived value of a urinary catheter self-management program in the home. Home Healthc Nurse 31:465–473 www.underactivebladder.org

Chapter 2
Evaluation and Diagnosis of Underactive Bladder

Ananias C. Diokno

Introduction

The hallmark manifestation of someone with an underactive bladder is a prolonged act of voiding usually associated with partial or complete urinary retention and confirmed with poor or absent detrusor contractility (Chancellor and Diokno 2014; Valente et al. 2014). This statement means that the symptoms and signs of underactive bladder must be recognized and then confirmed by demonstrating that the detrusor contractility is reduced in strength and/or duration (Abrams et al. 2002). Since underactive bladder and outlet obstruction may coexist, efforts must be made to document that indeed the detrusor is underactive regardless of whether there is obstruction or not. But first, we must identify the symptoms and/or signs of the patient who may be candidate for the underactive bladder condition. However, the diagnostician must also be aware that UAB may be completely silent, meaning that the person with UAB may be totally asymptomatic or may have symptoms but not recognizing the symptoms as a manifestation of UAB. Therefore, the health-care provider must be proactive in uncovering this entity.

Symptoms Related to UAB

The symptoms that may be suggestive of UAB include a potpourri of voiding or emptying symptoms. If one follows the premise that UAB is due to bladder muscle weakness, then one should consider UAB in all patients manifesting voiding or bladder emptying difficulties. Classic symptoms of voiding difficulties include:

A.C. Diokno, MD
Department of Urology, Oakland University William Beaumont School of Medicine, Rochester, MI, USA

Department of Urology, Beaumont Health System, Royal Oak, MI, USA
e-mail: adiokno@beaumont.edu

M.B. Chancellor, A.C. Diokno (eds.), *The Underactive Bladder*,
DOI 10.1007/978-3-319-23687-2_2

- Hesitancy or delay in passing urine or urine flow from the time the patient initiates voiding
- Weak or thin urine stream
- Urine flow that is either interrupted or continuous but weakens and tapers at the end
- Post-void dribbling of urine
- Feeling of having to go again after the stream has stopped
- Voiding a second or even multiple times after the initial voiding has completed
- Having to strain to facilitate voiding
- Frequent urination day and night in small volumes

Another common symptom that may be associated with underactive bladder is urinary incontinence associated with incomplete bladder emptying. UAB must be suspected when the urinary incontinence is considered an overflow type where patient has constant dribbling of small amounts, and further testing revealed that there is high post-void residual urine. Overflow urinary incontinence may be confused with the urge urinary incontinence because in both cases, urgency and urinary frequency are the hallmark symptoms. However, in urge urinary incontinence, the patient will have efficient bladder emptying capability such that the post-void residual urine will be negligible, whereas in overflow urinary incontinence, the post-void residual urine is excessive.

Underactive bladder may present with frequent urinary infections of the lower urinary tract. Although diagnosing and treating lower urinary tract infection is relatively a simple exercise, discovering the cause may be complex especially if the infection is associated with high post-void residual urine volume. In this instance, one must include UAB as a differential diagnosis in evaluating the cause of recurrent infections.

Another manifestation of UAB is a complaint of pressure or pain in the suprapubic infraumbilical area, and upon examination, the patient has a big suprapubic mass that turns out to be a huge distended bladder. Occasionally, flank pain may be the presenting symptom secondary to the development of bilateral hydronephrosis (Fig. 2.1).

Signs of UAB

UAB may exist without any of the symptoms described above. In this instance, the patient may have lost the sensory perception of bladder distention. Therefore, the health-care providers should be alert for signs that may suggest UAB such as a huge suprapubic mass that turns out to be a distended bladder. The chronically distended bladder with or without bilateral hydronephrosis may be discovered during a routine physical examination being performed for another unrelated complaint or as an incidental finding in abdominal ultrasound, CT scan of the abdomen, or MRI. In all these cases, UAB needs to be included in the differential diagnosis.

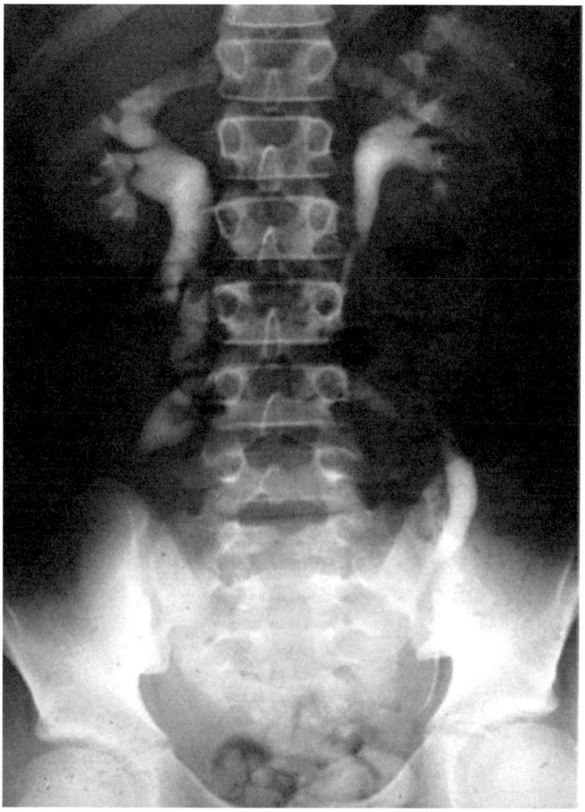

Fig. 2.1 Massively distended bladder with bilateral hydronephrosis

Identifying the UAB

Once a patient is suspected of having underactive bladder, it will be up to the healthcare provider to confirm that symptoms and/or signs that the patient is manifesting are due to an underactive bladder. The evaluation for confirming the UAB must be thorough and in a phased approach in order to arrive at an accurate diagnosis.

History

The history must detail the voiding symptoms and document the presence of hesitancy, weak stream, urine flow intermittency, post-void dribbling, straining to void, and feeling of incomplete voiding. For those who present with acute urinary retention, attempts should be made to obtain potential precipitating factors that led to urinary retention. In elderly men, one may suspect a long-standing obstructive uropathy on the basis of benign prostatic hypertrophy (BPH) or urethral stricture. Was it an associated surgery that led to postoperative retention? Was it the use of pharmacologic agents that can induce urinary retention such as the use of an alpha agonist to reduce upper respiratory tract congestion or the use of anticholinergic agents or sedatives that can inhibit bladder contractility? Is patient on chronic antidepressant medications that can cause depression of the detrusor function?

For those who present with an indwelling catheter or already on intermittent catheterization to drain the urinary bladder or just having significant voiding symptoms with high post-void residual urine, it is imperative that attempt should be made to determine any predisposing factors such as neurologic disorders including spinal cord injury, cerebrovascular accidents, Parkinson's disease, multiple sclerosis, spina bifida, and diabetic neuropathy (Miyazato et al. 2013).

There are also other non-neurologic conditions that can lead to UAB that one needs to explore. This includes habit and behavior towards fluid intake and toileting frequencies. A combination of excessive fluid intake of over the required daily requirements associated with infrequent voiding has been postulated to lead to chronic overdistention and detrusor underactivity. The infrequent voiding syndrome that is also referred to as the "lazy bladder" had been associated with the busy housewives, teachers, nurses, and people who are afraid to use public rest rooms (Purohit et al. 2008). Delay in voiding when the bladder is already full leads to overdistention of the bladder that could lead to detrusor muscle overstretching, and this overstretched detrusor could potentially lead to underactivity (Finkbeiner and Lapides 1974). This is the rationale for catheterizing women in prolonged labor so as not to encounter prolonged overdistention of the urinary bladder.

Another important history that should be obtained is previous surgical intervention related to the lower urinary tract. For women, history of radical hysterectomy could lead to detrusor underactivity due to disturbance of the motor nerves to the bladder (Seski and Diokno 1977). On the other hand, the various anti-incontinence surgeries for stress urinary incontinence could lead to increased urethral resistance that may produce obstructive phenomena to the outlet that may cause obstruction (Lemack 2006). If unattended, over time, the detrusor could fail and lead to urinary retention.

In men, because of high incidence of obstruction secondary to benign prostatic enlargement, transurethral resection of the prostate is a very common procedure performed in these men with significant voiding symptoms especially those with high post-void residual urine. Unfortunately, there are a few men where the urinary retention is not going to respond successfully to the TURP procedure because the basic pathology is underactive bladder, either as a primary condition or secondary to chronic obstructive uropathy (Ignjatovic 2001). Lastly, the use of drugs that can lead to detrusor weakness should be uncovered. Foremost, among these medications are the antidepressants, anticholinergic, alpha agonists, and narcotics.

Physical Examination

A focused physical examination is essential in a comprehensive evaluation of a patient suspected of having an UAB. This should include an overall general assessment of the physical and cognitive ability as this could impact the ability to control bladder function. Is the patient ambulatory or mobility impaired, and if so, is the patient needing support to ambulate? This is important because voiding may be inhibited by poor ambulation or lack of help to be able to micturate at appropriate places. Likewise, assessing the level of cognition is important to determine the ability of the person to pick up the queue to void on time and in appropriate place.

Physical examination should include assessment of neurologic signs that may point to the various neurologic conditions including Parkinson's disease, cerebrovascular accident, multiple sclerosis, spinal cord lesions, and spina bifida. Abdominal examination should include inspection and palpation of the suprapubic area to identify any signs of distended bladder especially for patients having frequent voiding with or without constant urinary dribbling that may suggest urine overflow. The lumbar area should also be palpated for any evidence of any masses or tenderness that may indicate hydronephrosis.

Genital and perineal examination is mandatory for suspected cases of UAB. The skin of the genitalia and the perineum may indicate significant irritation manifested by erythema or even excoriation and ulceration from chronic urinary leakage and wearing of undergarments/diapers. For men, the penis and scrotum and its content should be evaluated. Digital rectal examination should elicit the anal sphincter tone and the voluntary ability to contract the sphincter. The prostate is palpated to assess the size and evidence of any tenderness or masses or nodules. One should remember that the size of the prostate on digital rectal examination does not necessarily correlate to the voiding symptoms. A small size prostate may present with a more intense lower urinary tract symptoms than one with a large prostate palpated on digital examination.

For women, a vaginal inspection, speculum examination, and bimanual examination need to be performed. Inspection should identify the health of the vaginal mucosa to identify signs of atrophy and signs of skin irritation suggestive of atrophic vaginitis. Pelvic organ prolapse is identified visually for any organ protruding outside of the vaginal introitus and provoked by asking the patient to strain and cough to determine the extent of the prolapse. One should also look for evidence of urine leakage during coughing and straining. The lack of leakage does not eliminate urinary incontinence; however, the presence of urine leakage during straining or coughing is a positive sign for stress urinary incontinence. The vaginal speculum is used to inspect the cervix and the vaginal mucosa and to assess the level of the individual pelvic organ prolapse if one is present. The prolapsing organ should be identified such as cystocele (anterior), rectocele (posterior), uterus, or intestine/enterocele (central/vaginal vault). The severity of prolapse should be established using the pelvic organ quantification (POPQ) method (Diokno and Borodulin 2005). This is important because in severe vaginal prolapse, chronic obstruction from the prolapsing pelvic organ could lead to chronic urinary retention. Digital examination of the anal canal should also be performed to assess the anal tone and voluntary strength as well as assess the status of the rectovaginal wall.

In both men and women, the perineal sensation should be tested for sensory deficiency by testing the ability to perceive a gentle pinprick applied to the saddle and the perianal area. Without performing this maneuver, one may miss saddle perineal anesthesia that may be the only neurologic sign that may suggest sacral cord lesions that may be contributing to an underactive bladder.

Laboratory Test

Urinalysis should look for signs of pyuria and bacteriuria, and if infection is suspected, urine culture and sensitivity should be ordered. Urinalysis should also seek to check the presence of glucose as this may correlate to diabetes and its potential consequence, diabetic neuropathy, and for albumin for possible kidney disease. Specific gravity should also be tested to provide a hint of the ability of the kidney to concentrate the urine. Nephrogenic diabetes insipidus causing excessive diuresis can lead to chronic bladder overdistention and underactive bladder (Lemack 2006). Blood tests that may contribute to the overall assessment of UAB include the renal panel (BUN, creatinine, GFR rate), serum protein, electrolytes, and glucose/Hgb A1c levels.

Imaging Tests

The portable bladder scanner has made it easier to quickly measure post-void residual (PVR) urine volume and establish the efficiency of bladder emptying. It also obviates the risk of trauma, pain, and potential contamination with the use of catheter to measure the post-void residual urine (Fig. 2.2). It is important to remember that one-time PVR measurement may not be reliable if there is abnormal PVR volume and more than one measurement is therefore recommended. There is no one magic number that can be used to declare the PVR volume to be abnormal except of course if the PVR is more than the minimum normal bladder capacity of approximately 300 ml. In general, a PVR of less than 150 ml is considered acceptable however for patients with small capacity bladder such as those seen in radiation cystitis and interstitial cystitis where the bladder capacity may not be more than 200 ml. 150 ml PVR may be significant if the patient is symptomatic for the "distended bladder." On the other hand, in patients with very large capacity of over 500 ml, a residual of 200 ml may be insignificant for these patients. In other words, we must individualize the interpretation of the PVR volume.

Other imaging techniques that have led to identifying large distended bladder are the abdominal and pelvic ultrasound, CT, and MRI that may be performed for other indications. When a distended bladder is incidentally identified and reported by the radiologist, it is imperative that the patient be queried whether he/she voided prior to the study. Also, a confirmatory bladder scan should be performed post void to confirm that the PVR is abnormal.

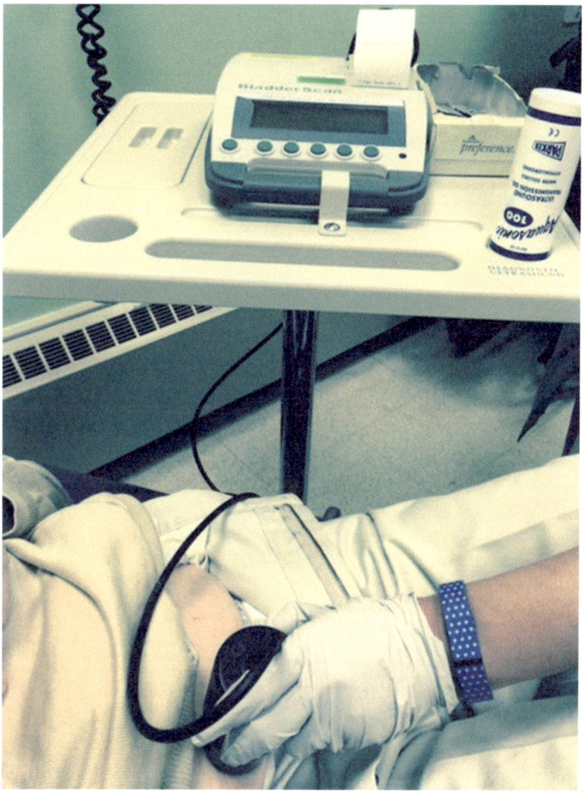

Fig. 2.2 Portable bladder scanner

Endoscopic Assessment

Cystourethroscopy is an optional procedure performed to confirm the presence or absence of anatomical obstruction including enlarged occluding prostate gland and bladder neck contracture or the presence of urethral strictures. The presence of obstruction may indicate that the underactive bladder may be secondary to the obstruction. Cystoscopy will confirm the presence of bladder wall trabeculations, cellule and even diverticula formations. If there is any evidence of detrusor contractility by pressure-flow study, consideration for the relief of obstruction to possibly enhance the detrusor function once the obstruction is relieved. If there is no evidence of any detrusor contractility, relieving the obstruction will be a futile effort. Time should be allowed after the relief of bladder overdistention (urinary retention) to allow the bladder to rest with the hope of the detrusor to recover its contractility.

In the absence of an outlet obstruction, the underactive bladder may be considered neurogenic or myopathic in origin. Endoscopy is helpful if the study revealed no evidence of any urethral stricture and the prostatic fossa appeared widely open especially after a previous TURP (Fig. 2.3). Likewise, in UAB not caused by chronic obstruction, cystoscopy may reveal a large bladder with smooth lining.

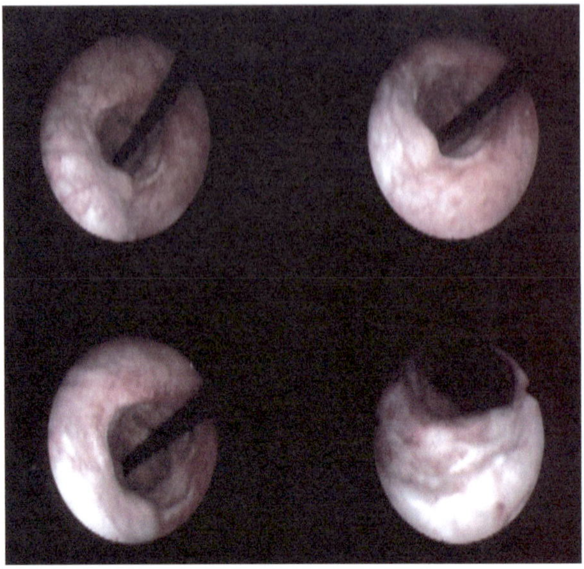

Fig. 2.3 Retroflexed flexible cystoscope view of the prostatic fossa showing a wide-open well-resected outlet

Confirming When UAB Is due to Detrusor Underactivity

The presence of symptoms and signs of underactive bladder is mainly suggestive of an underactive bladder. However, unless there is compelling evidence that the symptoms and signs are truly underactive as in the case of overt disease such as spinal cord injury to the cauda equina, the symptom/sign complex suggestive of an underactive bladder must be confirmed with urodynamic testing.

Urodynamic Tests

Uroflowmetry

Uroflowmetry is a noninvasive test that measures urine flow rates. Urine flow rates may be measured using a stopwatch, but most commonly, uroflowmetry uses an electronic machine that can record the speed of the urine stream over time, thereby abling to measure maximum peak flow and average flow rate. It can also ascertain if the flow is continuous or interrupted. Uroflowmetry alone will provide useful indirect information as to the strength of the detrusor contraction based on the measurement of the maximum or peak flow rate, the time it took to complete the act of voiding, and the average flow rate. However, it in itself will not be sufficient to make a diagnosis of underactive bladder.

Cystometry

Cystometry is a test that measures bladder capacity, bladder wall compliance, sensory perception of bladder distention, presence of involuntary detrusor contraction, and ability to voluntarily contract the detrusor. Cystometry is usually performed using a filling medium infused through the catheter that has the ability to measure pressures. Cystometry can provide a hint of underactive bladder with observation of a large capacity bladder, poor sensation or perception of bladder distention, abnormally high compliance, and lack of detrusor contractility. This last observation should be interpreted with caution as many patients subjected to cystometry are unable to develop a voluntary detrusor contraction at capacity because of the environment of testing that may inhibit the patient but not because of lack of intrinsic contractility. Although in underactive bladder, the post-void residual urine is usually abnormally elevated, the fact that the bladder is empty post-void does not rule out underactive bladder.

Multichannel Pressure-Flow Urodynamic

Combined pressure-flow test is the only legitimate test that can diagnose underactive detrusor and therefore confirmatory of the underactive bladder suspected on the basis of clinical manifestations described above. Unfortunately, caution should be exercised in accepting the one-time urodynamic diagnosis because currently, there is no way to predict which patient with detrusor underactivity will regain some detrusor contractility and be able to void successfully over time. The state of detrusor contractility could be evolving such that over time with rest, the muscle could regain its contractility. Another issue that one must remember when labeling a diagnosis of underactive detrusor is that there are varying levels of detrusor underactivity that has not been fully elucidated to date. There are detrusors that have permanently lost its contractility, and there are underactive detrusors that are transient or only partially underactive and could possibly be rehabilitated to regain its full contractility. This is certainly a fertile ground for research for students of urodynamics.

Combined pressure-flow abdominal pressure study utilizes either a three small caliber catheters (6–8 Fr) for inflow of fluid into the bladder or two other channels that are connected to external transducers to record pressures of the bladder and the sphincteric urethra. Another method is using multichannel microtransducers where the transducers are at the tip of small caliber catheter. The pressures being monitored such as bladder and urethra are transmitted into a recording machine. Concomitant to the bladder and sphincteric urethral pressure, intra-abdominal pressure is measured as well through an intrarectal balloon catheter that is connected to external transducer. In some cases, urethral sphincteric electromyography either using surface electrode imbedded in the catheter or using direct needle electrode into the periurethral striated muscle around the urethral sphincter is performed in conjunction with the above test. At times, urethral sphincter pressure measurement replaced the sphincter electromyography. The last measurement in this test is the uroflowmeter that measures all the parameters mentioned above regarding uroflowmetry.

The basic principle in this test is to simultaneously measure the intravesical pressure, the abdominal pressure, intraurethral pressure, bladder volume, urine flow rates, and post-void residual urine volume. When properly done, the detrusor pressure can be ascertained by subtracting the intravesical pressure from the abdominal pressure. The detrusor pressure at the height of the maximum urine flow rate will determine the presence of underactive, overactive, obstructive, or normal detrusor function. The most common accepted tenets of pressure-flow abdominal pressure diagnosis include the following results:

- Obstructed outlet when there is high detrusor pressure associated with poor urine flow rate.
- Underactive bladder when there is abnormal low or absent detrusor voiding pressure associated with poor urine flow rate.
- Overactive bladder may be diagnosed when involuntary detrusor contractions are noted during the filling phase of the study.
- Normal study when the detrusor pressure and the urine flow rate are within the limits of accepted normal rates.

Unfortunately, except for the obvious case of extreme pressures of high detrusor and poor flow or extremely low detrusor pressure and poor flow, there are many cases that are somewhere in between. This may be due to the severity of the dysfunction or technicalities of the procedure as performance of pressure-flow abdominal pressure test demands great precision and patient cooperation. Another problem is the lack of consensus about specific pressure-flow data that defines the bladder dysfunction. This once again is a fertile ground for further research. Others have attempted to move one more step in using the pressure-flow abdominal pressure data to develop indices or estimating isovolumetric contraction strength, the Watt factor. All these sophisticated advanced tests are currently needing further elucidation. Detailed discussion of these urodynamic tests, results, and interpretation will be presented in Chap. 3 on Urodynamics.

Potential Future Tests for UAB

There are reports that measurement of the detrusor wall thickness may be a helpful test to diagnose detrusor overactivity and obstructive uropathy especially those secondary to benign prostatic enlargement. Such diagnostic test of transabdominal ultrasonographic assessment of detrusor wall thickness could potentially be used to bladders with detrusor underactivity not only for diagnosis but also for prognosticating outcomes of management (Tokgoz et al. 2012).

The development of urine biomarkers that can identify underactive bladder will certainly solve the very complex way of diagnosing underactive detrusor or confirm the etiology of underactive bladder. There are reports that nerve growth factor (NGF) is associated with overactive bladder syndrome (Seth et al. 2013). Another recent observation is the ratio of ATP/nitric oxide (NO) release from the urothelium. Preliminary observation showed that ATP release has a positive correlation and NO release has a negative correlation with the bladder contraction frequency (Munoz et al. 2011). These are preliminary findings and will require further advanced studies. These types of research deserve further support considering the noninvasive nature of these studies.

One last area of potential test for diagnosing underactive bladder is the development of electron-microscopic histopathologic ultrastructural assessment of the detrusor/bladder wall. There was a glimmer of hope from the report of El-Badawi and Resnick when they described various electron-microscopic characteristics of detrusor dysfunctions including characteristic findings of detrusors with impaired contractility (Elbadawi et al. 1993). This test is invasive because it calls for bladder wall biopsy unless the biopsy is done concomitant to some indicated bladder surgery. Unfortunately, except for some follow-up studies, clinical application has been lacking which impedes widespread clinical adoption.

Conclusions

Underactive bladder has many forms of presentation with multiple etiologies. Accurately diagnosing this entity is a major challenge. In order to suspect the condition underactive bladder, the health-care provider must be familiar with symptoms and signs that are associated with underactive bladder syndrome.

References

Abrams P, Cardozo L, Fall M, Griffiths D, Rosier P, Ulmsten U, van Kerrebroeck P, Victor A, Wein A (2002) Sub-committee of the International Continence Society: The standardization of the terminology of lower urinary tract function: report from the Standardization Sub-committee of the International Continence Society. Neurol Urodynam 21:167–178

Chancellor MB, Diokno A (2014) CURE-UAB: shedding light on the underactive bladder syndrome. Int Urol Nephrol 46(Suppl 1):S1–S46

Diokno AC, Borodulin G (2005) A new vaginal speculum for pelvic organ prolapse quantification (POPQ). Int Urogynecol J Pelvic Floor Dysfunct 16:384–388

Elbadawi A, Yalla SV, Resnick NM (1993) Structural basis of geriatric voiding dysfunction II. Normal versus impaired contractility. J Urol 150:1657–1667

Finkbeiner A, Lapides J (1974) Effect of distension on blood flow in dog's urinary bladder. Invest Urol 12:210–227

Ignjatovic I (2001) Symptoms & urodynamics after unsuccessful transurethral prostatectomy. Int Urol Nephrol 32:655–658

Lalli AF, Thornbury JR, Lapides J (1971) Large capacity smooth-walled bladders as an indication of the infrequent voiding syndrome. J Urol 105:662–663

Lemack GE (2006) Urodynamic assessment of bladder outlet obstruction in women. Nat Clin Pract Urol 3:38–44

Miyazato M, Yoshimura N, Chancellor MB (2013) The other bladder syndrome: underactive bladder. Rev Urol 15:11–22

Munoz A, Smith CP, Boone TB, Somogyi GT (2011) Overactive and underactive bladder dysfunction is reflected by alteration in urothelial ATP and NO release. Neurochem Int 58:295–300

Purohit RS, Blaivas JG, Saleem KL, Sandhu J, Weiss JP, Redy B, Sidhu RK (2008) The pathophysiology of large capacity bladder. J Urol 179:1006–1011

Seski JC, Diokno AC (1977) Bladder dysfunction after radical abdominal hysterectomy. Am J Obstet Gynecol 128:643–651

Seth JH, Sahai A, Khan MS, van der Aa F, de Ridder D, Panicker JN, Dasgupta P, Fowler CJ (2013) Nerve growth factor (NGF): a potential urinary biomarkers for overactive bladder syndrome (OAB)? BJU Int 111:372–380

Tokgoz O, Tokgoz H, Unal I, Delibas U, Yildiz S, Voyvoda N, Erdem Z (2012) Diagnostic values of detrusor wall thickness, post void residual urine and prostate volume to evaluate lower urinary tract symptoms in men. Diagn Interv Radiol 18:271–281

Valente S, DuBeau C, Chancellor D, Odonski J, Vereecke A, Doo F, Lajiness M, Diokno A (2014) Epidemiology and demographics of the underactive bladder: a cross sectional survey. Int Urol Nephrol 46(Suppl 1):S7–S10

Chapter 3
Urodynamics Evaluation of Underactive Bladder

Michael B. Chancellor

Introduction

The UAB syndrome is a chronic, complex, and debilitating disease which affects the urinary bladder with serious consequences including urinary incontinence and urinary tract infections (Chancellor and Kaufman 2008; Chancellor and Diokno 2014). The symptoms and severity of underactive bladder vary from one person to another and the course of the disease is often unpredictable. Some of the established causes of UAB include neurogenic, myogenic, aging, and medication side effects (van Koeveringe et al. 2011; Osman et al. 2014). Symptoms are variable and don't predict the underlying pathophysiology. The symptoms may include urgency, frequency, nocturia, hesitancy, and straining to void. The International Continence Society (Abrams et al. 2002) recommends using the term detrusor underactivity (DU), defined as a contraction of reduced strength and/or duration, resulting in prolonged bladder emptying and/or failure to achieve complete bladder emptying within a usual time span. UAB is associated with excessively large bladder capacity that does not adequately empty and DU is a medical diagnostic term based on urodynamics testing of impaired detrusor contractility (Fig. 3.1a–d).

Noninvasive measurement of post-void residual urine (PVR) volume via either catheter or ultrasound and uroflowmetry are two first-line urodynamics assessment techniques available to most clinicians (Blaivas and Chancellor 1996). PVR measurement and uroflow testing are simple to learn and of modest expense and may be used before consideration of catheter-based cystometrogram and multichannel urodynamics.

M.B. Chancellor, MD
Department of Urology, Aikens Research Center, Oakland University William Beaumont School of Medicine, Rochester, MI, USA

Neurourology Program, Beaumont Health System, Royal Oak, MI, USA
e-mail: Michael.Chancellor@beaumont.edu

M.B. Chancellor, A.C. Diokno (eds.), *The Underactive Bladder*,
DOI 10.1007/978-3-319-23687-2_3

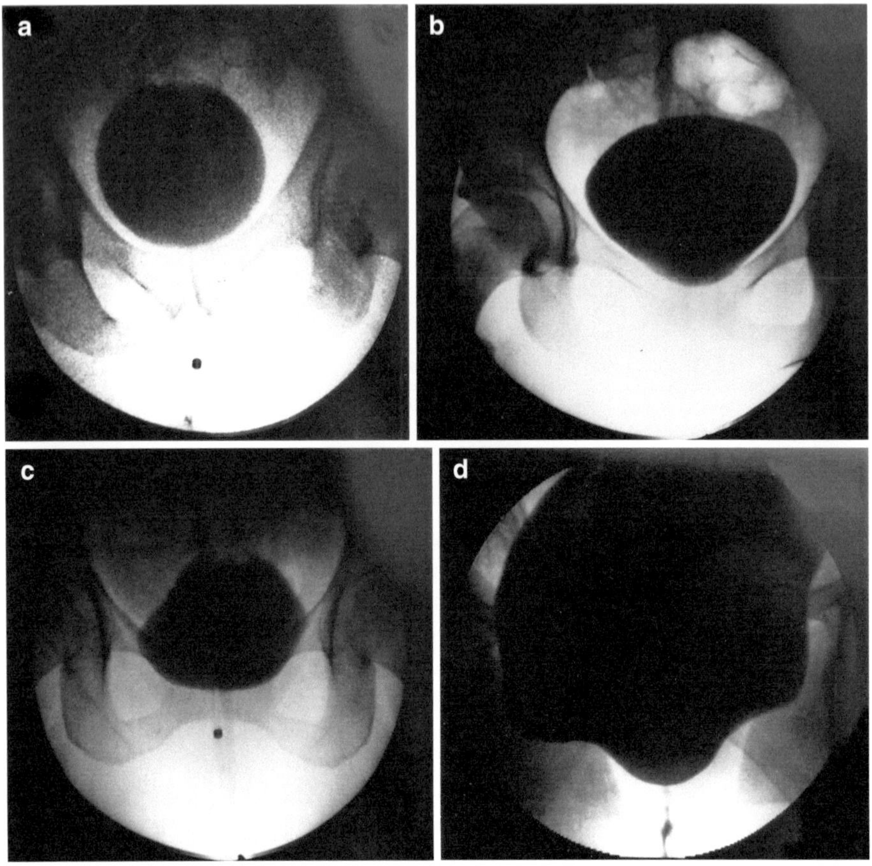

Fig. 3.1 (**a–c**) Normal-size bladder capacity in three patients on contrast-filled cystogram. (**d**) Cystogram of underactive bladder in a 54-year-old woman with bladder capacity over 1,200 ml and PVR of 750 ml

Post-void Residual Urine Volume

Post-void residual refers to the amount of urine left in the bladder after urination. Post-void residual testing is used to assess the degree of bladder dysfunction. There are two types of this test: in-and-out catheterization and transabdominal or pelvic ultrasound.

Acute urinary retention such as immediately after a surgical procedure with anesthesia and narcotics that resolves after a few hours and a single catheterization is not within the scope of UAB or DU. Chronic urinary retention has been defined by the International Continence Society as a PVR >300 mL or rather committing to an absolute volume, stating that it is "non-painful bladder, which remains palpable after the patient has passed urine" (Abrams et al. 2002).

European Urology's UAB working definition is "the underactive bladder is a symptom complex suggestive of detrusor underactivity and is usually characterized by prolonged urination time with or without a sensation of incomplete bladder emptying, usually with hesitancy, reduced sensation on filling, and a slow stream (Chapple et al. 2015)."

Other definitions of urinary retention and elevated residual urine volume one should be aware of include the National Library of Medicine's definition of urinary retention as "inability to empty the urinary bladder with voiding (urination)." In the United States the standard medical diagnosis code, ICD-10-CM, has the diagnosis code R33.9 *Retention of Urine* as:

- A disorder characterized by accumulation of urine within the bladder because of the inability to urinate
- Inability to empty the urinary bladder with voiding (urination)
- Incomplete emptying of the bladder

The Underactive Bladder Foundation (www.underactivebladder.org) working terminology of underactive bladder syndrome is "urinary symptoms including hesitancy, straining and incomplete bladder emptying in the absence of anatomic obstruction."

Ultrasound Measurement

This test is performed to measure the amount of urine that is left in a patient's bladder immediately after the patient made attempt to empty it completely. The test is done with ultrasound in the supine position. The clinician will place gel on the skin over the patient's bladder and then place an ultrasound probe over this area and make a recording (Figs. 3.2 and 3.3). There is no special preparation for this test and the patient may resume usual daily activities immediately following the ultrasound.

Catheterization Measurement

The test is done with a small thin, flexible tube (catheter). After going to the bathroom, the patient will lie flat on the exam table. The entrance to the urethra will be sterilely prepped and the clinician will insert the catheter into the bladder through the urethra. The volume of any urine remaining in the bladder will be drained and measured. There is no special preparation for this study.

Other than complete urinary retention and inability to void, there is no definite consensus between what is normal and abnormal nor a value above which clean intermittent catheterization must be implemented. In older people with less effective bladder emptying, most clinicians even tolerate a greater value for PVR if the

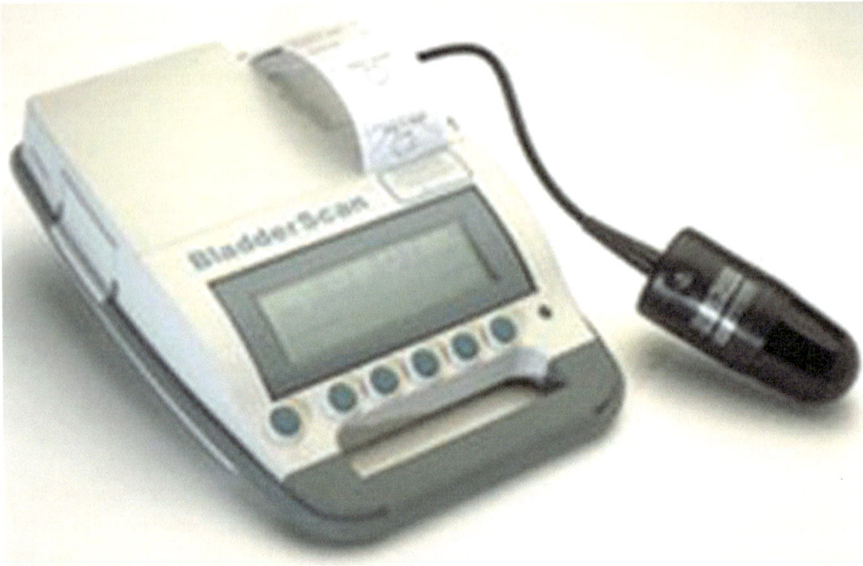

Fig. 3.2 Ultrasound post residual urine volume measurement machine

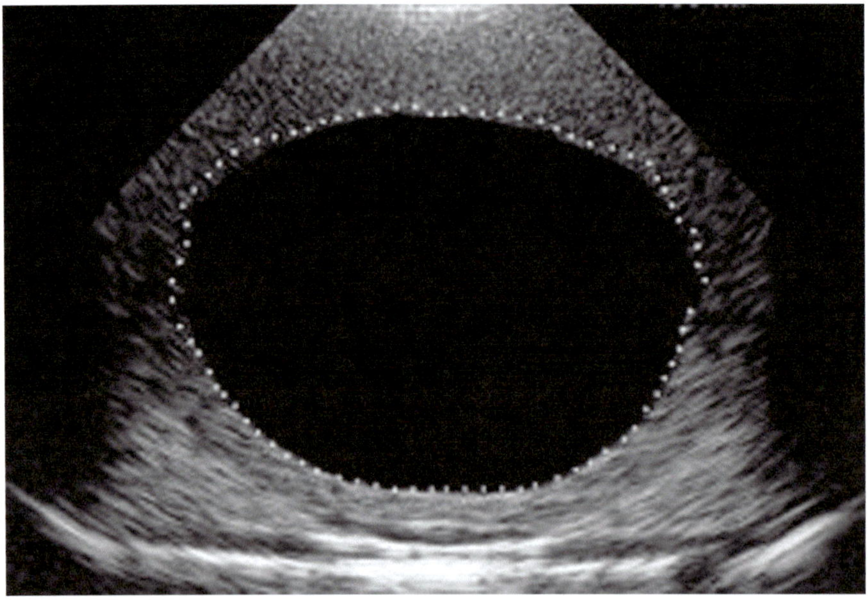

Fig. 3.3 Ultrasound image of bladder being measured for PVR with bladder outlined

patient does not have urinary tract infection and not significantly symptomatic. In general, 150–250 ml is considered by many experts as the threshold and cutoff for being abnormal. There is also a rational argument that PVR should not base not on a single number but rather as a percent of functional bladder capacity. Even for a value of >150–250 ml, further assessment and treatment may not necessarily be undertaken especially if someone would not be a surgical candidate or would not be able to handle catheter care.

Recent ICS guideline (Asimakopoulos et al. 2014) recommends that the interval between voiding and PVR measurement should be short and preferably via ultrasound instead of urethral catheterization. There is no universally accepted definition of a significant residual urine volume. Large PVR >200–300 ml may indicate marked bladder dysfunction and may predispose to unsatisfactory treatment results if, for example, invasive treatment for bladder-outlet obstruction is undertaken. The ICS guideline also concluded that PVR does not seem to be a strong predictor of acute urinary retention and does not specifically indicate the presence of BOO.

Practical Pearls of Post-void Residual Measurement

- The time interval between voiding and residual urine estimation should be recorded: this is particular important if the patient is in a diuretic phase.
- Poorly drained bladder diverticulum or vesicoureteral reflux offers a problem of interpretation and may indicate a need for surgical treatment if the patient is symptomatic.
- The absence of elevated residual urine is clinical valuable, but does not exclude obstruction or bladder dysfunction.
- An isolated finding of elevated residual urine volume requires confirmation before being considered significant.

Uroflow

Urinary flow rate represents the net interaction of detrusor contractility and outlet resistance (Fig. 3.4). The flow rate remains an extremely sensitive indicator of lower urinary tract dysfunction, but the Achilles heel of uroflow measurement is that a low flow may be due to UAB, bladder-outlet obstruction, or both (Chancellor et al. 1991). A slow downstream low flow in itself cannot distinguish the cause of upstream bladder dysfunction or outlet obstruction.

Consistently low flow rates despite adequate voided volumes generally indicate increased outlet resistance, decreased bladder contractility, or both. The minimum voided volume adequate for interpretation of an accurate uroflow is generally considered to be 125 ml (Blaivas and Chancellor 1996). Therefore, in an adult, flow events of less than 125 ml should be interpreted with caution. Nomenclature and some basic concepts bear defining prior to further discussion of different types of flow rates and patterns (Fig. 3.5):

- Voided volume: The total volume of urine expelled from the bladder.
- Flow time: The time over which measurable flow actually occurs.
- Maximum flow rate (Qmax): The maximum measured value of the flow rate.

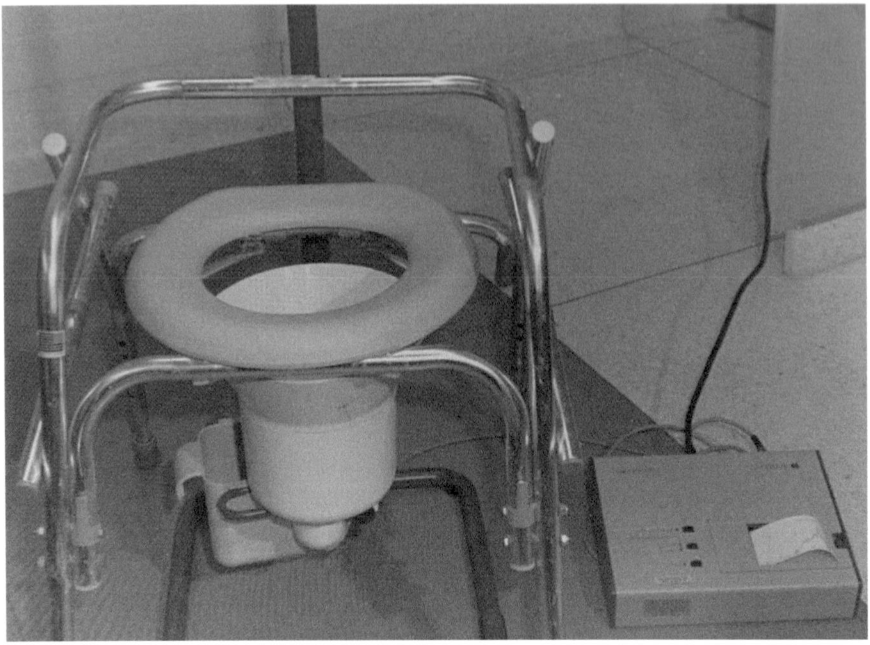

Fig. 3.4 Flowmeter

- Mean flow rate (Qmean): Volume voided divided by flow time. It is important to note that the average flow rate is only interpretable if flow is continuous and without aberrancy, either at the initiation or termination of voiding.
- Flow pattern: Subjective description of the regularity of voiding.
- Intermittent flow: Flow pattern where interruptions of varying duration occur between episodes of voiding. The same parameters used to characterize continuous flow may be used to describe intermittent flow only if caution is exercised. In order to quantify flow time, however, the time intervals between flow episodes should be disregarded. Conversely, the voiding time refers to the total duration of micturition, including the intervals between flow episodes.

Maximum Flow Rate

Among the many parameters provided by uroflowmetry, the maximum urinary flow rate (Qmax: ml/s) is regarded by most experts as most useful not only in assessing the degree of impairment but also in monitoring treatment effects. There have been multiple attempts to normalize uroflow parameters for age, sex, and voided or total bladder volume; however, none of the proposed methods have been universally accepted. It is currently assumed that correction or adjustment of the maximum flow rate value is unnecessary if voided volume exceeds 125 ml.

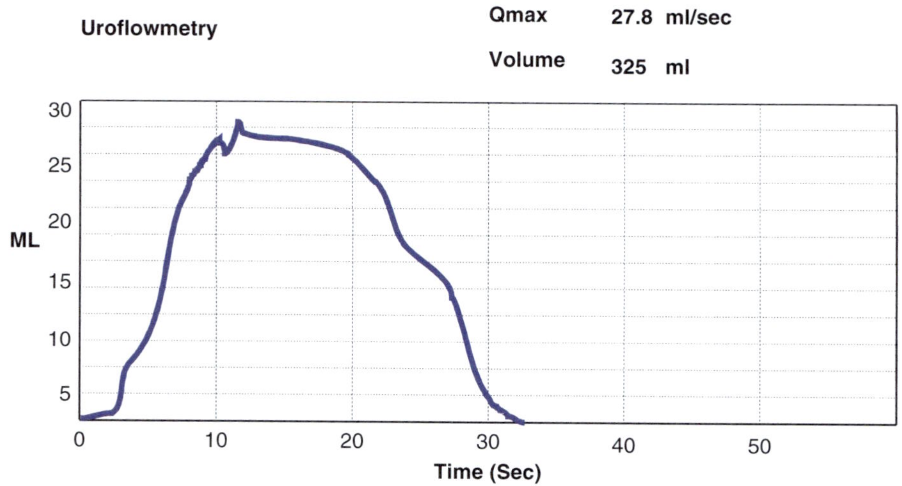

Fig. 3.5 Normal uroflow in a 63-year-old man without voiding symptoms. The patient voided 325 ml over 32 s duration and his maximum flow rate (Qmax) was 27.8 ml/s

Uroflow Patterns

A normal flow pattern is represented by a bell-shaped curve (Fig. 3.5). Upon comparison, women tend to have a higher mean and maximum flow rate than men. The urinary flow pattern of the patient with bladder-outlet obstruction is typically recognizable by a prolonged flow time accompanied by a sustained, substandard flow rate (Fig. 3.6).

Patients with outlet obstruction or impaired detrusor contractility (or both) may in fact eliminate urine by increasing intra-abdominal pressure until outlet resistance is overcome. This pattern of "Valsalva voiding" can often be identified by the urinary flow pattern (Fig. 3.7). In such instances, frequent sharp increases and decreases in the urinary flow rate are noted during the voiding period. Despite a Qmax which may approach normal values, this voiding method is not physiologic and can be detrimental. Valsalva voiding pattern exemplifies the importance of examining not only the flow parameters Qmax, Qmean, and voided volume but also the flow pattern. The parameters in such a case may not accurately reflect the severe nature of voiding dysfunction present in those utilizing Valsalva maneuvers to accomplish voiding (Blaivas and Chancellor 1996).

The pattern of bladder-outlet obstruction may indeed be more variable and not clearly indicative of obstruction. For example, refer to the equivocal flow rate seen in Fig. 3.8 of a 67-year-old man with moderate voiding symptoms and a PVR of 125 ml. He voided 250 ml with maximum flow rate of 12.5 ml/s. The uroflow in this

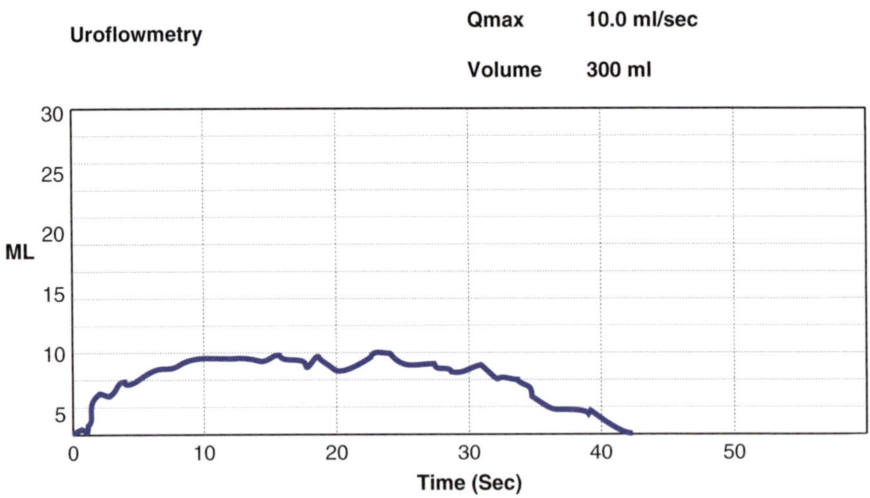

Fig. 3.6 Decreased flow rate in a 79-year-old diabetic woman with urgency, frequency, recurrent urinary tract infections, and a PVR of 150 ml. The flow pattern notes a low Qmax of 10.0 ml/s over 42 s and a voided volume of 300 ml. She has a grade 3 cystocele and a previous pelvic prolapse surgery 15 years ago. The impaired uroflow pattern is abnormal but it cannot differentiate among progressive impaired detrusor contractility with aging or diabetes, urethral obstruction from prolapse or previous surgery, or a combination of the conditions that can contribute to her UAB

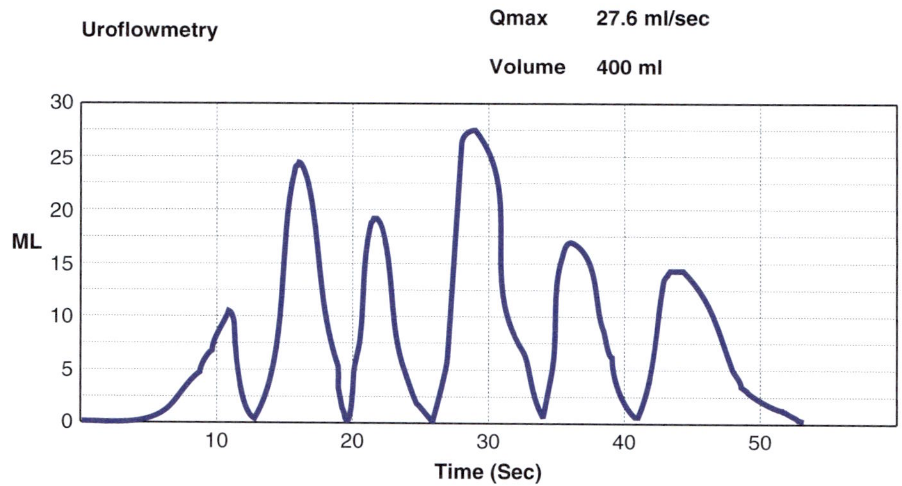

Fig. 3.7 Normal Qmax of 27.6 ml/s on this uroflow readout and the patient did not have any residual urine volume. But from the tracing, the voiding can be seen to be due to abdominal straining. The urinary stream occurs in spurts with complete interruption between the spurts. This pattern of "Valsalva voiding" points out the value of looking at the flow pattern in addition to just the numeric values of uroflowmetry

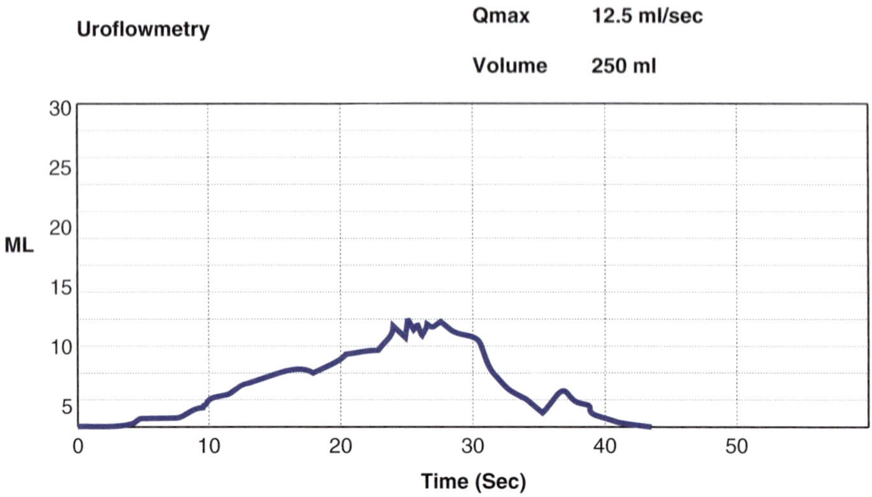

Fig. 3.8 Equivocal flow rate of Qmax at 12.5 ml/s in a 67-year-old man with moderate irritable and obstructive voiding symptoms. He voided 250 ml but had a PVR of 125 ml. The uroflow in this clinical situation is not diagnostic and multichannel pressure-flow urodynamics evaluation would be recommended

clinical situation is not diagnostic. Therefore, formal urodynamics evaluation would be necessary in order to determine whether either outlet obstruction or impaired contractility was responsible for the abnormal flow pattern in this patient.

It is most useful to ensure that the flow event depicted by the uroflow examination closely approximates the usual voiding event for that patient. Urodynamics evaluation, therefore, ideally should include at least two flow events. In individuals who can initiate voluntary micturition, one event should be at the initiation of the study prior to instrumentation, ideally when the patient arrives with a comfortably, but not excessively, full bladder.

Future Flow

The future of uroflowmetry is already here in Japan. Toto Corporation (Kokura, Japan) the world leader in smart toilet that Japan is famous for have embedded the sensors of flowmeter into top of the line smart toilet (i-Step Newsletter 2013) (Fig. 3.9). The toilet when commanded will sense the volume and flow rate and in a normal sitting or standing positions for women and men and provide readout. The build in flow toilets has been installed in some of the physician's offices in Japan and provides a more natural flow reading on a regular toilet rather than special urodynamics commode.

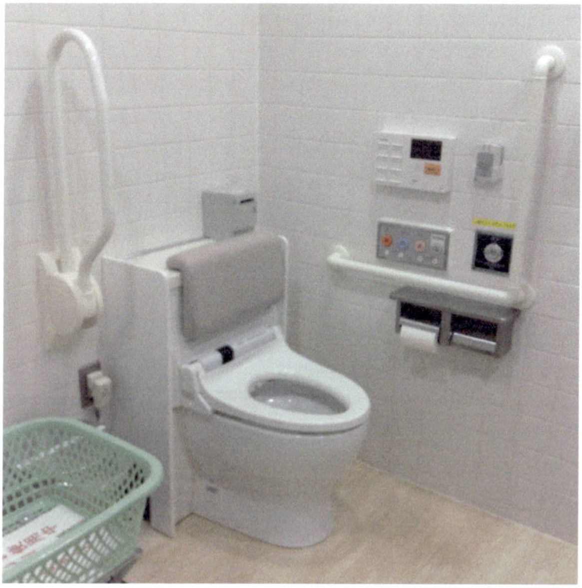

Fig. 3.9 Future flowmeter (Toto, Kokura, Japan). The next-generation uroflowmeter build into normal patient bathroom toilet in Doctor Tomohiro Ueda's specialty clinic in Kyoto, Japan

Practical Pearls of Uroflow

- Urinary flow rate varies significantly with the voided volumes. The minimum voided volume adequate for interpretation of an accurate uroflow is generally considered to be ≥125 ml.
- It may be helpful to have a urinary flow rate nomogram available in the laboratory for comparison of measured flow rate and voided volume (Siroky et al. 1979).
- Because urinary flow rates can vary in an individual from one voiding episode to another, more than one flow rate study should be done when first flow test is equivocal.
- In circumstances where doubt remains following an uroflow study, further urodynamics studies are essential to identify the etiology of voiding dysfunction.

Cystometrogram

Cystometry is the method by which the pressure/volume relationship of the bladder is measured. Cystometry (CMG) is used to assess detrusor activity, sensation, capacity, and compliance. Before starting to fill the bladder, the residual urine should be measured. Certain cystometric parameters may be significantly altered by the speed of bladder filling so filling should not be faster than 50 ml/min in most cases. The patient should be awake, unanesthetized, and neither sedated nor taking drugs that affect bladder function (Blaivas and Chancellor 1996; Schafer et al. 2002). Any variations should be specified and recorded (Fig. 3.10).

Definitions of Pressure Measurements

- Intravesical pressure (Pves) is the pressure within the bladder.
- Abdominal pressure (Pabd) is taken to be the pressure surrounding the bladder. In current practice it is estimated from rectal or, less commonly, extraperitoneal vaginal pressure measurement.
- Detrusor pressure (Pdet) is that component of intravesical pressure that is created by forces in the bladder wall (passive and active). It is estimated by subtracting abdominal pressure from intravesical pressure (Pdet = Pves–Pabd).
- The simultaneous measurement of abdominal pressure is essential for the interpretation of the intravesical pressure trace. However, artifacts on the detrusor pressure trace may be produced by intrinsic rectal contractions.

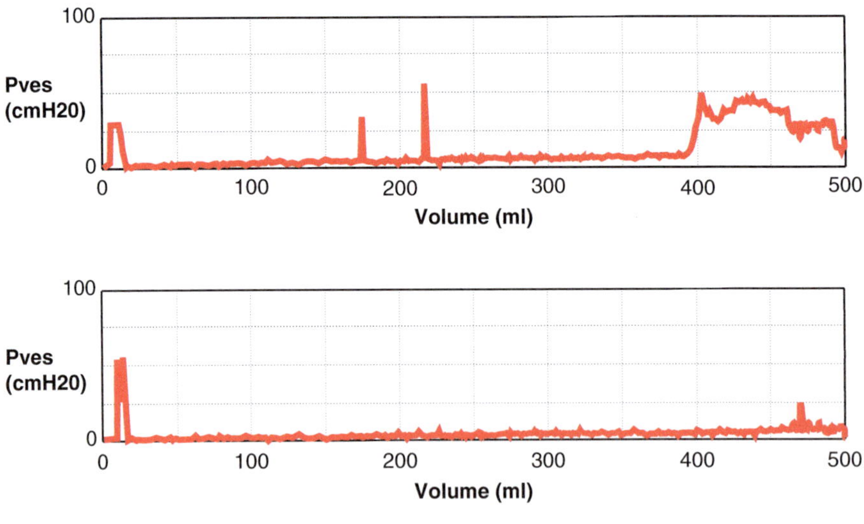

Fig. 3.10 Cystometrograms illustrating the filling and voiding phases of normal (*top*) versus UAB bladders (*bottom*). The normal patient had sensation of filling and fullness and at approximately 400 ml initiated a voluntary bladder contraction with maximum Pves of approximately 50 cmH20 and voiding to completion (*top*). The UAB patient did not have any sensation of filling and was not able to generation any intravesical pressure (*bottom*)

- Bladder sensation. Sensation is difficult to evaluate because of its subjective nature. It is usually assessed by questioning the patient in relation to the fullness of the bladder during cystometry.
- Maximum cystometric capacity, in patients with normal sensation, is the volume at which the patient feels he/she can no longer delay micturition.
- Compliance indicates the change in volume for a change in pressure. Compliance is calculated by dividing the volume change by the change in detrusor pressure during that change in bladder volume (Fig. 3.11). Compliance is expressed as ml/cmH2O.

Phases of the CMG: The normal adult cystometrogram is divided into four phases (Fig. 3.11).

- The initial pressure rise in phase 1 represents the initial response to filling, and the level at which the bladder trace stabilizes is known as the initial filling pressure. The designation "resting pressure," though often used, is incorrect. The first phase of the curve is contributed to by the initial myogenic response to filling and by the elastic and viscoelastic response of the bladder wall to stretch, factors previously discussed. With more rapid rates of filling, there may be an initially higher peak, which then levels off.
- Phase 2 is called the tonus limb, and compliance is normally high and uninterrupted by phasic rises. In practice, the compliance seen in the urodynamics laboratory is always lower than that existing during physiologic bladder filling. Normally, the rise is less than 10 cmH20.

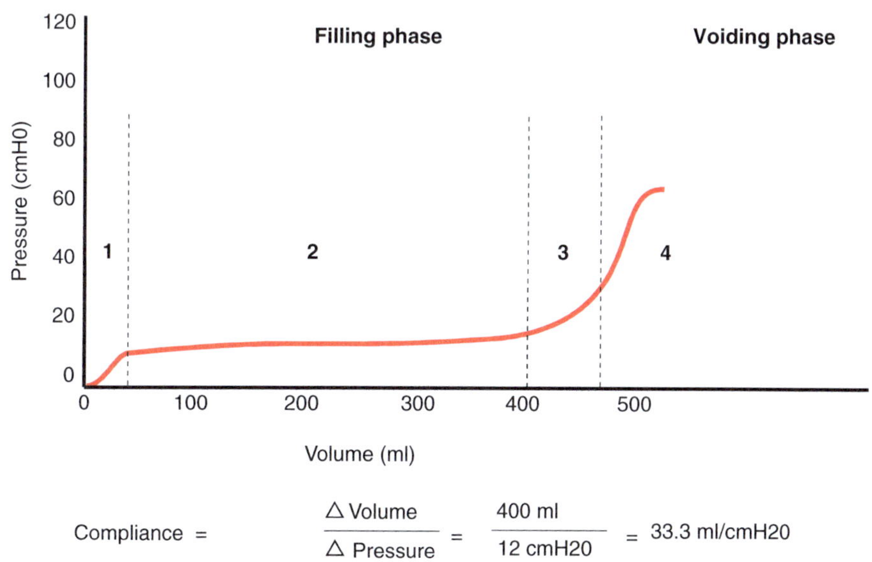

Fig. 3.11 Idealized normal adult cystometrogram illustrating phases 1 through 4 and calculation of compliance

- Phase 3 is reached when the elastic and viscoelastic properties of the bladder wall have reached their limit. Any further increase in volume generates a substantial increase in pressure. This increase in pressure is not the same as a detrusor contraction. If a voluntary or involuntary contraction occurs, phase III may be obscured by the rise in pressure so generated.
- Phase 4 consists of the initiation of voluntary micturition. Many patients are unable to generate a voluntary detrusor contraction in the testing situation, especially in the supine position. This should not be called detrusor areflexia but, simply, absence of a detrusor contraction during cystometry, a finding that is not considered abnormal unless other clinical or urodynamics findings are present that substantiate the presence of neurologic or myogenic disease.

Bethanechol Supersensitivity Test

Bethanechol supersensitivity test was considered in the 1970s and 1980s as a helpful adjunct during urodynamics testing to determine if detrusor areflexia is neurogenic in etiology. The patient receives a subcutaneous injection of bethanechol 0.035 mg/kg, after which the cystometrogram is repeated 15 min later. A bladder afflicted by denervation will demonstrate a 15 cmH2O increase in intravesical pressure at 100 ml of filling, whereas a primary detrusor myopathy, such as from overdistention, will exhibit no such increase in pressure (Fig. 3.12). In patients with evidence of decentralization, a steady rise in intravesical pressure with filling will be noted, especially if the sphincteric mechanism is unimpaired, and high-pressure urinary storage will result.

Validity of the bethanechol supersensitivity test has mostly been abandoned. Wheeler et al. (1988) studied 7 women who strained to void and high residual urines and had detrusor areflexia, with a borderline or positive bethanechol supersensitivity test, ranging from 19 to 55 cmH2O change in intravesical pressure after 5 mg of subcutaneous bethanechol. However, all patients had a normal neurologic workup.

Blaivas et al. (1980) studied the bethanechol supersensitivity test in 33 patients who demonstrated detrusor areflexia during urodynamics. The presence or absence of a neurologic lesion was documented carefully by complete neurologic evaluation. Of the 21 patients with a neurogenic bladder, there was a falsely negative rate of 24 %. Of the 12 patients without a neurogenic bladder, the falsely positive rate was 50 %. The authors concluded that a positive bethanechol test is not by itself indicative of neurogenic bladder nor does a negative test exclude this diagnosis. The bethanechol test is not commonly used in urodynamics testing today because false-positive and false-negative results can frequently occur.

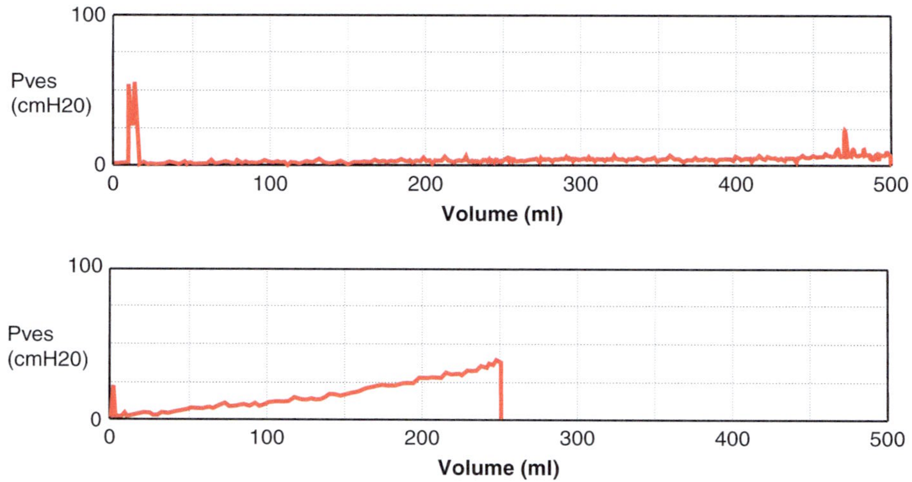

Fig. 3.12 Illustration of the bethanechol test in a 43-year-old man status post pelvic fracture with detrusor areflexia managed with intermittent catheterization. (*Top*) CMG demonstrated a compliant filling curve to capacity over 500 ml without voluntary or involuntary bladder contraction (*bottom*). CMG was repeated 15 min after subcutaneous injection of bethanechol 0.035 mg/kg. There was a 14 cmH2O increase in intravesical pressure at 100 ml of filling. The study was stopped at 250 ml due to patient discomfort

Pressure-Flow Multichannel and Video-Urodynamics

Intravesical pressure, intra-abdominal pressure (generally reflected by rectal pressure), and flow are often measured simultaneously. The purpose of pressure/flow studies is to be able to assess detrusor contractility more precisely and to better define whether obstruction is present (Ouslander et al. 1983; Chancellor and Kiilholma 1992). The normal adult male generally voids with a detrusor pressure of between 40 and 60 cmH20; the normal adult female voids at a lower pressure (Diokno et al. 1990) (Fig. 3.13). Indeed, many women void with almost no detectable rise in detrusor pressure. This does not indicate that contraction is not occurring but simply that outlet resistance, lower in the female to begin with, drops to very low levels during bladder contraction. Urodynamically, obstruction is defined by the relationship between detrusor pressure and flow-high pressure and low flow. Once obstruction is diagnosed, it is necessary to determine the site, and in order to do this, simultaneous fluoroscopy is often used (Figs. 3.14 and 3.15).

Multichannel detrusor pressure subtracted cystometry is performed by filling the bladder through a double- or triple-lumen, 8–10 Fr urodynamics catheters with normal saline at 30–50 ml/min. Rectal pressure is recorded with a fluid-filled catheter. Post-void residual urine volume will be recorded before the start of infusion. Infused volume and time are recorded automatically. The volume at first sensation of filling, first desire to void, urgency, and pain will be recorded in those patients with sensation. The volume at which involuntary bladder and urine leaks per meatus occur is equal to urodynamics bladder capacity.

Video-Urodynamics

Video-urodynamics is a technique utilizing synchronously recorded urodynamics studies and cystourethrography for the evaluation of complex lower urinary tract problems. The advantages of such a system are that by measuring and displaying all of the parameters simultaneously, one obtains a much clearer understanding of normal and abnormal physiology. The ability to obtain spot films from the recordings without interrupting the study permits the study to be performed in a much more physiologic manner. Video-urodynamics is considered the "gold standard" for the evaluation of voiding abnormalities. The whole event can be videotaped for later review and for documentation (Blaivas and Chancellor 1996).

Video-urodynamics adds an anatomic dimension to the urodynamics study that is complimentary to the pressure study. One of the key advantages of video-urodynamics study is that it can identify and localize the level of bladder-outlet obstruction (Figs. 3.16 and 3.17). While multichannel bladder and urethral pressure studies can identify the presence of obstruction, its anatomic level always remains

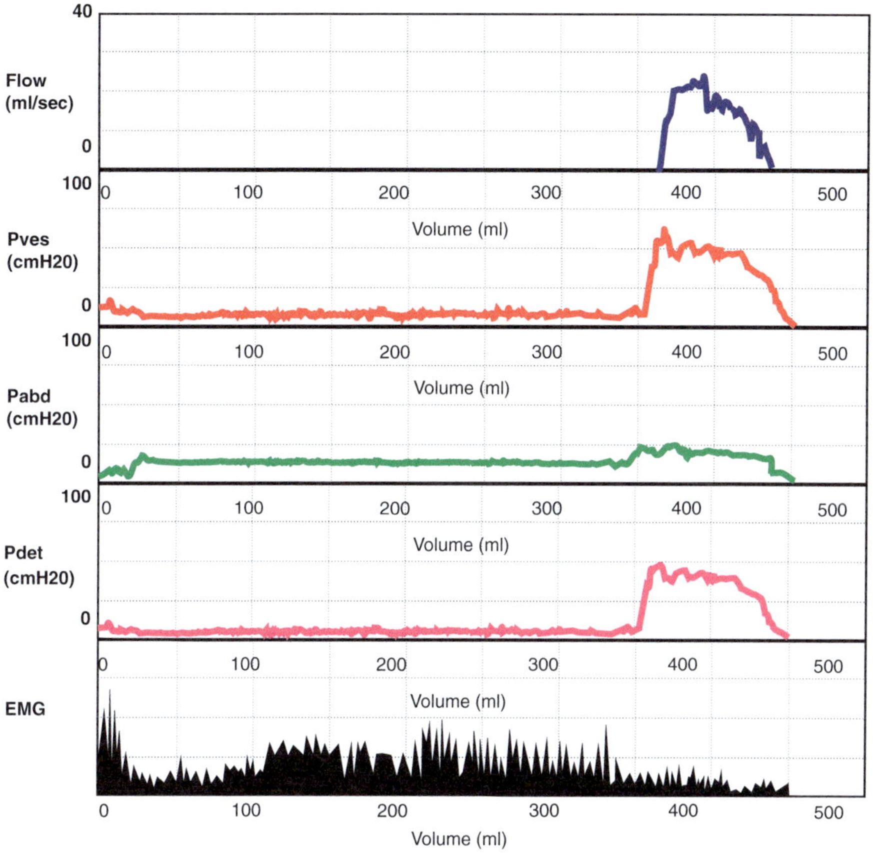

Fig. 3.13 Normal pressure-flow urodynamics in a 32-year-old. Urodynamics tracing demonstrates a voluntary detrusor contraction with detrusor voiding pressure of 46 cmH20 at 360 ml. Her maximum flow rate was 22 ml/s

in doubt. Cystogram or voiding cystourethrogram done in the absence of simultaneous bladder pressure measurement may be helpful, but cannot be certain the circumstance where the bladder neck or sphincter opening or closure is and if the high PVR with low voiding Pdet may be due to less common problems such as vesicoureteral reflux or bladder diverticulum (Fig. 3.18).

Another advantage of video-urodynamics is in the diagnosis of incontinence. Fluoroscopy is helpful to separate between urethral hypermobility and intrinsic sphincteric deficiency types of stress incontinence. Video-urodynamics helps identify bladder neck and urethral incompetence and confirm rotational descent of the bladder neck and urethra during stress maneuvers. The major disadvantage of video-urodynamics is that it requires a major investment in equipment.

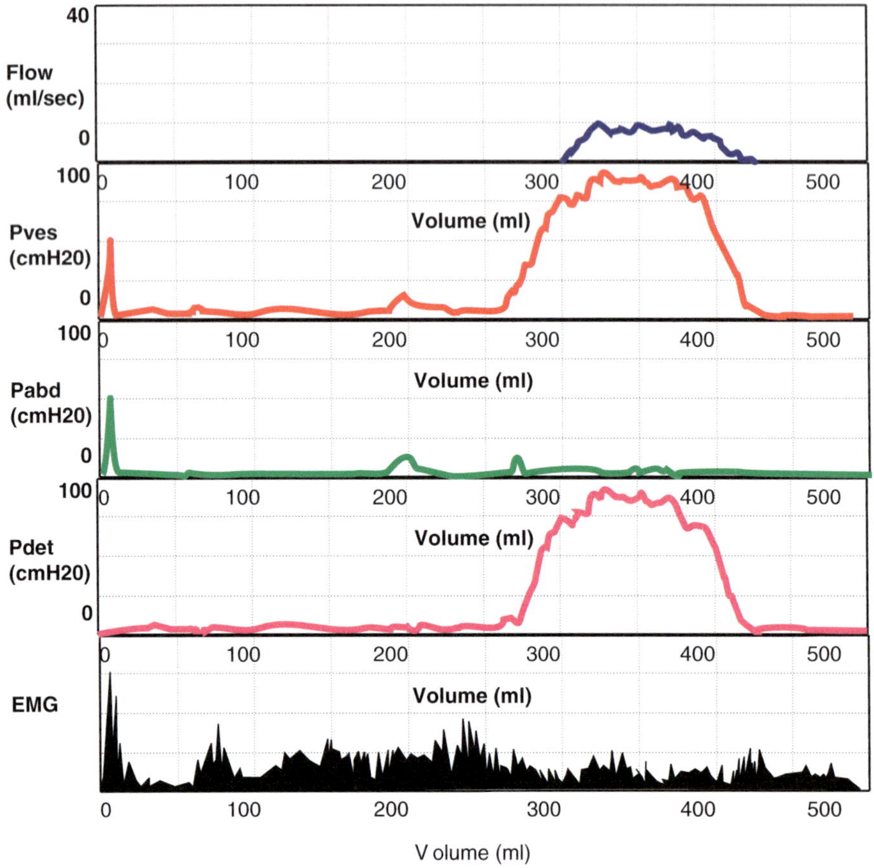

Fig. 3.14 Pressure-flow urodynamics in a 68-year-old man with obstructed voiding symptoms. Urodynamics tracing demonstrates an involuntary detrusor contraction starting at 275 ml that the patient could not inhibit, and he voided with a Pdet of 92 cm H20 and a Qmax of only 10 ml/s

Urodynamics Pitfalls in Assessment of UAB

- What are the precise criteria for outlet obstruction? Most authorities would agree that bladder-outlet obstruction is diagnostic as Qmax <10 ml/s with a sustained Pdet greater than 80 cmH20. Qmax between 10 and 15 ml/s and Pdet between 60 and 80 cmH20 are controversial for determining obstruction.
- Low pressure, low flow: There is a gray zone in which all the urodynamics parameters and computer assistant calculations presently available still cannot differentiate if low pressure, low flow (Qmax <10 ml/s in the presence of a detrusor contraction of <30 cmH2O) is due to outlet obstruction, impaired contractility, or a combination of both (Fig. 3.19). Impaired bladder emptying is often associated

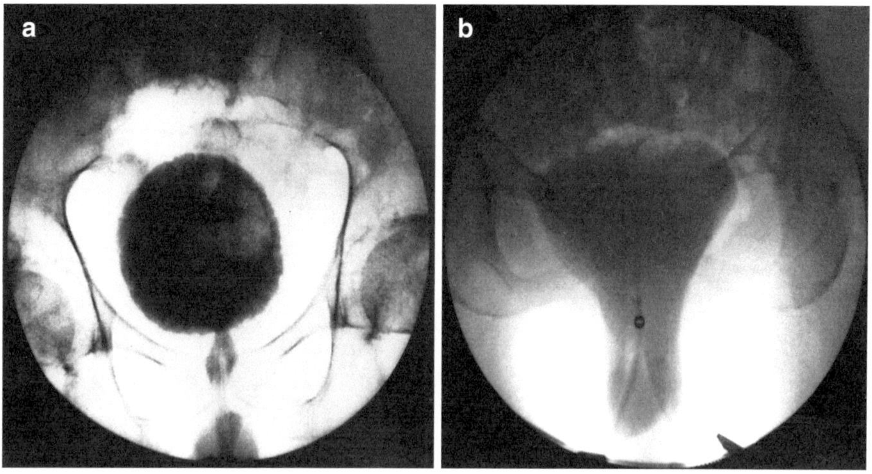

Fig. 3.15 Fluoroscopy imaging during the voiding phase demonstrating bladder-outlet obstruction at the (**a**) bladder neck and (**b**) grade 4 cystocele prolapse

with detrusor overactivity with or without bladder outflow obstruction (Blaivas and Chancellor 1996). Detrusor hyperreflexia impaired contractility (DHIC) is a common and important finding based on urodynamics studies in both healthy and symptomatic elderly (Ameda et al. 1999). Griffiths (2004) noted the coincidental occurrence and overlap of OAB and UAB with different etiological factors. Histological studies including electron microscopic analysis detected age-related change in the bladder in DHIC patients (Resnick and Yalla 1995) (Fig. 3.20).

- Concomitant neuropathy and obstruction: A difficult question in the urological management of an elderly man with Parkinson disease with detrusor hyperreflexia is whether this patient also has a bladder-outlet obstruction. Prostatectomy can be considered to relieve outlet obstruction but urgency and urge incontinence may persist or worsen after prostatectomy. Despite doing urodynamics on many of these men, we have no reliable method of predicting who will improve with prostatectomy. The patient must therefore have a clear understanding beforehand of the risks and benefits of surgery. He should be informed that he may remain incontinent and that, if anticholinergic medications fail, condom catheter drainage may be a possibility. If obstruction is ruled out, initial treatment with anticholinergic is recommended. Decreased bladder compliance is another important pathology that is associated with UAB and incontinence that requires urodynamics for diagnosis (Fig. 3.21).
- Testing anxiety: Anxiety during an urodynamics study is common. A person who cannot void during an urodynamics test does not imply obstruction or detrusor areflexia. Sometimes the study needs to be rescheduled after the patient is more familiar with the setup. At other times uroflow and residual urine is all the urodynamics testing we can ever get out of a particularly nervous patient who cannot tolerate a catheter.

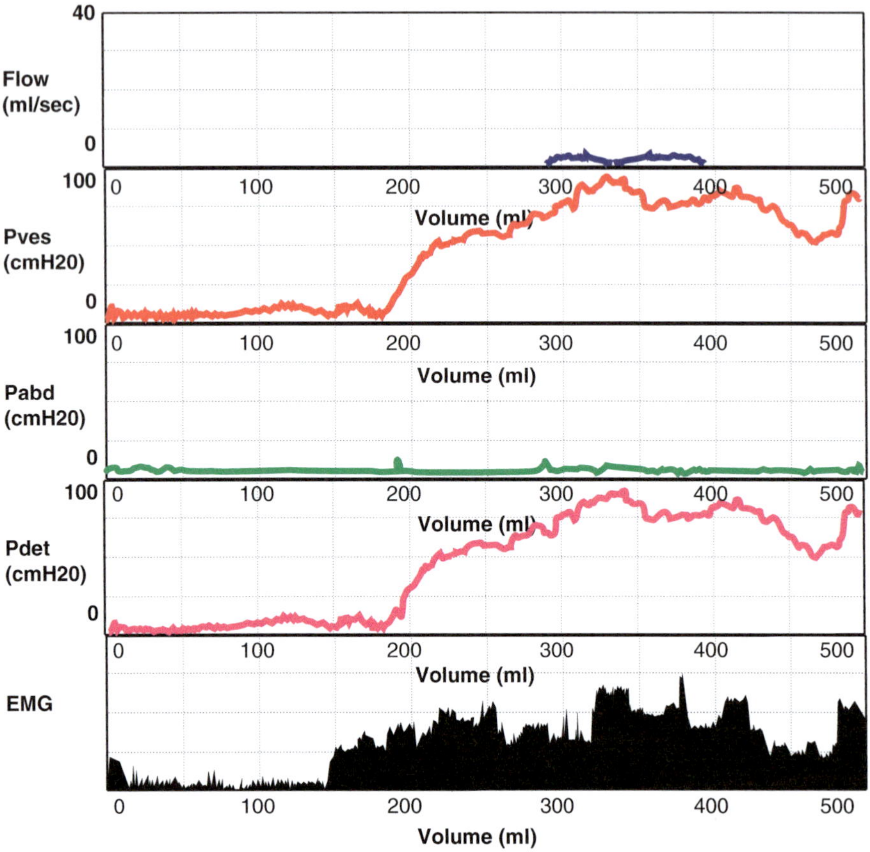

Fig. 3.16 Detrusor hyperreflexia with detrusor-external sphincter dyssynergia in a 33-year-old man with T1-level spinal cord injury. He performs intermittent self-catheterization and is taking antimuscarinic agents but still has refractory urge incontinence. Involuntary detrusor contraction occurred at low volume with elevated voiding pressure of 90 cmH20. Note the increased EMG activity during involuntary bladder contraction

Parameters of Detrusor Power and Work in UAB

There is a wide variation in the urodynamics criteria considered as diagnostic of DU in clinical studies (Osman et al. 2014). Measurement of detrusor contraction strength and sustainability of contraction have been proposed (Schafer 1991). For both contraction strength and sustainability of contraction, normal range is mostly derived from men undergoing surgery to relieve bladder-outlet obstruction (Schafer 1991). These ranges may not be applicable to women.

Multichannel Urodynamics Parameters: Pdet at Qmax (<40 cmH20); Qmax (<15 ml/s)

The urodynamics estimation of detrusor contractile function is based upon the detrusor pressure required to expel urine through the urethra. Measurement of

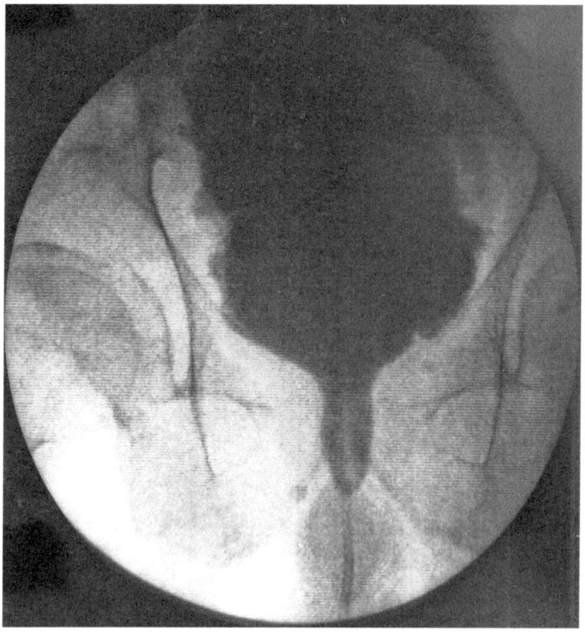

Fig. 3.17 Fluoroscopic imaging during voiding of the patient in Fig. 3.16 demonstrated a significantly trabeculated bladder with open bladder neck and prostatic urethra but closed membranous urethral sphincter

detrusor contractile function may underestimate true detrusor contractility, as the contraction generates both flow and pressure (Griffiths 2004). To compensate, methods attempting to estimate isovolumetric detrusor pressure during uninterrupted or interrupted voiding have been developed. Most methods are based on the inverse relation between pressure and flow. The bladder-outlet relationship (BOR) states that in any given bladder if outflow is stopped, the detrusor pressure reaches its highest possible value (isovolumetric pressure), and when increasing flow is allowed, pressure decreases reaching a minimum when flow reaches a maximum. On this basis, measuring detrusor pressure at the time of highest flow (i.e., Pdet at Qmax) does not correlate to the peak of contraction strength. Consequently, methods that assess isovolumetric detrusor pressure have been suggested and are either based on mathematical analysis of urodynamics data or real-time interruption of urine flow (Osman et al. 2014).

Occlusion Testing

Noninvasive techniques assessing contraction strength have been explored. One technique is to use condom catheters. The pressure is measured by a continuous column of fluid from the catheter via condom to the urethra and bladder.

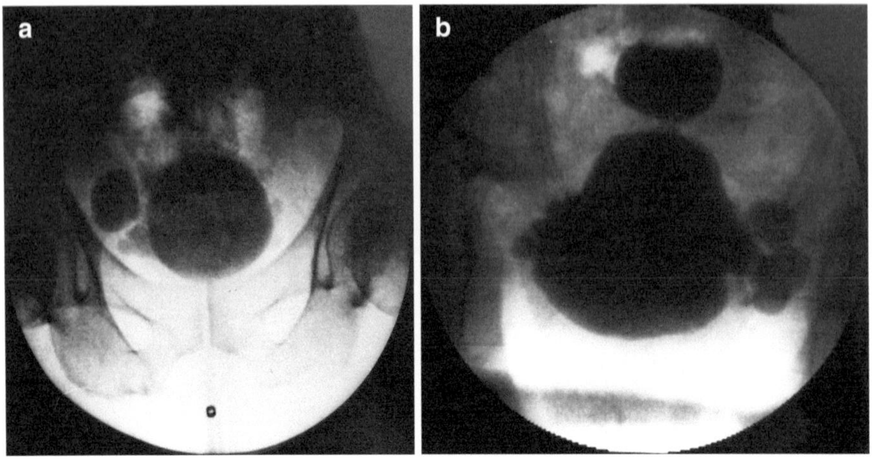

Fig. 3.18 Two examples where video-urodynamics were helpful in diagnosis of UAB symptoms. Two women with symptoms of urgency, frequency, sensation incomplete bladder emptying, recurrent urinary tract infections, and elevated PVR >200 ml. On pressure-flow studies, there were involuntary detrusor contraction but Pdet at maximum flow of less than 20 cmH20. Fluoroscopic imaging during voiding demonstrated a large right bladder side wall diverticulum with narrowed neck (**a**) and multiple diverticula in (**b**). Both women underwent surgical resection of their diverticula with resolution of symptoms and complete bladder emptying postoperatively

Measurements of Pdet-iso correlate with invasive pressure-flow urodynamics in nonobstructed patients but less so in bladder-outlet obstruction (Pel and van Mastright 1999). Several problems can lead to artifacts such as leakage around the condom, closure of the external sphincter in response to line occlusion, and increased compliance within the system (Blake and Abrams 2004). McIntosh et al. (2004) used an inflatable penile cuff to interrupt voiding but noted that this method overestimates Pdet-iso by approximately 16 cmH_2O. The occlusion test can only be applied to men and may be painful. Abdominal straining cannot be diagnosed by the occlusion urodynamics test.

Ambulatory Urodynamic

Ambulatory urodynamics may have a role in the diagnosis of UAB when a person cannot void or generate detrusor contraction on filling CMG in the urodynamics laboratory (Osman et al. 2014). van Koeveringe et al. (2010) found that in 71 % of patients whom no detrusor contraction during office filling CMG did have detrusor contractility in ambulatory urodynamics studies. Filling CMG is conducted at

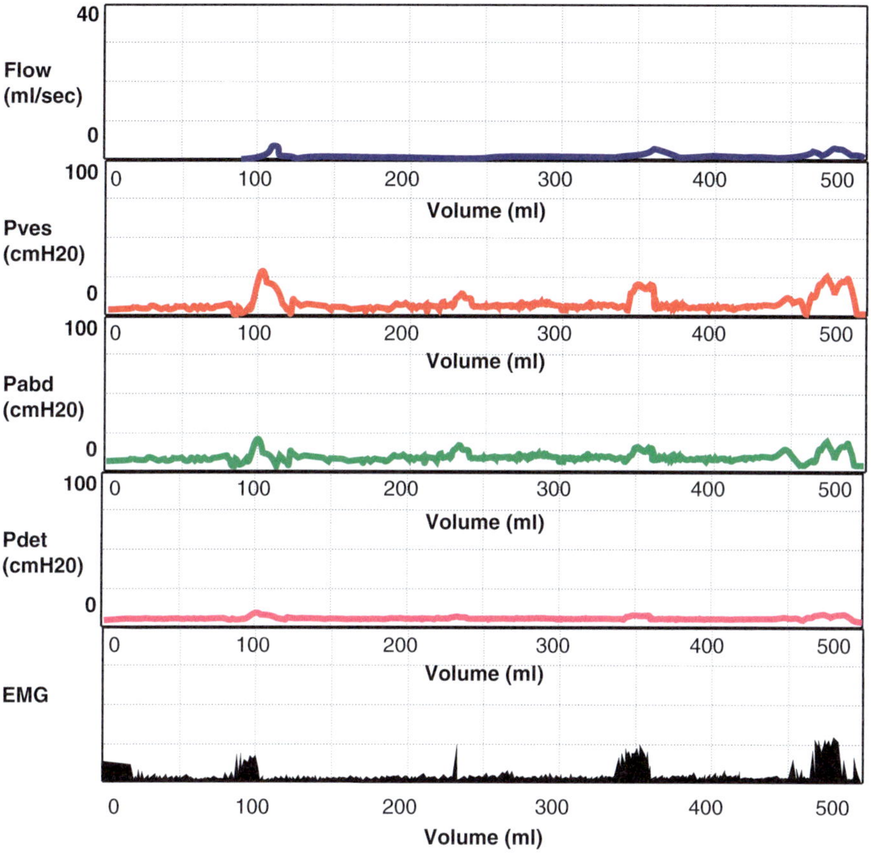

Fig. 3.19 UAB acontractile bladder on multichannel urodynamics. Detrusor areflexia in this case was secondary to acute bilateral herniated lumbar intervertebral disks in an otherwise healthy 54-year-old man without prior urological history. The bladder is areflexic to over 500 ml without voluntary or involuntary detrusor contractions

nonphysiological filling rates and so its validity as a modality for assessing detrusor contractility can be questioned. This is likely due to patient anxiety with catheter and observers that pelvic floor/sphincter contraction triggers the guarding reflex impairing detrusor contraction. Despite the potential advantages of ambulatory urodynamics, it remains a research tool as it is time consuming to setup, download, and interpret. The catheters can dislodge or fall out or are prone to artifacts of daily activity. Moreover, the frequent observation of involuntary detrusor contractions in normal patients without overactive bladder raises questions about value and interpretation of results. Advances in telemedicine and miniaturization may revolutionize ambulatory urodynamics in the future.

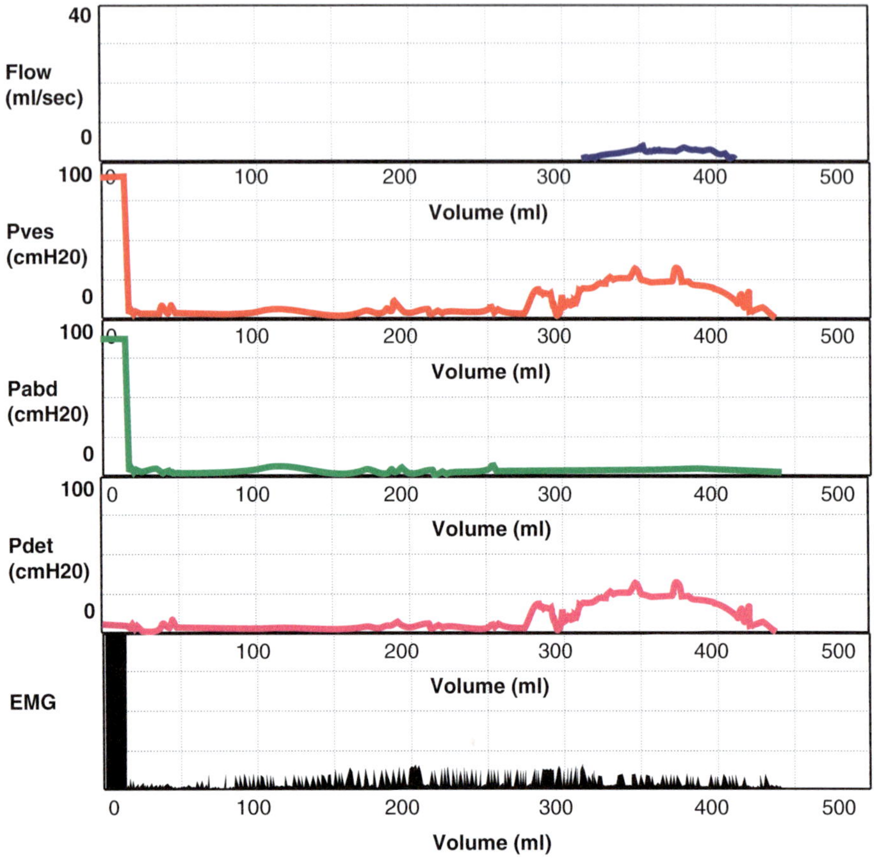

Fig. 3.20 Detrusor hyperreflexia with impaired contractility on pressure/flow urodynamics testing in a 75-year-old woman with urgency, frequency, and post-void residual urine volume of 225 ml. Urodynamics tracing demonstrates small-magnitude involuntary detrusor contraction with maximum Pdet of only 28 cmH20 and a Qmax of only 4 ml/s

Conclusions

Urodynamics testing for UAB starts with widely available office-based noninvasive urodynamics of post-void residual urine measurement and uroflowmetry. The fundamental rationale for multichannel pressure-flow urodynamics testing is that underactive bladder and detrusor underactivity is difficult to differentiate from bladder-outlet obstruction on the basis of symptoms, elevated residual urine volume, or impaired flow rate. However, diagnosis relies upon invasive pressure-flow studies that have methodological limitations and lack wide availability and clinical expertise. There is a need for biomarker and noninvasive methods of screening for

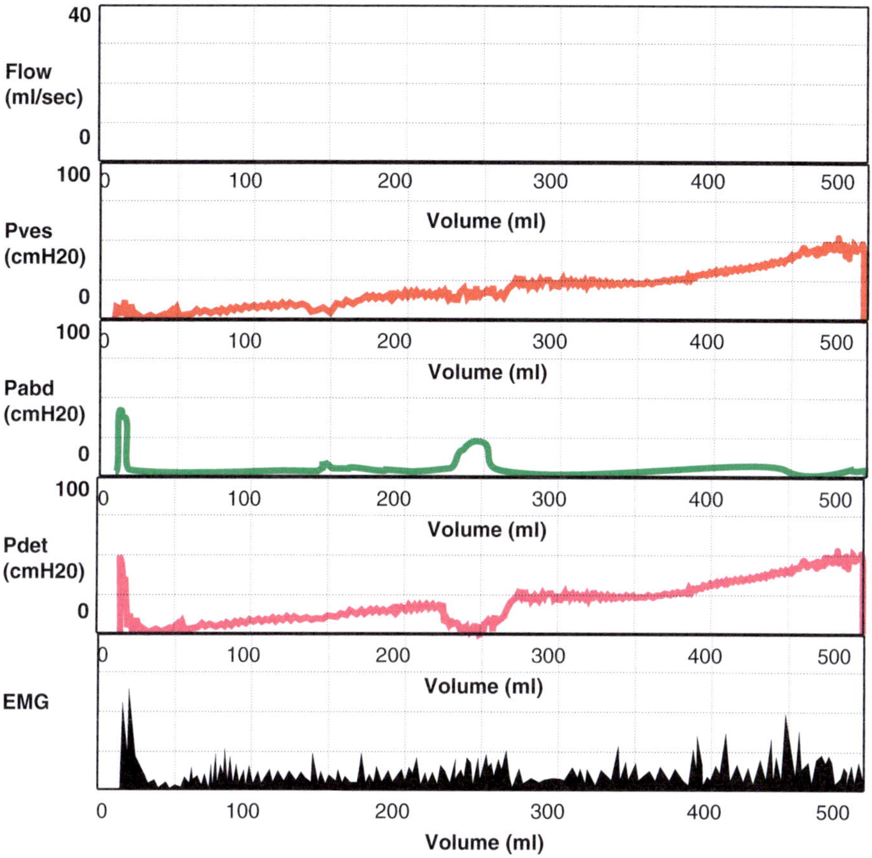

Fig. 3.21 Detrusor areflexia with poor compliance in a 31-year-old woman with pelvic fracture. She does careful intermittent self-catheterization and yet has incontinence and several bouts of febrile urinary tract infections. Urodynamics tracings demonstrated an areflexic bladder with detrusor leak point pressure of 50 cmH20

and diagnosing of underactivity bladder. Reliable and noninvasive method of determining detrusor contractility would be a priority for the large number of patients at risk for underactive bladder.

References

Abrams P, Cardozo L, Fall M et al (2002) The standardization of terminology of lower urinary tract function: report from the Standardisation Subcommittee of the International Continence Society. Neurourol Urodyn 22:167–178

Ameda K, Sullivan MP, Bae RJ, Yalla SV (1999) Urodynamic characterization of nonobstructive voiding dysfunction in symptomatic elderly men. J urology 162:142–146

Asimakopoulos AD, De Nunzio C, Kocjancic E, Tubaro A, Rosier PF, Finazzi-Agrò E (2014) Measurement of post-void residual urine. Neurourol Urodyn. doi:10.1002/nau.22671

Blaivas JG, Chancellor MB (1996) Atlas of urodynamics. Williams and Wilkins, Philadelphia

Blaivas JG, Labib KB, Michalik SJ, Zayed AA (1980) Failure of bethanechol denervation supersensitivity as a diagnostic aid. J Urol 123:199–201

Blake C, Abrams P (2004) Noninvasive techniques for the measurement of isovolumetric bladder pressure. J Urol 171:12–19

Chancellor MB, Kaufman J (2008) Case for pharmacotherapy development for underactive bladder. Urology 72:966–967

Chancellor MB, Diokno A (2014) CURE-UAB: shedding light on the underactive bladder syndrome. Int Urol Nephrol 46(Suppl 1):S1–S46

Chancellor MB, Kaplan SA, Axelord D, Blaivas JG (1991) Bladder outlet obstruction versus impaired detrusor contractility: role of uroflow. J Urol 145:810–812

Chancellor MB, Kiilholma P (1992) Urodynamic evaluation of patients following spinal cord injury. Semin Urol 10:83–94

Chapple CR, Osman NI, Birder L et al (2015) The underactive bladder: a new clinical concept. Eur Urol 68:351–353. http://dx.doi.org/10.1016/j.eurouro.2015.02.030

Diokno AC, Normolle DP, Brown MB, Herzog AR (1990) Urodynamic tests for female geriatric urinary incontinence. Urology 36:431–439

Griffiths D (2004) Detrusor contractility – order out of chaos. Scand J Urol Nephrol Suppl 215:93–100

i-Step newsletter (2013) http://istep.ifmefector.com/2013/04/09/intelligent-toilet-monitors-your-health/

McIntosh SL, Drinnan MJ, Griffiths CJ, Robson WA, Ramsden PD, Pickard RS (2004) Noninvasive assessment of bladder contractility in men. J Urol 172:1394–1398

Osman NI, Chapple CR, Abrams P et al (2014) Detrusor underactivity and the underactive bladder: a new clinical entity? A review of current terminology, definitions, epidemiology, aetiology, and diagnosis. Eur Urol 65:389–398

Ouslander J, Leach G, Abelson S, Staskin D, Blaustein J, Raz S (1983) Simple versus multichannel cystometry in the evaluation of bladder function in an incontinent geriatric population. J Urol 140:1482–1486

Pel JJ, van Mastrigt R (1999) Non-invasive measurement of bladder pressure using an external catheter. Neurourol Urodyn 18:455–469; discussion 69–75

Resnick NMEA, Yalla SV (1995) Age and the lower urinary tract: what is normal? Neurourol Urodyn 14:577–579

Schafer W (1991) Analysis of active detrusor function during voiding with bladder working function. Neuorurol Urodyn 10:19–35

Schafer W, Abrams P, Liao L, Mattiasson A, Pesce F, Spangberg A, Sterling AM, Zinner NR, van Kerrebroeck P (2002) Good urodynamic practices: uroflowmetry, filling cystometry, and pressure-flow studies. Neurourol Urodyn 21:261–274

Siroky MB, Olsson CA, Krane RJ (1979) The flow rate nomograms: I development. J Urol 122:665–668

van Koeveringe GA, Rahnama'i MS, Berghmans BC (2010) The additional value of ambulatory urodynamic measurements compared with conventional urodynamic measurements. BJU Int 105:508–513

van Koeveringe GA, Vahabi B, Andersson KE, Kirschner-Herrmans R, Oelke M (2011) Detrusor underactivity: a plea for new approaches to a common bladder dysfunction. Neurourol Urodyn 30:723–728

Wheeler JS Jr, Culkin DJ, Canning JR (1988) Positive bethanechol supersensitivity test in neurologically normal patients. Urology 31:86–89

The underactive bladder foundation (2015) www.underactivebladder.org

Chapter 4
Pathophysiology and Animal Modeling of Underactive Bladder

Naoki Yoshimura, Pradeep Tyagi, and Michael B. Chancellor

Introduction

The International Continence Society defines detrusor underactivity/underactive bladder as a detrusor contraction of inadequate strength and/or duration, resulting in prolonged bladder emptying and/or a failure to achieve complete bladder emptying in the absence of urethral obstruction (Jeong et al. 2012; Miyazato et al. 2013). This is a great starting point but does not describe what can cause UAB and what we can do to improve it. To understand the pathology of UAB, we need to first understand the normal physiology of the lower urinary tract during filling and voiding.

Neurons from the spinal cord and brain are connected to form a neural control system which coordinates the reciprocal activity during bladder emptying where the detrusor contracts and the sphincter relaxes (de Groat 2006). To fully empty the bladder during micturition, relaxation of the internal smooth muscle and external striated muscle sphincters are both required. After initial sphincter relaxation, detrusor smooth muscle contraction occurs with increased intravesical pressure. This switch from filling to emptying phase is under voluntarily control in healthy adults (Fig. 4.1).

Neuron reflexes guiding the voiding are mediated by a spinobulbospinal pathway passing through the pontine micturition center in the brainstem (Tyagi et al. 2009).

N. Yoshimura, MD, PhD (✉)
Departments of Urology and Pharmacology & Chemical Biology, University of Pittsburgh School of Medicine, Pittsburgh, PA, USA
e-mail: nyos122@hotmail.com

P. Tyagi, PhD
Department of Urology, University of Pittsburgh School of Medicine, Pittsburgh, PA, USA

M.B. Chancellor, MD
Department of Urology, Oakland University William Beaumont School of Medicine, Royal Oak, MI, USA

Neurourology Program, Beaumont Health System, Royal Oak, MI, USA

M.B. Chancellor, A.C. Diokno (eds.), *The Underactive Bladder*,
DOI 10.1007/978-3-319-23687-2_4

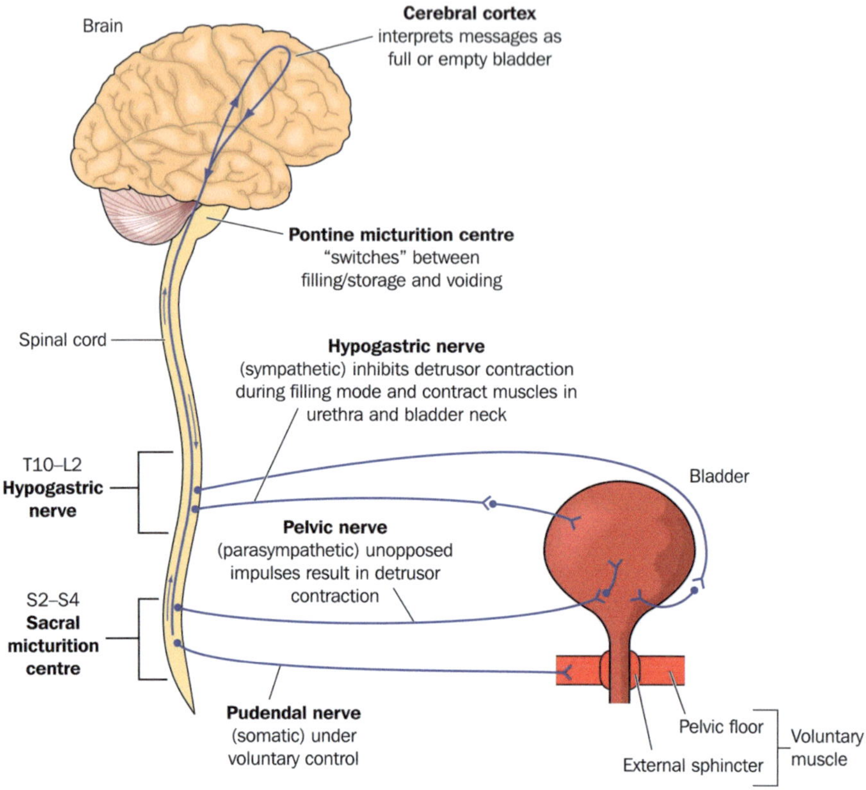

Fig. 4.1 Neurophysiology of the lower urinary tract

Afferent neuronal signals from the bladder activate and maintain the micturition reflex to the central nervous system. Afferent nerves carry the sensation of bladder fullness via Aδ-fiber afferents during filling. These afferents also signal the magnitude of detrusor contractions during the emptying phase (Tyagi et al. 2004; de Groat 1993, 1997; de Groat et al. 1998).

A number of important neurotransmitters are involved in the control of micturition including acetylcholine, norepinephrine, serotonin, dopamine, adenosine triphosphate, excitatory and inhibitory amino acids, nitric oxide, and neuropeptides (de Groat 2006). Acetylcholine is the primary neurotransmitter effecting bladder emptying through its action on the muscarinic receptors on detrusor muscle (Tyagi et al. 2004), and the storage phase is mediated by norepinephrine released from sympathetic nerve terminals (Tyagi et al. 2006). Efficient voiding is also dependent on the activity of urethral afferents responding to urine flow in the urethral lumen. Signal from urethral afferent is fed back to the central nervous system to facilitate detrusor contraction when there is urine in the urethra and inhibit detrusor contraction when urine stop flowing through the urethra lumen (de Groat et al. 2001).

Pathophysiology of UAB

Multiple etiology factors has been implicated in its pathogenesis of UAB including aging, bladder outlet obstruction, diabetes mellitus contributing in myogenic UAB, Parkinson's disease resulting in neurogenic UAB, spinal cord injury, multiple sclerosis, infectious neurological problems (e.g., AIDS, herpes zoster infection), and pelvic surgery and radical prostatectomy that can lead to iatrogenic UAB (Miyazato et al. 2013). Iatrogenic UAB could also be caused by side effects of drugs including neuroleptics, calcium channel antagonists, and α-receptor agonists. Although the prevalence of UAB is higher in the aged population, UAB is not part of the normal aging process.

Underactive bladder includes both functional and anatomical causes (Fig. 4.2). The following are the factors that alone or in combination contribute to UAB:

- Functional and/or anatomical changes result from BOO or reduced detrusor contractility.
- Abnormalities of sensory and motor neural pathways and cognitive function.

It may be helpful to consider the two tradition hypotheses on underactive bladder pathophysiology: myogenic and neurogenic. The classic myogenic hypothesis focuses on the ability of the detrusor to adequately contract. More recently, the neurogenic hypothesis focuses on defect in bladder afferent innervation, micturition control at spinal and supraspinal center, or both that may also lead to UAB (Tyagi et al. 2014).

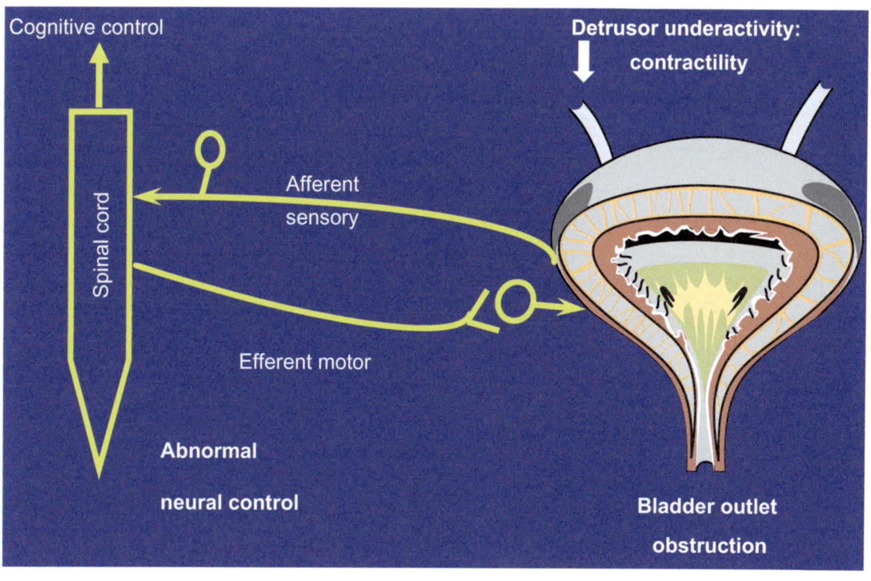

Fig. 4.2 Functional and anatomical causes of UAB

Myogenic UAB

The myogenic hypothesis suggests that UAB results from changes within the bladder smooth muscle that lead to reduced excitability and loss of intrinsic muscle contractility. Detrusor ultrastructural studies have revealed characteristic changes associated with UAB (Brierly et al. 2003a), which could hinder adequate contraction of the detrusor muscle (Blatt et al. 2012).

Neurogenic UAB

Given the importance of an intact afferent system to voiding function, UAB may arise when the levels of afferent activity are decreased during bladder filling (Smith et al. 2012). There can be age-dependent loss of bladder volume sensitivity due to changes in neurotransmitter release from the urothelium and coupling of the suburothelial interstitial cell-afferent network. Afferents in the bladder and urethra can be damaged through an effect of aging or ischemia (Azadzoi et al. 2008). Urethral afferent dysfunction as a late consequence of diabetes (Yang et al. 2010) can also reduce or prematurely end the micturition reflex, leading to loss of voiding efficiency, as seen in diabetic cystopathy. Autonomous detrusor activity during bladder filling generates bladder sensation, and absence of spontaneous contractions can hinder the initiation of afferent signals and lead to UAB (Andersson 2010).

It is quite possible that many patients with UAB have both myogenic and neurogenic components and it can be difficult to isolate the contribution of each component. In such cases, decreased detrusor contractility may lead to reduced neuronal activity of the bladder, which can reduce the afferent signal to the central nervous system leading to incomplete micturition and UAB.

Smith and associates (2012) have recently proposed an exciting new integrative hypothesis for UAB. The integrative hypothesis proposes that complex interactions among smooth muscle, connective tissue, urothelium, and supportive structures with peripheral nerves contribute to normal generation of localized spontaneous activity that is observed as localized contractions and stretches (micromotions) in the human bladder (Drake et al. 2005). These findings suggest that the detrusor muscle is functionally modular in arrangement.

Importance of Animal Models

Since direct human experimentation on UAB subjects is not possible for ethical reasons, hypotheses stated for UAB will require alternatives to test the derived predictions. Animal models can be used to generate novel directions of research and

Table 4.1 Animal models of underactive bladder

Animal models of underactive bladder
Aging model
Myogenic injury models
Bladder outlet obstruction (BOO) models
Ischemia and hyperlipidemia models
Peripheral neurogenic models of UAB
Diabetic bladder dysfunction (DBD)
Diabetes-induced urethral dysfunction
Central neurological models of UAB
Lumbar canal stenosis (LCS)
Pelvic nerve injury
Ventral avulsion
Transgenic models of UAB
Prostaglandin receptor knockout
Purinergic receptor knockout

corroborate findings obtained in case studies or other methods. Animals who share similar integrative physiology of the lower urinary tract and the neural control of micturition as humans provide a suitable tool to dissect the underlying mechanisms in clinical features of UAB. Animal models can be used to reproduce some or all of the facets of UAB seen clinically as a consequence of myogenic or neurogenic dysfunction to help identify suitable interventions (Table 1). Animal models provide suitable platforms of intact biological systems for assessing results from simpler in vitro research. The clinical context of animal studies can help build a confidence in a new treatment approach before clinical testing.

Development of an animal model for UAB is hindered by the lack of a surrogate that predicts treatment outcome. A number of animal models have been proposed to study UAB and they are discussed next.

Aging models of UAB

UAB is often seen in aged patients (Zimmern et al. 2014); therefore, aged animals would be an appropriate model to study UAB. Aged mouse (Lai et al. 2007; Smith et al. 2012) or rat models reproduce some of the UAB features, with age-dependent loss of bladder volume sensitivity manifesting as increased intercontractile interval (Fig. 4.3). Cystometry of young and old mice shows that detrusor contractility is preserved, but the response to rise in bladder volume is diminished in 26-month-old animals. Similar findings were observed in aged rats with increased volume and pressure thresholds for voiding (Chai et al. 2000). Age-dependent loss of bladder volume sensitivity in aged rats may be explained by the decreased response to intravesical capsaicin which is suggestive of reduced C-fiber afferent activity in aged rat

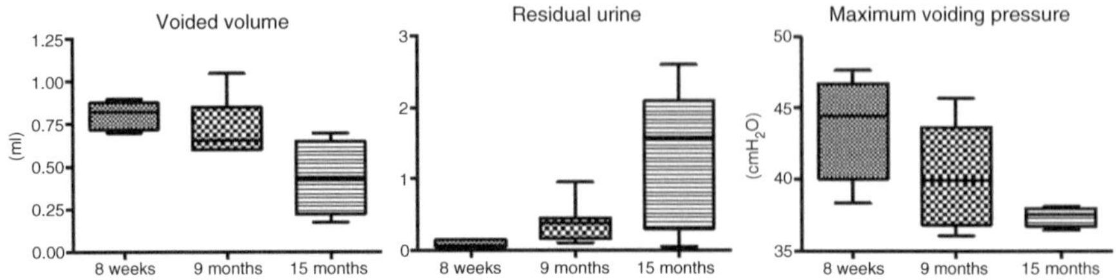

Fig. 4.3 Parameters of cystometrogram in 8-week, 9-month, and 15-month aged rats. (*Left*) Voiding volume (*ml*), (*middle*) residual urine volume (*ml*), and (*right*) maximum voiding pressure (*cmH$_2$0*). There was significant increase in residual urine volume in 15-month aged rats compared with 8-week and 9-month aged rats. Maximum voiding pressure and voided volume were significant decreased in 15-month aged rats compared with 8-week and 9-month aged rats

(Chai et al. 2000). Intravesical capsaicin is expected to increase detrusor contractility because of neurokinins released from afferent nerves following activation of transient receptor potential (TRP) channels. Aged rats also exhibit a reduction in the maximal bladder pressure generated during pelvic nerve stimulation (Hotta et al. 1995; Hotta and Uchida 2010). Staining for calcitonin gene-related peptide, substance P in lumbosacral dorsal root ganglion neurons (Mohammed and Santer 2002), and density of pituitary adenylate cyclase-activating peptide innervation of the bladder base are also decreased in aged rats (Mohammed et al. 2002).

Significant decreases in the amplitude of neurogenic contractions were associated with fibrosis but without accompanying a decrease in nerve density in the bladder neck. These findings from aged rats implicate impairment of both afferent and efferent transmission results in incomplete voiding. There may also be an upregulation of purinergic receptors in the urothelium and bladder nerve bundles compared to control rats. This may correspond to the increased non-adrenergic and noncholinergic innervation seen in aging humans. Upregulation of β-adrenoceptors (Iaina et al. 1988) has also reported in aged rat bladder (Lluel et al. 2003b).

Aged male rats exhibited urethral dysfunction and impairment of the urethrovesical coordination (Lluel et al. 2000, 2003a, b). Decrease in resting urethral pressure at voiding threshold and a significant delay in urethral relaxation that leads to increased post-void residual urine volume was observed in aged male rats. The responses to carbachol in the bladder body and to phenylephrine and carbachol in the urethra have also been observed in the aged male rat bladder.

Myogenic Models of UAB

Decreased detrusor contractility in UAB can result from a lack of contractile stimulus (acetylcholine and ATP) (Yoshida et al. 2004) and/or a lack of tissue responsiveness due to irreversible changes in the bladder wall. Similar decrease in muscle function has been described as sarcopenia (loss of muscle tissue, increased collagen deposition) (Brierly et al. 2003a, b). Several factors may contribute to altered excitation and contraction coupling mechanisms in UAB including changes in the properties and density of calcium (Gomez-Pinilla et al. 2011) and potassium channels, gap junctions, and receptors in detrusor smooth muscles.

Bladder Outlet Obstruction (BOO) Models of UAB

Effects similar to BOO in humans have been well documented in a variety of animal species including pig, rat, guinea pig, and rabbit. Most typical BOO model is one created by inducing partial obstruction of the urethra using some form of ligature that either obstruct the urethra immediately or does so gradually as the animal grows (Murakami et al. 2008). Partial BOO can be created in female rats by ligating the proximal urethra over a 1 mm catheter. The obstructed animals are followed and evaluated from 2 weeks up to 6 months. Prolonged BOO caused a decrease in electrical field stimulation, acetylcholine release, and the number of nerves in the rat urinary bladder. The amount of acetylcholine can be measured in the dialysate fraction obtained from a microdialysis probe inserted into the muscle strips during electrical field stimulation. The reduced density of acetylcholinesterase-positive nerves in obstructed bladders may play an important role in insufficient efferent activation that can lead to UAB.

Ischemia and Hyperlipidemia Models of UAB

Epidemiological studies have suggested bladder ischemia and metabolic syndrome as potential etiological factors of UAB. Evidence suggests that there is likely to be both vascular and neurogenic components and that chronic bladder ischemia (Fu and Longhurst 1998) secondary to atherosclerosis may induce UAB. Cystometry of myocardial infarction-prone Watanabe heritable hyperlipidemic rabbits shows significantly shorter micturition intervals, smaller voided volume with non-voiding contractions, and lower micturition pressure (Yoshida et al. 2010), as compared to control animals. The carbachol and electrical field stimulation-induced contractions of these rabbit's detrusor strips were also significantly decreased. Also, a rat model of bladder ischemia induced by balloon endothelial injury of the common iliac arteries shows the progressive vascular damage resulting in bladder dysfunction that develops from OAB to UAB conditions (Nomiya et al. 2014). These animal models may serve well to screen for drugs that seek to improve detrusor contractility.

Peripheral Neurogenic Models of UAB

Animal models of neurogenic UAB can be broadly divided into peripheral and central models based on the predominant site of the deficit. Peripheral models are those resulting from direct damage to the bladder and its peripheral innervation or blood supply, whereas central models are developed following injuries to the spinal cord or brainstem.

Diabetic Bladder Dysfunction (DBD) Models of UAB

Diabetic bladder dysfunction includes both storage and voiding problems such as decreased sensation and increased bladder capacity in both type I and II diabetes mellitus DM (Goins et al. 2001; Gray et al. 2008; Sasaki et al. 2002, 2003, 2004). Streptozotocin injection is the classic model for induction of DM in rats, which is confirmed by increases in blood glucose and urine production. After streptozotocin animals will initially show time-dependent changes in cystometry with initial compensated changes similar to detrusor overactivity. The decompensated stage at 12 weeks shows features of UAB that are the result of long-term hyperglycemia-related oxidative stress and polyuria. The streptozotocin-induced DBD is associated with increased bladder weight and residual urine, which indicate the incomplete bladder emptying. Streptozotocin-induced DBD affects Aδ-fiber afferent-dependent conscious voiding, which was evaluated in metabolic cage measurements and awake cystometry (Goins et al. 2001; Gray et al. 2008; Sasaki et al. 2002, 2003, 2004). The impairment of C-fiber-mediated bladder nociceptive responses in the DBD bladder has been shown by reduced sensitivity of C-fiber afferent pathways to nociceptive stimuli during acetic acid cystometry of rats with DBD under urethane anesthesia (Sasaki et al. 2002).

Genetically engineered mouse models have also been developed that display salient features of DBD relevant to UAB. Liver-specific deletion of insulin receptor substrate 1 (IRS1) and IRS2 leads to hyperglycemia by 5 weeks of life (Dong et al. 2008; Cheng et al. 2009) and development of DBD that models pathologic changes in humans with type II diabetes mellitus (Wang et al. 2012) The IRS1/IRS2 double knockout model displays bladder overactivity in young mice, but bladder underactivity in older animals. Detrusor underactivity was characterized by decreased force generation in muscle strips from older diabetic mice compared to age-matched controls in response to electrical field stimulation, carbachol, and KCl-mediated depolarization (Yang et al. 2010).

Diabetes Induced Urethral Dysfunction

Urethral dysfunction is believed to cause changes in voiding behavior of aged male rats (Lluel et al. 2000, 2003a, b) which results in decreased resting urethral pressure at voiding threshold and the occurrence of a significant delay in urethral relaxation. Therefore, impaired urethral relaxation can also prolong the bladder emptying during voiding phase. Urethral dysfunction is also a consequence of diabetes (Fig. 4.4) (Torimoto et al. 2004, 2005; Christ et al. 2009; Yang et al. 2010). Nitric

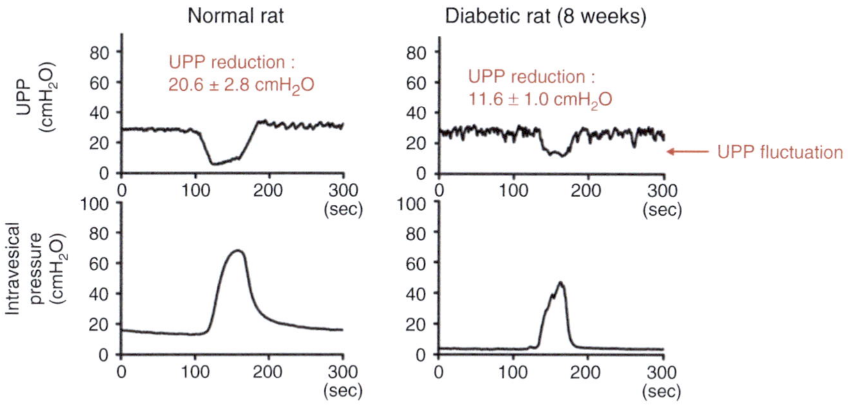

Fig. 4.4 Diabetes-induced urethral dysfunction contributes to incomplete voiding. In these experiments, striated sphincter activity was suppressed by α-bungarotoxin and NO-mediated urethral relaxation was suppressed by L-NAME. Diabetic rat shows significantly reduced urethral pressure profile (*UPP*) compared to normal rat (With permission Tyagi et al. 2014)

oxide-mediated relaxation of the urethra is considered to be impaired in diabetes. Other studies have reported damage to urethral afferents, which reduces or prematurely ends the micturition reflex, leading to loss of voiding efficiency, as in diabetic cystopathy. DBD is also associated with altered receptor expression (Li et al. 2013) and changes in non-adrenergic and non-cholinergic transmission (Bschleipfer et al. 2012; Philyppov et al. 2012).

Central Neurological Models of UAB

Dysfunction of the central control of the voiding reflex can lead to UAB by impacting upon key processes in perception, integration, and outflow. Considering that voluntary voiding is a learned phenomenon, age-related decline of dopamine binding has been reported in brain areas involved in cognition (MacDonald et al. 2012). Brain areas involved in cognition overlap with areas involved in processing afferent input from the bladder, which implicate the dopamine role in central transmission as key for UAB.

A number of central nervous system disorders can cause voiding dysfunction in humans, including cerebrovascular events, dementia, Parkinson's disease, multiple sclerosis, and stroke. The coordination between the detrusor smooth muscle and the sphincter mechanism of the bladder occurs in the pontine region of the brainstem. Neurological models improve our understanding of the complex pathways controlling micturition.

Lumbar Canal Stenosis (LCS) Model for UAB

LCS induces mechanical compression of the cauda equina by insertion of silicon rubber pieces into the L6 epidural space in female rats (Sekido et al. 2012). The mechanical compression causes degeneration of both afferent and efferent spinal nerves involved in voiding. The animal model exhibits both decreased voiding efficiency and reduced detrusor contractility (Wang et al. 2015) (Figs. 4.5 and 4.6).

Pelvic Nerve Injury Model for UAB

Iatrogenic UAB is may be associated with pelvic nerve injury at time of pelvic surgery. The animal model can be developed for UAB by performing a bilateral pelvic nerve crush in adult female rats with a straight micro mosquito clamp as illustrated

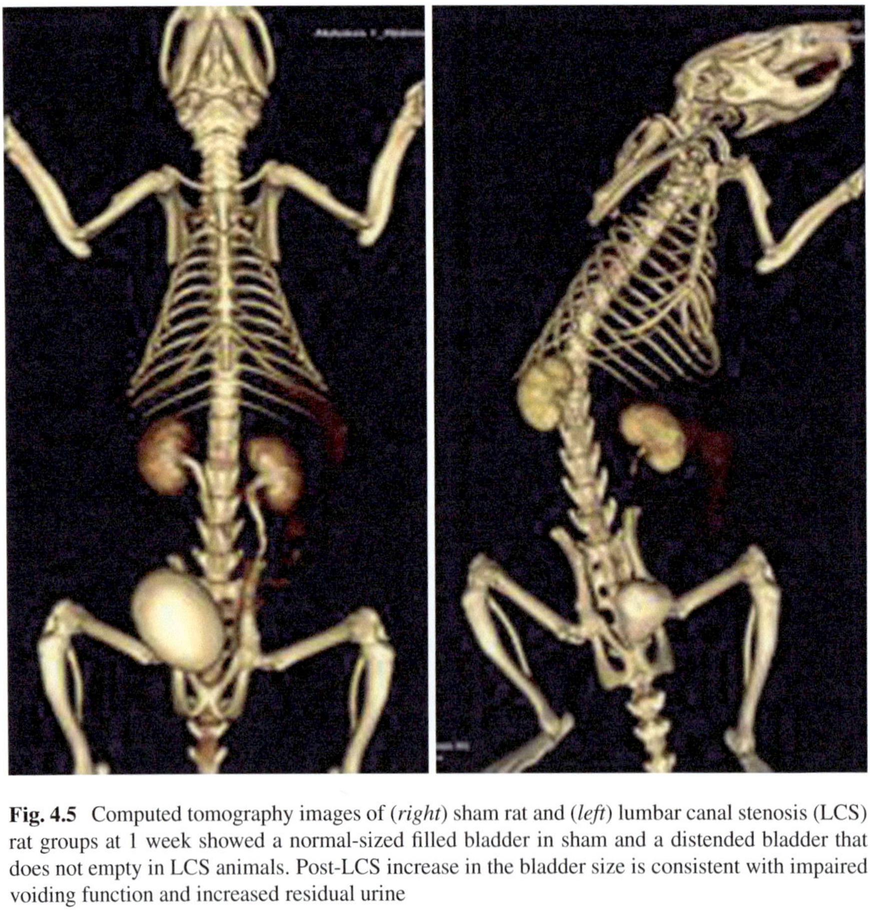

Fig. 4.5 Computed tomography images of (*right*) sham rat and (*left*) lumbar canal stenosis (LCS) rat groups at 1 week showed a normal-sized filled bladder in sham and a distended bladder that does not empty in LCS animals. Post-LCS increase in the bladder size is consistent with impaired voiding function and increased residual urine

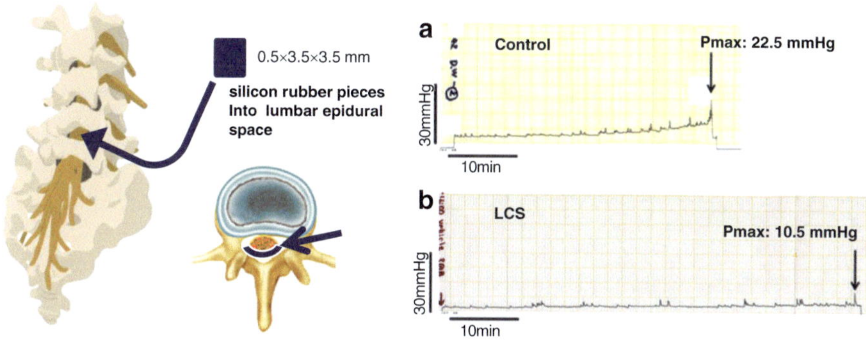

Fig. 4.6 Lumbar canal stenosis (*LCS*) rat model. (*Left*) LCS induces mechanical compression of the cauda equine via insertion of silicon rubber piece into the L6 epidural space in female rats. (*Right*) Cystometrogram demonstrating difference in bladder capacity and contractility between control (**a**) and LCS animals (**b**) consistent with degeneration of afferent and efferent nerves

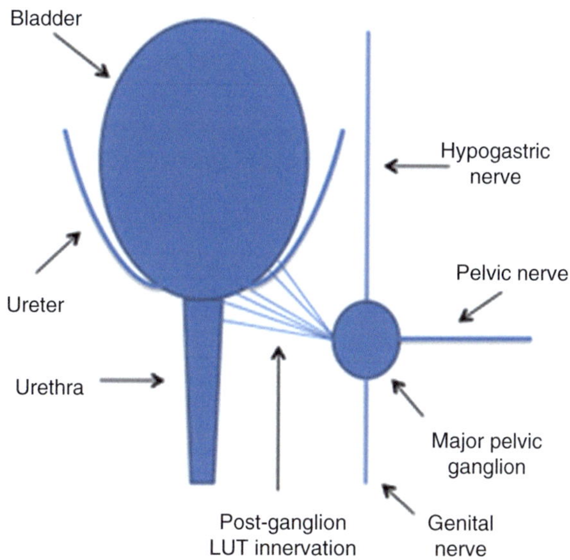

Fig. 4.7 Schematic illustration for rat model of iatrogenic UAB induced by bilateral pelvic nerve crush in adult female rats (With permission Tyagi et al. 2014)

in Fig. 4.7. The clamp was used to crush each pelvic nerve for a total of 30 s. The crush was performed proximal to each pelvic nerve's entry into the major pelvic ganglion. Pelvic nerve crush injury caused significant increases in bladder capacity in cystometry performed 1 week after nerve injury as shown in Fig. 4.8. The model shows increased PVR and decreases in maximum voiding pressure and voiding efficiency in cystometry. The pelvic nerve injury model includes afferent and efferent nerve dysfunction and may be useful for pharmacotherapy studies.

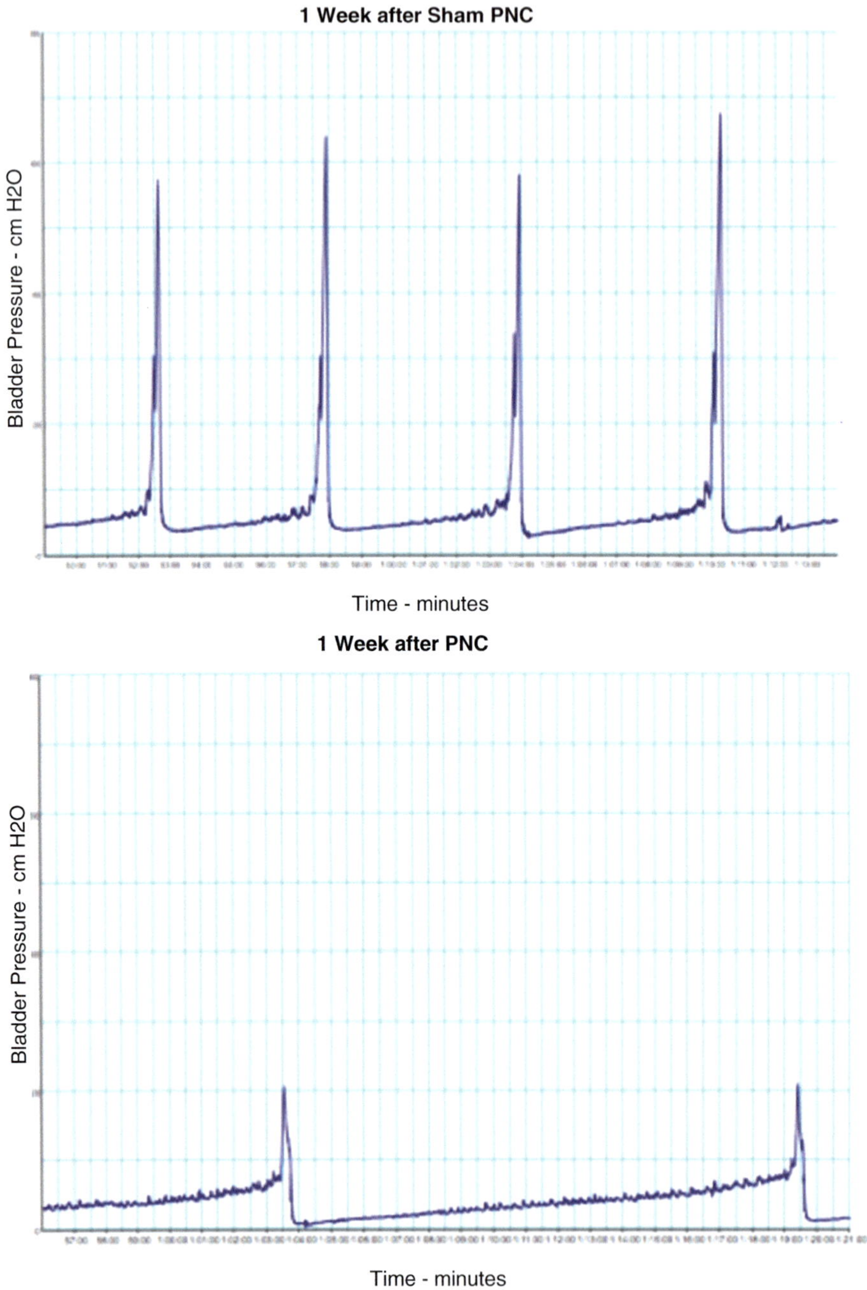

Fig. 4.8 Cystometric outcomes of bilateral pelvic nerve crush (*PNC*) in female rats. Compared to sham group, the crush injury of pelvic nerves exhibited increases in PVR and decreases in maximum voiding pressure and voiding efficiency (With permission Tyagi et al. 2014)

Ventral Avulsion Model for UAB

Trauma to the thoracolumbar spine commonly results in injuries to the cauda equina and the lumbosacral portion of the spinal cord. A unilateral L5–S2 ventral root avulsion injury in rats mimics a partial lesion to the cauda equina and conus medullaris (Chang and Havton 2013). Detailed cystometrogram studies found that a markedly reduced voiding efficiency was noted at 12 weeks after the ventral avulsion injury with decreased maximum amplitude to indicate reduced contractile stimuli. Concurrent external urethral sphincter electromyography demonstrated shortened burst and prolonged silent periods associated with the elimination phase. (Chang and Havton 2013). The animal model demonstrated that a 5HT1A receptor agonist, 8-hydroxy-2-(di-n-propylamino)-tetralin (8-OH-DPAT), administered intravenously, elicited the supraspinal micturition reflex during cystometry.

Transgenic Models of UAB

Several transgenic mouse models have demonstrated that molecular alterations in the urothelium, peripheral innervation, and smooth muscle lead to significant changes in voiding function (Schnegelsberg et al. 2010)

Prostaglandin Receptor Knockout Mouse of UAB

Prostaglandins are produced by the constitutively expressed cyclooxygenase (COX)-1 enzyme and, an inducible isozyme, COX-2 in urothelium (Rahnama'i et al. 2010, 2011, 2012a, b). Prostaglandin E_2 (PGE_2) produced by this enzyme is decreased in the urine of UAB patients (Kim et al. 2005). PGE_2 mediates its effects by activating the EP family (EP_1–EP_4 isoforms) of G-protein-coupled receptors. PGE_2 have a physiological role as it is produced by detrusor muscle in response to stretch. Mouse knockout models of the EP_3 receptor showed enlarged bladder capacity (McCafferty et al. 2008), which could be used to screen drugs and test new hypothesis for UAB. Since, EP_3 knockout mice do not exhibit bladder overactivity after instillation of an EP_3 receptor agonist; therefore changes in peripheral afferent sensitivity in this model cannot be ruled out.

Purinergic Receptor Knockout Mouse of UAB

ATP is released from human and animal urothelium in response to mechanical stretch. Prostaglandins were shown to be involved in the stretch-evoked ATP release from the urothelium (Tanaka et al. 2011). ATP acts as a sensory neurotransmitter by binding to purinergic receptors (P_2X) on suburothelial afferent nerve endings. P_2X_3

receptor knockout mice appear to have reduced bladder sensation, with reduced urinary frequency and larger voided volumes (Apostolidis et al. 2005; Cockayne et al. 2000, 2005; Vlaskovska et al. 2001).

Limitations of Animal Models of UAB

An ideal disease model would be one which replicates the symptoms, etiology, and natural history of clinical UAB. Most of the animal models presented in this chapter here do not mimic all the aspects of UAB, but bear enough similarities to make them relevant for a limited number of aspects of the human condition. It is unlikely that any single animal model will replicate all the symptoms and complications observed in UAB patients. More realistically, animal models need to be viewed as research tools to answer a particular experimental hypothesis. Studies using rodents and small laboratory animals are relatively simpler to perform and maintain than studies done using larger animals. Rodents can adapt to surgery through neural plasticity and cellular adaptations. Results in rodents may represent compensatory changes or collateral effects rather than having pathophysiological relevance for UAB.

We should remember that there are significant differences in the composition of the urinary bladder wall between small and large animal bladders and between animals and human. The location of postganglionic parasympathetic cell bodies innervating the rat bladder is entirely in the pelvic ganglia, whereas a substantial proportion of these cell bodies are located in the bladder wall of humans and other animal species (McMurray et al. 2006). Therefore, the outcomes following partial BOO differ among species (Gabella 1999; Gabella and Davis 1998). Unlike rats, long-term untreated BOO does not appear to result in significant clinical decompensation of detrusor function in human (Chang et al. 2008).

The structural and functional differences discussed above are but a few examples of the interspecies variability (Insel 2007). The interspecies variability lends different strengths and weaknesses to each model and makes them suitable for studying different aspects of UAB. Regardless of the type of model used, careful validation of both the model itself and the results that it generates ensures that any findings are correctly extrapolated from animals to humans.

Conclusions

Research into the pathogenesis of detrusor underactivity and underactive bladder is hampered by a lack of adequate and accepted animal model for the disease. Despite the difficulties associated with animal modeling, there is no substitute for their use as tools to advance understanding and develop medical interventions for UAB. The models that have been used to date have different strengths and weaknesses, and the findings should be reproduced in more than one mammalian species before extrapolating data to human subjects. A number of leading research laboratories from around the world are now starting to work on UAB and we are excited to see groundbreaking research report on improved understanding of the pathophysiology and suitable animal modeling of underactive bladder.

References

Andersson KE (2010) Detrusor myocyte activity and afferent signaling. NeurourolUrodyn 29:97–106, 2009/12/22 edn.29

Apostolidis A, Popat R, Yiangou Y, Cockayne D, Ford AP, Davis JB, Dasgupta P, Fowler CJ, Anand P (2005) Decreased sensory receptors P2X3 and TRPV1 in suburothelial nerve fibers following intradetrusor injections of botulinum toxin for human detrusor overactivity. J Urol 174:977–982, 2005/08/12 edn.174; discussion 982–973

Azadzoi KM, Radisavljevic ZM, Siroky MB (2008) Effects of ischemia on tachykinin-containing nerves and neurokinin receptors in the rabbit bladder. Urology 71:979–983, 2008/03/04 edn.71

Blatt AH, Brammah S, Tse V, Chan L (2012) Transurethral prostate resection in patients with hypocontractile detrusor – what is the predictive value of ultrastructural detrusor changes? J Urol 188:2294–2299, 2012/10/23 edn.188

Brierly RD, Hindley RG, McLarty E, Harding DM, Thomas PJ (2003a) A prospective controlled quantitative study of ultrastructural changes in the underactive detrusor. J Urol 169:1374–1378, 2003/03/12 edn.169

Brierly RD, Hindley RG, McLarty E, Harding DM, Thomas PJ (2003b) A prospective evaluation of detrusor ultrastructural changes in bladder outlet obstruction. BJU Int 91:360–364, 2003/02/27 edn.91

Bschleipfer T, Nandigama R, Moeller S, Illig C, Weidner W, Kummer W (2012) Bladder outlet obstruction influences mRNA expression of cholinergic receptors on sensory neurons in mice. Life Sci 91:1077–1081, 2012/05/29 edn.91

Chai TC, Andersson KE, Tuttle JB, Steers WD (2000) Altered neural control of micturition in the aged F344 rat. Urol Res 28:348–354, 2000/12/29 edn.28

Chang HH, Havton LA (2013) Serotonergic 5-HT(1A) receptor agonist (8-OH-DPAT) ameliorates impaired micturition reflexes in a chronic ventral root avulsion model of incomplete cauda equina/conus medullaris injury. Exp Neurol 239:210–217, 2012/10/27 edn.239

Chang SJ, Chiang IN, Yu HJ (2008) The effectiveness of tamsulosin in treating women with voiding difficulty. Int J Urol 15:981–985, 2008/08/30 edn.15

Cheng Z, Guo S, Copps K, Dong X, Kollipara R, Rodgers JT, Depinho RA, Puigserver P, White MF (2009) Foxo1 integrates insulin signaling with mitochondrial function in the liver. Nat Med 15:1307–1311, 2009/10/20 edn.15

Christ GJ, Bushman W, Fraser MO (2009) Impact of diabetes and obesity on the prostate and urethra: implications to improved bladder dysfunction understanding and treatment. J Urol 182:S38–S44, 2009/10/23 edn.182

Cockayne DA, Hamilton SG, Zhu QM, Dunn PM, Zhong Y, Novakovic S, Malmberg AB, Cain G, Berson A, Kassotakis L, Hedley L, Lachnit WG, Burnstock G, McMahon SB, Ford AP (2000) Urinary bladder hyporeflexia and reduced pain-related behaviour in P2X3-deficient mice. Nature 407:1011–1015, 2000/11/09 edn.407

Cockayne DA, Dunn PM, Zhong Y, Rong W, Hamilton SG, Knight GE, Ruan HZ, Ma B, Yip P, Nunn P, McMahon SB, Burnstock G, Ford AP (2005) P2X2 knockout mice and P2X2/P2X3 double knockout mice reveal a role for the P2X2 receptor subunit in mediating multiple sensory effects of ATP. J Physiol 567:621–639, 2005/06/18 edn.567

de Groat WC (1993) Anatomy and physiology of the lower urinary tract. Urol Clin North Am 20:383–401, 1993/08/01 edn.20

de Groat WC (1997) A neurologic basis for the overactive bladder. Urology 50:36–52, 1998/01/14 edn.50; discussion 53–36

de Groat WC (2006) Integrative control of the lower urinary tract: preclinical perspective. Br J Pharmacol 147(Suppl 2):S25–S40, 2006/02/09 edn.147 Suppl 2

de Groat WC, Araki I, Vizzard MA, Yoshiyama M, Yoshimura N, Sugaya K, Tai C, Roppolo JR (1998) Developmental and injury induced plasticity in the micturition reflex pathway. Behav Brain Res 92:127–140, 1998/06/25 edn.92

de Groat WC, Fraser MO, Yoshiyama M, Smerin S, Tai C, Chancellor MB, Yoshimura N,Roppolo JR (2001) Neural control of the urethra. Scand J Urol Nephrol Suppl 207:35–43. 2001/06/21 edn., discussion 106–125

Dong XC, Copps KD, Guo S, Li Y, Kollipara R, DePinho RA, White MF (2008) Inactivation of hepatic Foxo1 by insulin signaling is required for adaptive nutrient homeostasis and endocrine growth regulation. Cell Metab 8:65–76, 2008/07/02 edn.8

Drake MJ, Harvey IJ, Gillespie JI, Van Duyl WA (2005) Localized contractions in the normal human bladder and in urinary urgency. BJU Int 95:1002–1005, 2005/04/21 edn.95

Fu LW, Longhurst JC (1998) Role of 5-HT3 receptors in activation of abdominal sympathetic C fibre afferents during ischaemia in cats. J Physiol 509(Pt 3):729–740, 1998/05/23 edn.509 (Pt 3)

Gabella G (1999) Structure of the intramural nerves of the rat bladder. J Neurocytol 28:615–637, 2000/06/14 edn.28

Gabella G, Davis C (1998) Distribution of afferent axons in the bladder of rats. J Neurocytol 27:141–155, 2000/01/20 edn.27

Goins WF, Yoshimura N, Phelan MW, Yokoyama T, Fraser MO, Ozawa H, Bennett NJ, de Groat WC, Glorioso JC, Chancellor MB (2001) Herpes simplex virus mediated nerve growth factor expression in bladder and afferent neurons: potential treatment for diabetic bladder dysfunction. J Urol 165:1748–1754, 2001/05/09 edn.165

Gomez-Pinilla PJ, Pozo MJ, Camello PJ (2011) Aging differentially modifies agonist-evoked mouse detrusor contraction and calcium signals. Age (Dordr) 33:81–88, 2010/07/03 edn.33

Gray MA, Wang CC, Sacks MS, Yoshimura N, Chancellor MB, Nagatomi J (2008) Time-dependent alterations of select genes in streptozotocin-induced diabetic rat bladder. Urology 71:1214–1219, 2008/02/19 edn.71

Hotta H, Uchida S (2010) Aging of the autonomic nervous system and possible improvements in autonomic activity using somatic afferent stimulation. Geriatr Gerontol Int 10(Suppl 1):S127–S136, 2010/07/16 edn.10 Suppl 1

Hotta H, Morrison JF, Sato A, Uchida S (1995) The effects of aging on the rat bladder and its innervation. Jpn J Physiol 45:823–836, 1995/01/01 edn.45

Iaina A, Serban I, Kapuler S, Gavendo S, Lindner A, Eliahou HE (1988) Beta-adrenergic receptors in the urinary bladder of adult and developing rats. Isr J Med Sci 24:237–240, 1988/04/01 edn.24

Insel TR (2007) From animal models to model animals. Biol Psychiatry 62:1337–1339, 2007/12/07 edn.62

Jeong SJ, Kim HJ, Lee YJ, Lee JK, Lee BK, Choo YM, Oh JJ, Lee SC, Jeong CW, Yoon CY, Hong SK, Byun SS, Lee SE (2012) Prevalence and clinical features of detrusor underactivity among elderly with lower urinary tract symptoms: a comparison between men and women. Korean J Urol 53:342–348, 2012/06/07 edn.53

Kim JC, Park EY, Hong SH, Seo SI, Park YH, Hwang TK (2005) Changes of urinary nerve growth factor and prostaglandins in male patients with overactive bladder symptom. Int J Urol 12:875–880, 2005/12/06 edn.12

Lai HH, Boone TB, Thompson TC, Smith CP, Somogyi GT (2007) Using caveolin-1 knockout mouse to study impaired detrusor contractility and disrupted muscarinic activity in the aging bladder. Urology 69:407–411, 2007/02/27 edn.69

Li Y, Sun Y, Zhang Z, Feng X, Meng H, Li S, Zhu Y, Chen S, Wang Y, Wang J, Zhang D, Jiang X, Li N, Shi B (2013) Cannabinoid receptors 1 and 2 are associated with bladder dysfunction in an experimental diabetic rat model. BJU Int 112:E143–E150, 2013/06/26 edn.112

Lluel P, Palea S, Barras M, Grandadam F, Heudes D, Bruneval P, Corman B, Martin DJ (2000) Functional and morphological modifications of the urinary bladder in aging female rats. Am J Physiol Regul Integr Comp Physiol 278:R964–R972, 2000/04/06 edn.278

Lluel P, Deplanne V, Heudes D, Bruneval P, Palea S (2003a) Age-related changes in urethrovesical coordination in male rats: relationship with bladder instability? Am J Physiol Regul Integr Comp Physiol 284:R1287–R1295, 2002/12/31 edn.284

Lluel P, Palea S, Ribiere P, Barras M, Teillet L, Corman B (2003b) Increased adrenergic contractility and decreased mRNA expression of NOS III in aging rat urinary bladders. Fundam Clin Pharmacol 17:633–641, 2004/01/06 edn.17

MacDonald SW, Karlsson S, Rieckmann A, Nyberg L, Backman L (2012) Aging-related increases in behavioral variability: relations to losses of dopamine D1 receptors. J Neurosci 32:8186–8191, 2012/06/16 edn.32

McCafferty GP, Misajet BA, Laping NJ, Edwards RM, Thorneloe KS (2008) Enhanced bladder capacity and reduced prostaglandin E2-mediated bladder hyperactivity in EP3 receptor knockout mice. Am J Physiol Renal Physiol 295:F507–F514, 2008/05/30 edn.295

McMurray G, Casey JH, Naylor AM (2006) Animal models in urological disease and sexual dysfunction. Br J Pharmacol 147(Suppl 2):S62–S79, 2006/02/09 edn.147 Suppl 2

Miyazato M, Yoshimura N, Chancellor MB (2013) The other bladder syndrome: underactive bladder. Rev Urol 15:11–22, 2013/05/15 edn.15

Mohammed HA, Santer RM (2002) Distribution and changes with age of calcitonin gene-related peptide- and substance P-immunoreactive nerves of the rat urinary bladder and lumbosacral sensory neurons. Eur J Morphol 40:293–301, 2004/04/23 edn.40

Mohammed H, Hannibal J, Fahrenkrug J, Santer R (2002) Distribution and regional variation of pituitary adenylate cyclase activating polypeptide and other neuropeptides in the rat urinary bladder and ureter: effects of age. Urol Res 30:248–255, 2002/08/31 edn.30

Murakami S, Yoshida M, Masunaga K, Maeda Y, Ueda S (2008) Change in acetylcholine release from rat bladder with partial outlet obstruction. BJU Int 101:633–639, 2007/12/12 edn.101

Nomiya M, Yamaguchi O, Akaihata H, Hata J, Sawada N, Kojima Y, Andersson KE (2014) Progressive vascular damage may lead to bladder underactivity. J Urol 191(5):1462–1469

Philyppov IB, Paduraru ON, Andreev YA, Grishin EV, Shuba YM (2012) Modulation of TRPV1-dependent contractility of normal and diabetic bladder smooth muscle by analgesic toxins from sea anemone Heteractis crispa. Life Sci 91:912–920, 2012/09/18 edn.91

Rahnama'i MS, van Koeveringe GA, Essers PB, de Wachter SG, de Vente J, van Kerrebroeck PE, Gillespie JI (2010) Prostaglandin receptor EP1 and EP2 site in guinea pig bladder urothelium and lamina propria. J Urol 183:1241–1247, 2010/01/26 edn.183

Rahnama'i MS, de Wachter SG, van Koeveringe GA, van Kerrebroeck PE, de Vente J, Gillespie JI (2011) The relationship between prostaglandin E receptor 1 and cyclooxygenase I expression in guinea pig bladder interstitial cells: proposition of a signal propagation system. J Urol 185:315–322, 2010/11/16 edn.185

Rahnama'i MS, Biallosterski BT, de Wachter SG, Van Kerrebroeck PE, van Koeveringe GA (2012a) The distribution of the prostaglandin E receptor type 2 (EP2) in the detrusor of the guinea pig. Prostaglandins Other Lipid Mediat 99:107–115, 2012/09/11 edn.99

Rahnama'i MS, van Kerrebroeck PE, de Wachter SG, van Koeveringe GA (2012b) The role of prostanoids in urinary bladder physiology. Nat Rev Urol 9:283–290, 2012/03/14 edn.9

Sasaki K, Chancellor MB, Phelan MW, Yokoyama T, Fraser MO, Seki S, Kubo K, Kumon H, Groat WC, Yoshimura N (2002) Diabetic cystopathy correlates with a long-term decrease in nerve growth factor levels in the bladder and lumbosacral dorsal root Ganglia. J Urol 168:1259–1264, 2002/08/21 edn.168

Sasaki K, Yoshimura N, Chancellor MB (2003) Implications of diabetes mellitus in urology. Urol Clin North Am 30:1–12, 2003/02/13 edn.30

Sasaki K, Chancellor MB, Goins WF, Phelan MW, Glorioso JC, de Groat WC, Yoshimura N (2004) Gene therapy using replication-defective herpes simplex virus vectors expressing nerve growth factor in a rat model of diabetic cystopathy. Diabetes 53:2723–2730, 2004/09/28 edn.53

Schnegelsberg B, Sun TT, Cain G, Bhattacharya A, Nunn PA, Ford AP, Vizzard MA, Cockayne DA (2010) Overexpression of NGF in mouse urothelium leads to neuronal hyperinnervation, pelvic sensitivity, and changes in urinary bladder function. Am J Physiol Regul Integr Comp Physiol 298:R534–R547, 2009/12/25 edn.298

Sekido N, Jyoraku A, Okada H, Wakamatsu D, Matsuya H, Nishiyama H (2012) A novel animal model of underactive bladder: analysis of lower urinary tract function in a rat lumbar canal stenosis model. NeurourolUrodyn 31:1190–1196, 2012/04/05 edn.31

Smith PP, DeAngelis A, Kuchel GA (2012) Detrusor expulsive strength is preserved, but responsiveness to bladder filling and urinary sensitivity is diminished in the aging mouse. Am J Physiol Regul Integr Comp Physiol 302:R577–R586, 2011/12/30 edn.302

Tanaka I, Nagase K, Tanase K, Aoki Y, Akino H, Yokoyama O (2011) Modulation of stretch evoked adenosine triphosphate release from bladder epithelium by prostaglandin E(2). J Urol 185:341–346, 2010/11/16 edn.185

Torimoto K, Fraser MO, Hirao Y, De Groat WC, Chancellor MB, Yoshimura N (2004) Urethral dysfunction in diabetic rats. J Urol 171:1959–1964, 2004/04/13 edn.171

Torimoto K, Hirao Y, Matsuyoshi H, de Groat WC, Chancellor MB, Yoshimura N (2005) alpha1-Adrenergic mechanism in diabetic urethral dysfunction in rats. J Urol 173:1027–1032, 2005/02/16 edn.173

Tyagi P, Chancellor MB, Li Z, De Groat WC, Yoshimura N, Fraser MO, Huang L (2004) Urodynamic and immunohistochemical evaluation of intravesical capsaicin delivery using thermosensitive hydrogel and liposomes. J Urol 171:483–489, 2003/12/11 edn.171

Tyagi S, Tyagi P, Van-le S, Yoshimura N, Chancellor MB, de Miguel F (2006) Qualitative and quantitative expression profile of muscarinic receptors in human urothelium and detrusor. J Urol 176:1673–1678, 2006/09/06 edn.176

Tyagi P, Thomas CA, Yoshimura N, Chancellor MB (2009) Investigations into the presence of functional Beta1, Beta2 and Beta3-adrenoceptors in urothelium and detrusor of human bladder. Int Braz J Urol 35:76–83, 2009/03/04 edn.35

Tyagi P, Smith PP, Kuchel GA, de Groat WC, Birder LA, Chermansky CJ, Adam RM, Tse V, Chancellor MB, Yoshimura N (2014) Pathophysiology and animal modeling of underactive bladder. Int Urol Nephrol 46(Suppl 1):S11–S21, 2014/09/23 edn.46 Suppl 1

Vlaskovska M, Kasakov L, Rong W, Bodin P, Bardini M, Cockayne DA, Ford AP, Burnstock G (2001) P2X3 knock-out mice reveal a major sensory role for urothelially released ATP. J Neurosci 21:5670–5677, 2001/07/24 edn.21

Wang Z, Cheng Z, Cristofaro V, Li J, Xiao X, Gomez P, Ge R, Gong E, Strle K, Sullivan MP, Adam RM, White MF, Olumi AF (2012) Inhibition of TNF-alpha improves the bladder dysfunction that is associated with type 2 diabetes. Diabetes 61(61):2134–2145

Wang HJ, Tyagi P, Chuang YC, Yoshimura N, Huang CC, Chancellor MB (2015) Pharmacologic and molecular characterization of underactive bladder induced by lumbar canal stenosis. Urology 85:1284–1290, 2015/03/17 edn.85

Yang Z, Dolber PC, Fraser MO (2010) Differential vulnerabilities of urethral afferents in diabetes and discovery of a novel urethra-to-urethra reflex. Am J Physiol Renal Physiol 298:F118–F124, 2009/10/30 edn.298

Yoshida M, Miyamae K, Iwashita H, Otani M, Inadome A (2004) Management of detrusor dysfunction in the elderly: changes in acetylcholine and adenosine triphosphate release during aging. Urology 63:17–23, 2004/03/12 edn.63

Yoshida M, Masunaga K, Nagata T, Satoji Y, Shiomi M (2010) The effects of chronic hyperlipidemia on bladder function in myocardial infarction-prone Watanabe heritable hyperlipidemic (WHHLMI) rabbits. Neurourol Urodyn 29:1350–1354, 2010/02/04 edn.29

Zimmern P, Litman HJ, Nager CW, Lemack GE, Richter HE, Sirls L, Kraus SR, Sutkin G, Mueller ER (2014) Effect of aging on storage and voiding function in women with stress-predominant urinary incontinence. J Urol 192(2):464–468

Chapter 5
Nonsurgical Therapy; Catheters; Devices

Michelle J. Lajiness

Introduction

The treatment for under bladder (UAB) is to protect the upper urinary tract, to improve continence and quality of life, and whenever possible to improve lower tract functioning (Stohrer et al. 2009). Regular bladder emptying reduces intravesical bladder pressure and overdistention, which improves blood flow to the bladder and reduces the risk of infection (Lapides et al. 1972).

Nonsurgical therapy in the underactive bladder patient includes catheters, behavioral management, various devices that promote bladder emptying, and incontinence products. There is a paucity of information in the literature that discusses nonsurgical therapy for underactive bladder, other than discussing catheters and incontinence products. A PubMed search in March of 2015 utilizing the term "underactive bladder" revealed 134 articles available for review, utilizing "behavioral interventions" found 149,240 articles available for review, but these terms combined yielded only 2 articles for review.

Indwelling vs. Intermittent Catheterization (IC)

The optimal treatment for neurogenic bladder remains controversial. Clean intermittent catheterization (CIC) was first introduced in 1972 by Lapides and colleagues. The authors concluded that CIC will help the treatment of and prevention of urinary tract infections. Prevention is a direct result of reducing intravesical bladder pressure and improving blood flow to the bladder wall (Lapides et al. 1972).

M.J. Lajiness, FNP-BC
Department of Urology, Aiken Neurourology Research Center,
Urology Associates, Beaumont Health, Royal Oak, MI, USA
e-mail: mlajiness@beaumont.edu

M.B. Chancellor, A.C. Diokno (eds.), *The Underactive Bladder*,
DOI 10.1007/978-3-319-23687-2_5

Tubaro et al. (2012) in a comprehensive review discussed the importance of bladder emptying but were unable to make a recommendation on IC vs. indwelling catheter and felt the decision should be based on lifestyle. Weld and Dmochowski (2000) retrospectively reviewed medical records, upper tract imaging, and videourodynamic of 316 posttraumatic spinal cord-injured patients looking at their rate of urologic complications. They compared indwelling catheters, IC, spontaneous voiding, and suprapubic catheterization. Their results indicated that IC is the safest management option for spinal cord-injured patients (Weld and Dmochowski 2000).

Cochrane reviews concluded that there is a lack of compelling evidence from clinical trials that the incidence of UTI is affected by use of aseptic or clean technique, coated or uncoated catheters, single- (sterile) or multiple-use (clean) catheters, self-catheterization or catheterization by others, or any other strategy (Jamison et al. 2013; Prieto et al. 2013). There is no evidence to support any method above another; however, patient preference is noted throughout the clinical trials. More well-designed trials are strongly recommended and should include analysis of cost-effectiveness data, because there are likely to be substantial differences associated with the use of different catheter designs, catheterization techniques, and strategies (Jamison et al. 2013; Prieto et al. 2013). Evidence-based guidelines suggest CIC is preferable to indwelling or suprapubic catheters for patients with bladder-emptying dysfunctions (AUA 2015).

Indwelling Catheters

Indwelling catheters are utilized for both short- and long-term management of the underactive bladder. We will focus on the long-term use of indwelling catheters for UAB. Indwelling catheters can be urethral or suprapubic (Figs. 5.1 and 5.2). The complications of indwelling catheters include bacteriuria, catheter-associated urinary tract infections (CAUTI), and catheter-associated biofilms, encrustations, sepsis, and urethral damage (Table 5.1). Indwelling catheters should be considered when anatomical, functional, or familial limitations prohibit intermittent catheterizations.

Intermittent Catheterization (IC)

IC is the insertion of a catheter several times daily to empty the bladder. Once the bladder is empty, the catheter is immediately removed. There is no evidence that recommends frequency of IC, other than to prevent overdistention of the bladder. See Appendix 1 for a discussion on teaching catheterization to patients.

According to the European Association of Urology (EAU) Guidelines on Neurogenic Lower Urinary Tract Dysfunction, the gold standard for management is intermittent catheterization. The guidelines recommend using a 12–14 French catheter four to six times per day (Stohrer et al. 2009). CIC is also the preferred method of patients who have neurogenic bladder (Tubaro et al. 2012; Newman and Wilson 2011).

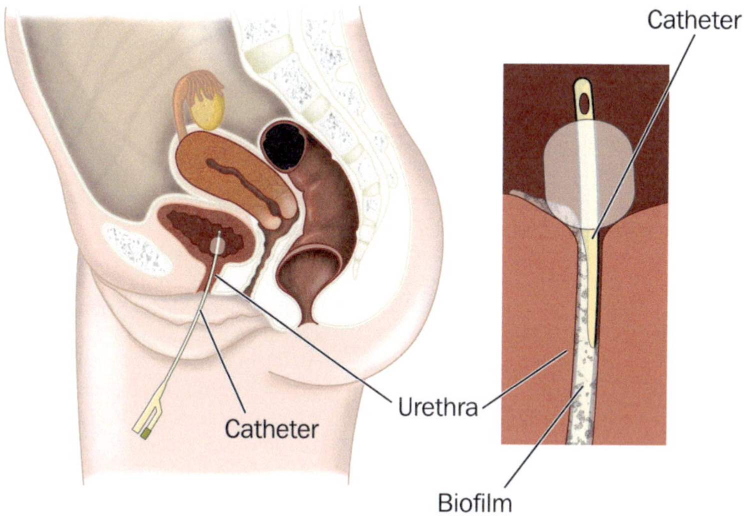

Fig. 5.1 Urethral indwelling catheter

Fig. 5.2 Suprapubic indwelling catheter

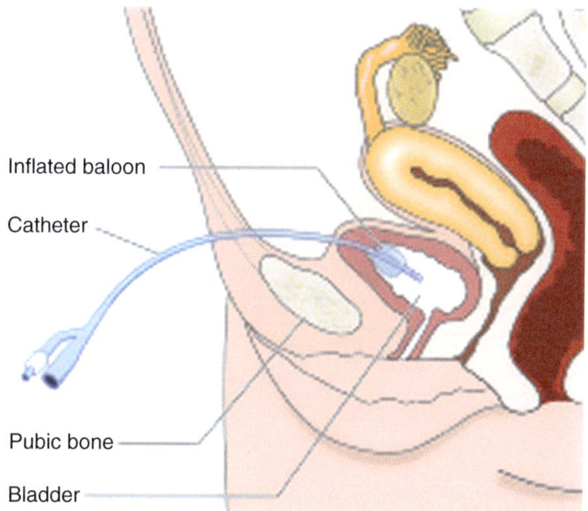

Newman and Wein (2009) stated that the advantages of CIC over indwelling included improved self-care and independence, reduced need for equipment, less barriers for intimacy and sexual activities, and potential for reduced lower urinary tract symptomology. According to evidence-based guidelines, CIC is preferable to indwelling or suprapubic catheters in patients with bladder-emptying dysfunction (AUA 2015).

Cochrane review discusses the complications of CIC that include bleeding, urethritis, stricture, creation of false passage, epididymitis, UTIs, and formation of bladder stones (Jamison et al. 2013) (Table 5.2). Maintaining low intravesical pressure and avoidance of bladder over distention are key components in successful CIC.

Table 5.1 Complications of indwelling catheterization

Complication	Prevention
Bacteriuria – most patients with long-term catheterizations develop bacteriuria. The incidence is 3–8 % per day and duration of catheter is the most important risk factor	Ensure sterile technique Maintain a closed system Do not treat unless patient is symptomatic
Catheter-associated urinary tract infections (CAUTI) – incidence varies based on definitions used. The Center for Disease Control (CDC) has come out with new definitions for use http://www.cdc.gov/nhsn/PDFs/pscManual/7pscCAUTIcurrent.pdf	Ensure proper insertion technique (see Appendix 1) Use sterile technique Use ample lubrication Following aseptic insertion, maintain a closed drainage system Maintain unobstructed urine flow Practice good hand hygiene
Biofilms and encrustations – biofilms are a result of colonization with uropathogens creating adhesions and adhering to the catheter wall. Encrustations are formed by organisms in biofilms and usually associated with alkaline urine. Encrustation can cause catheter blockage	Maintain natural pH Ensure sterile technique Maintain a closed system Change catheters when blockage occurs; it is not recommended to irrigate
Urethral damage – occurs primarily in men. Risk increases with the length of catheterization	Ensure proper technique is used Ensure liberal lubrication Ensure stability of catheter to leg May use antibiotic ointment at tip of meatus

Sterile vs. Clean Catheterization

One question that always comes up with IC is if the technique needs to be performed with sterile technique with new catheter each time or can clean technique be used with reusable catheter. This remains a controversial topic and most experts probably agree that clean intermittent catheterization (CIC) is appropriate for the majority of patients. Sterile catheterization is required for those with immunosuppression, those at risk for developing UTIs, and patients in acute or long-term care facilities (Stohrer et al. 2009; AUA 2015; Newman and Wein 2009).

Preventing Infections

There are no consistent guidelines available on the rationale or method for obtaining urine for culture from a chronically catheterized patient. Once urine is obtained, there are no consistent guidelines on what constitutes a true urinary infection versus asymptomatic bacteriuria. Using the white count on a urinalysis to predict infection in the underactive bladder is not predictive due to the low correlation with symptoms (AUA 2015). Patients with underactive bladder frequently do not experience typical symptoms of a UTI due to an altered afferent nervous system. When evaluating these patients for UTIs, a thorough understanding of their baseline bladder sensation is imperative (Newman and Wein 2009). See Table 5.3 for a list of symptoms associated with UTIs in the neurologically compromised patient (AUA 2015).

Table 5.2 Complications of clean intermittent catheterization

Complication	Prevention
Bleeding – more frequently seen in new patients and prevalence is about 1/3 of patients	Ensure patient is using proper technique (see Appendix 1) Encourage liberal lubrication
Urethritis – prevalence varies widely but is below 8 %	Ensure patient is using proper technique Change catheter material
Stricture –the incidence of stricture increases with longer follow-up with most events occurring 5 years after initiation. Prevalence is around 4 %	Ensure gentle introduction of the catheter Use of hydrophilic catheters may benefit
False passage – creation of a false passage. Trauma especially in men can create false passages; however incidence is rare	Ensure patient is using proper technique Gentle slow introduction of catheter
Epididymitis and prostatitis – both are rare and can be related to recurrent UTI	Ensure patient is using proper technique Ensure adequate hydration Ensure bladder is being emptied frequently to maintain residuals less than 500 ml Treat only when symptomatic
UTI – prevalence is between 12 and 88 % secondary to definition used and patient populations	Ensure patient is using proper technique Ensure adequate hydration Ensure bladder is being emptied frequently to maintain residuals less than 500 ml Treat only when symptomatic
Bladder stone – incidence of stone formation is rare and is usually related to introduction of a foreign body into the bladder such as a pubic hair or prolonged catheterization	Ensure patient is using proper technique Ensure adequate hydration

Table 5.3 Signs and symptoms associated with UTIs in the neurologically compromised patient

Signs and symptoms associated with a UTI include:
New onset or worsening of fevers
Rigors
Altered mental status changes
Malaise or lethargy with no other identified cause
Flank pain
Costovertebral angle tenderness
Acute hematuria
Pelvic discomfort
In patients with spinal cord injury
Increased spasticity
Autonomic dysreflexia
Pyuria is not diagnostic of a UTI in catheterized patients; however the absence of pyuria in a symptomatic patient suggests a diagnosis other than UTI
The absence or presence of odorous urine or cloudy urine should not be used to diagnose a UTI

Table 5.4 Preventing UTIs in patients undergoing catheterization

Treat only symptomatic UTIs
Do not do routine urinalysis or culture
Maintain good hygiene
Maintain adequate hydration
Do not routinely irrigate
Ensure adequate emptying of the bladder
In CIC catheterize to maintain 500 ml or less in the bladder
In indwelling catheters secure to leg and ensure no kinking of dislodgement of tubing
Although controversial acidification of the urine with use of cranberry pills has shown to be useful in preventing UTI
Cranberry pills cannot be used on patients with anticoagulant therapy
Change patient catheter based on patient tolerance

Until more data is available, the need for urine cultures must be individualized and based on the clinical suspicion of a progressively symptomatic urinary tract infection (AUA 2015). Although there is little evidence to support patient self-diagnosis of UTIs, many patients with a long-term history of neurogenic bladder are able to accurately identify their particular symptoms and note when treatment is necessary. Treatment of UTIs is outside the scope of this chapter; however prevention of UTIs is a key component in working with this population (Table 5.4).

Catheters

Catheters come in many sizes, materials (latex, silicone, Teflon™), and types (Foley, straight, Coude tip) (Figs. 5.3, 5.4, 5.5, and 5.6). One should always ask if the patient has latex allergy before selection of catheter and associated supplies. There are three main types of catheters:

- Indwelling catheter
- Intermittent (short-term) catheter
- Male external catheter collection systems

Indwelling Catheters

Commonly referred to as a Foley catheter, indwelling catheters can be classified as short term or long term based on the length of time utilized. Most indwelling catheters have two lumens: one for draining the urine and one for inflating the balloon. The most common standard catheters include polyvinyl chlorine (PVC), plain latex, polytetrafluoroethylene (PTFE) or Teflon, silicone coated, 100 %

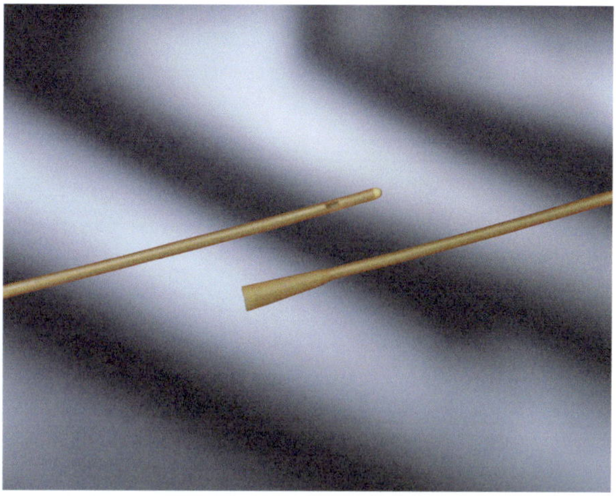

Fig. 5.3 Straight tip catheter (© 2015 C.R. Bard Used with Permission)

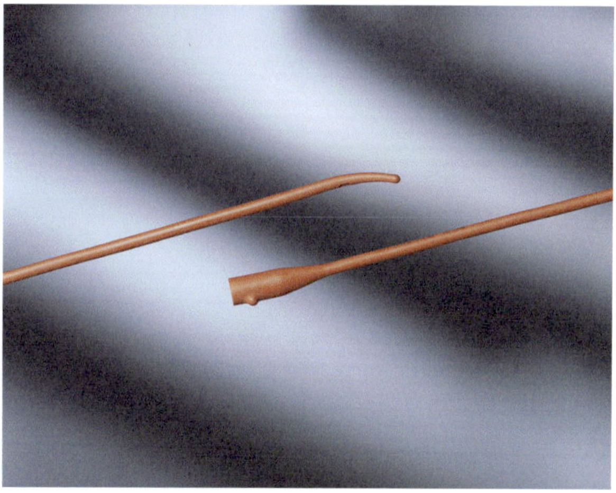

Fig. 5.4 Coude tip catheter (© 2015 C.R. Bard Used with Permission)

silicone, hydrogel coated, or catheters impregnated with antibacterial or antiseptic agents (Fig. 5.7). The most common bactericidal agent is silver (AUA 2015; Jahn et al. 2012).

Patil et al. (2012) reported that there have been claims that silver-alloyed catheters may decrease complications and increase patient comfort. However, it was felt that after review the studies were too small to make generalizations. They found a single randomized trial of 12 patients that compared silver-alloyed, hydrogel-coated, and silicone-coated catheters. It was determined that the trial was too small to make conclusions (Jahn et al. 2012). There is some controversial data to suggest that silicone is nonreactive and possibly associated with less bacterial adherence than other catheters (AUA 2015). A recent Cochrane review concluded that the lack of evidence and methodological weakness in the trials was not sufficient to make recommendations for practice.

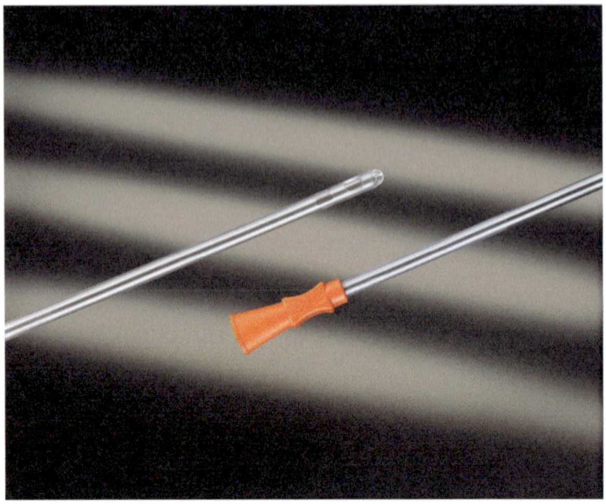

Fig. 5.5 Polyvinyl chlorine (PVC) catheter is the most common material used for intermittent catheters (© 2015 C.R. Bard Used with Permission)

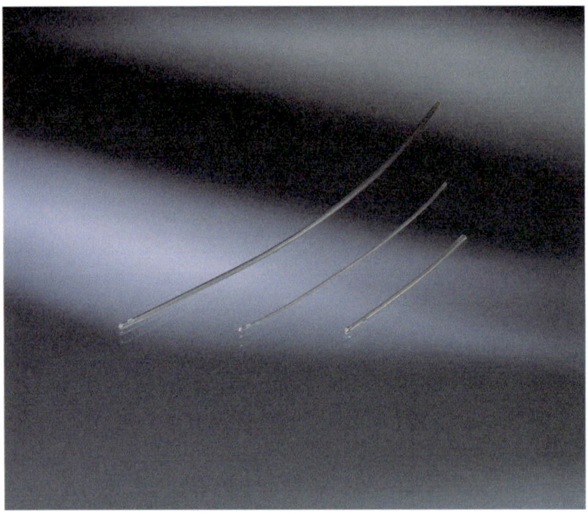

Fig. 5.6 Various lengths of catheters. Longer ones for men and shorter catheter for women are often easier to use (© 2015 C.R. Bard Used with Permission)

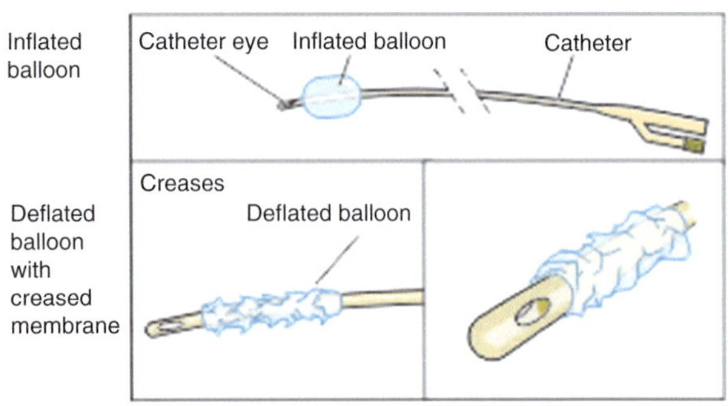

Fig. 5.7 Design of indwelling catheter with inflation balloon

Suprapubic tubes are utilized in this population when CIC is not an option and is preferable to a transurethral catheter (Fig. 5.2). This is especially necessary in meatal or urethral erosions, limited mobility, and those patients that would like to remain sexually active.

Male External Catheter Collections Systems

Male external catheters are condom-type sheaths that are placed over the penis and connected to urinary drainage bags for collection of urine. Common names for these devices are condom catheters, Texas catheters, or external male catheters (Fig. 5.8).

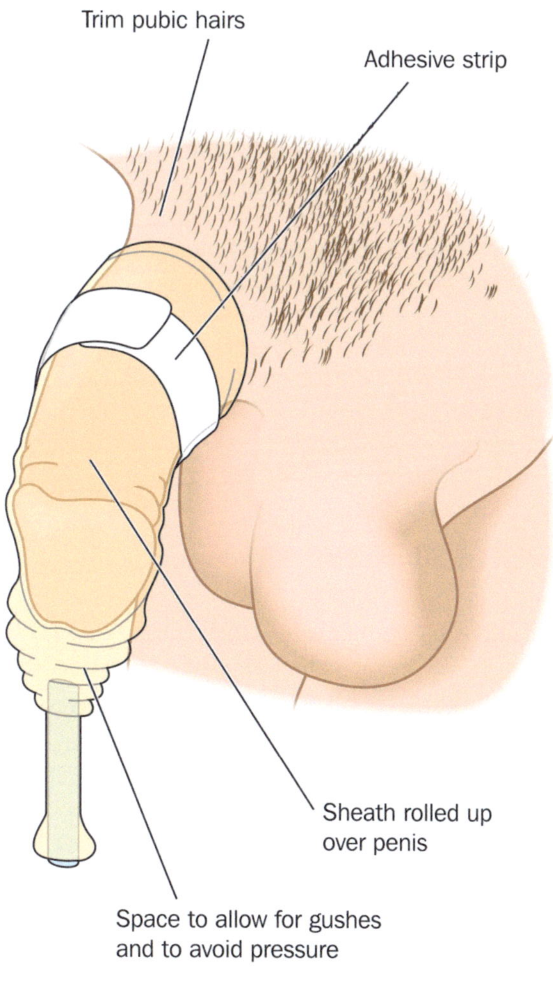

Fig. 5.8 Male external condom catheter

These are more useful for a patient with urinary incontinence than underactive bladder, as it does not empty the bladder but collects the urine. The EAU guidelines state that male external catheters such as condom catheters or Texas catheters can offer a "reliable solution" for the incontinent patient as long as these men are closely monitored for infection (Stohrer et al. 2009). The biggest challenge with external catheters is preventing unintentional dislodgment. Complications are generally irritative, allergic, or compressive in nature (AUA 2015).

Intermittent Catheters

There are many different sizes and configurations of catheters for CIC use. CIC for neurogenic bladder implies there is no obstruction or stricture; as such this catheter discussion will not include catheters to maintain urethral patency.

The CIC catheters can be simplified into two categories, those requiring lubrication and self-lubricating catheters. It has been proposed that the use of self-lubricating catheters produces less urethral trauma and lower infections rates than traditional catheters. The studies supporting the use of self-lubricating catheters have been small in number and have not had a head to head trial with traditional catheters (AUA 2015; Jahn et al. 2012).

Catheters come in many sizes and lengths. Adult use for CIC are generally between 14 and 22 French (Fr) and around 12 inches long for men and 6 inches long for women (Fig. 5.6). The catheters for CIC are made from the same material as discussed in indwelling. The most common catheter used for CIC is PVC. Depending on patient preference and rationale for catheterizing, there are various tips (Coude, olive, 1 eye, 2 eyes). CICs are made with various types of tips including blunt straight tips, curved tips (Coude), and tips with lumens designed for placement of guide wires (Council tip). See Figs. 5.3, 5.4, 5.5, and 5.6.

Reuse vs. Single Use

The current standard of care is that catheters are for single use only. This remains controversial; several authors support this level of care (Stohrer et al. 2009; AUA 2015; Jamison et al. 2013).

Patient Preference

Often the patient's clinical condition will influence the type of catheter utilized. Patient factors to consider include manual dexterity, urethral sensation, visual acuity, gender, and age (Jahn et al. 2012). Patients may need to try several catheters before finding one that suits their individual needs and circumstances.

Behavioral Interventions

According to the European Association of Urology Guidelines on Neurogenic Lower Urinary Tract Dysfunction, there are few prospective, randomized, controlled studies supporting conservative treatment. The guidelines state that lower urinary tract rehabilitation might be beneficial. Rehabilitation techniques include prompted voiding, timed voiding (bladder training), and lifestyle modifications (Stohrer et al. 2009).

The EAU guidelines do not recommend assisted bladder emptying such as Valsalva maneuver, Crede, or triggered reflux. The authors state these procedures may create high pressures and are potentially hazardous (Stohrer et al. 2009).

Tubaro et al. (2012) completed a systemic review on the treatment of lower urinary tract symptoms in patients with multiple sclerosis. A meta-analysis could not be performed secondary to the multiple and differing outcome criteria. The authors concluded the nature of bladder dysfunction and the course of the disease make it difficult to standardize treatments or create guidelines.

Patil and associates (2012) completed an open-arm pre-post study on eleven patients with multiple sclerosis (MS). The MS patients underwent a 21-day yoga intervention with statistical improvement noted in post-void residual, total micturition, and quality of sleep (McClurg et al. 2008). Prior to that McClurg and colleagues (2006) compared electromyography feedback, and neuromuscular electrical stimulation, alone or in combination with pelvic floor muscle training, and were able to reduce the amount of leakage in the MS population. Later McClurg (2009) taught 11 patients with MS pelvic floor training for lower urinary dysfunction and found the participants' quality of life was enhanced after completing the 9-week training course.

Behavioral therapy has been extensively studied in the overactive bladder population and authors have concluded that it may work in the UAB population. Other than those discussed above, no clinical studies are available to determine the effectiveness of behavioral therapy in the UAB population.

Other Devices

The EAU guidelines discourage the use of the penile clamp, as it is associated with high pressure on the urethral tissue and will reduce penile blood flow; it should not be used routinely (Stohrer et al. 2009). The American Urological Association (AUA 2015) states that penile clamps should be used only in those patients with normal bladder compliance, sensation of fullness, and reasonable bladder capacity.

Tubaro and associates (2012) determined after a comprehensive review that peripheral tibial nerve stimulation (PTNS) was inconclusive, with some authors demonstrating effectiveness in suppressing detrusor over activity and others unable to suppress the overactive bladder. Regarding quality of life, many authors were able to report subjective improvement in patients as high as 73 %. These studies were interested in treating overactive bladder and did not include patients with UAB.

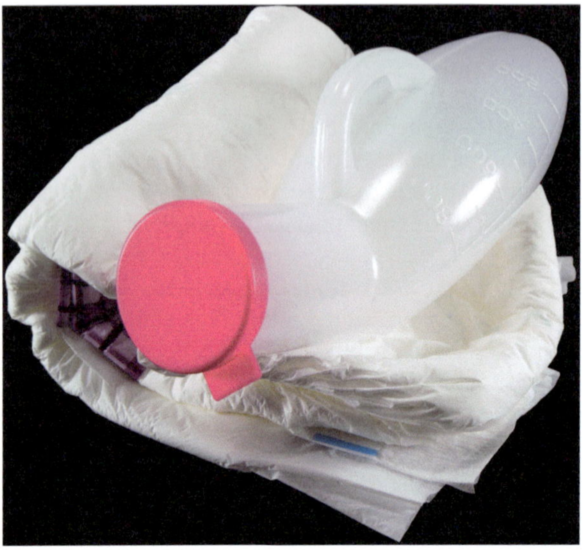

Fig. 5.9 Incontinence absorbent products and urinal may be used for patient and caregiver comfort and convenience

Incontinence Products

Patients may choose incontinence pads or diapers as their first initial method to remedy the loss of urine or may use them as a last resort. These items tend to be for long-term usage with UAB patients. The main goal of incontinence products is to minimize, conceal, and control urinary leakage. There are a variety of options available from pads to undergarments (Fig. 5.9). Patient preference, comfort, and level of incontinence, shape, and contour of the product will determine which products to use (AUA 2015; Newman and Wein 2009). Patients should be counseled that incontinence products are *management strategies* and not treatment options (Stohrer et al. 2009; Newman and Wein 2009).

Conclusions

There are more questions than answers when it comes to the "best" management of patients with underactive bladder. The literature has many case studies and small studies to support one method of care compared to another. However, randomized controlled studies need to be encouraged and funded to support evidence-based practice development.

Providers need to work with patients, families, caregivers, and other providers to individualize the care for each patient. Considerations include self-catheterization teaching, catheter selection, incontinence products, arranging home care, and coordination of durable medical equipment to optimize patient quality of life. The goal is to provide evidence-based care to this population

References

American Urological Association (2015) White paper on catheter-associated urinary tract infections: definitions and significance in the urologic patient 2014. Downloaded from https://www.auanet.org/common/pdf/education/clinical-guidance/Catheter-Associated-Urinary-Tract-Infections-WhitePaper.pdf on 29 June 2015

Jahn P, Beutner K, Langer G (2012) Types of indwelling urinary catheters for long-term drainage in adults (review). Cochrane Database Syst Rev 10:1–43

Jamison J, Maquire S, Mcann J (2013) Catheter policies for management of long term voiding problems in adults with neurogenic bladder disorders (review). Cochrane Database Syst Rev 11:1–59

Lapides J, Diokno A, Silber S, Lowe B (1972) Clean Intermittent Self-Catheterization in the Treatment of Urinary Tract Disease. J Urol 107(3):458–461

McClurg D (2009) Pelvic Floor Training for Lower Urinary Tract Dysfunction in MS. Nurs Times 105(7):45–47

McClurg D, Ashe RG, Marshall K, Lowe-Strong AS (2006) Comparison of Pelvic Floor Muscle Training, Electromyography Biofeedback and Neuromuscular Electrical Stimulation for Bladder Dysfunction in People with Multiple Sclerosis: A Randomized Pilot Study. NeurourolUrodyn 25:337–348

McClurg D, Ashe RG, Lowe-Strong AS (2008) Neuromuscular Electrical Stimulation and the Treatment of Lower Urinary Tract Dysfunction in Multiple Sclerosis-A Double Blind, Placebo Controlled, Randomised Clinical Trial. NeurourolUrodyn 27:231–237

Newman D, Wilson M (2011) Review of Intermittent Catheterization and Current Best Practices. Urol Nurs 31(1):12–28

Newman D, Wein A (2009) Managing and Treating Urinary Incontinence, 2nd edn. Health Professions Press, Baltimore, pp 365–483

Patil NJ, Nagaratna R, Garner C, Raghurman NV (2012) Effect of Integrated Yoga on Neurogenic Bladder Dysfunction in Patients with Multiple Sclerosis – A Prospective observational Series. Compliment Ther Med 20:424–430

Prieto J Murphy CL, Moore KN, Fader M (2013) Intermittent catheterisation for long-term bladder management. Cochrane Database Syst Rev. 9:1–97

Stohrer M, Blok B, Castro-Diaz D, Chartier-Kastler E, Del Popolo G, Kramer G, Pannek J, Piotr R, Wyandaele J (2009) EAU Guidelines on Neurogenic Lower Urinary Tract Dysfunction. Eur Urol 56:81–88

Tubaro A, Puccini F, De Nunzio C, Diggesu GA, Elneil S, Gobbi C, Khullar V (2012) The treatment of Lower Urinary Tract Symptoms in Patients with Multiple Sclerosis: A Systemic Review. Curr Urol Rep 13:335–342

Weld K, Dmochowski R (2000) Effect of Bladder Management on Urological Complications in Spinal Cord Injured Patients. J Urol 163:768–772

Chapter 6
Current Drug Therapy for Underactive Bladder

Michael B. Chancellor

Introduction

Lower urinary tract symptoms (LUTS) are usually associated with either failures of the bladder to store and empty normal volumes of urine and/or urethral dysfunction such as obstruction or sphincteric incompetence. For many of these disorders, effective therapies are available. However, symptoms attributable to a failure of the bladder to empty effectively in the absence of urethral obstruction have been difficult to address without resorting to intermittent or indwelling catheterization. The term underactive bladder (UAB) is applied to this condition and its associated symptoms (Chancellor and Diokno 2014; Osman et al. 2014).

Efforts to treat UAB are focused on improving detrusor output and decreasing urethral resistance. Improvements in detrusor output include enhanced stimulation of existing contractile elements, increases in muscle mass, and improvements in muscular work efficiency. Reduction in urethral resistance includes medication or surgery to decrease bladder outlet (bladder neck, prostate, and sphincter) or bypassing the obstruction with catheterization.

Detrusor underactivity (DU) is defined only with urodynamic evaluation as a detrusor contraction of reduced strength and/or duration, resulting in incomplete bladder emptying (Abrams et al. 2002). This definition suggests an inherent deficiency of detrusor smooth muscle. Therefore, therapies for UAB have focused only on increasing detrusor smooth muscle contractility. Paradoxically, pharmacologic agents that enhance cholinergic stimulation to treat the UAB have largely been ineffective (Smith et al. 2014; Krishnamoorthy and Kekre 2009). Some of the etiologies of UAB and DU

M.B. Chancellor, MD
Department of Urology, Aikens Research Center, Oakland University William Beaumont School of Medicine, Rochester, MI, USA

Neurourology Program, Beaumont Health System, Royal Oak, MI, USA
e-mail: Michael.Chancellor@beaumont.edu

M.B. Chancellor, A.C. Diokno (eds.), *The Underactive Bladder*,
DOI 10.1007/978-3-319-23687-2_6

are not attributable to a smooth muscle detrusor defect and it is not surprising that effective therapies for UAB have continued to prove elusive (Smith 2010).

Parasympathetic and Muscarinic Receptors

The primary contractile stimulus for normal detrusor contractions is the parasympathetic neurotransmitter acetylcholine. Acetylcholine acts on muscarinic receptors in the bladder (Hegde 2006; Yoshimura and Chancellor 2011). Deficient neurostimulation that results in non-sustained detrusor contraction may be due to reduced parasympathomimetic nerve fibers transmitter release, an increased degradation of transmitters in the synaptic cleft by acetylcholinesterase, or a combination of both. UAB could also result from impaired tissue responsiveness toward contractile stimuli such as acute urinary retention after surgical anesthesia and narcotics (Tyagi et al. 2014; Barendrecht et al. 2007) (Fig. 6.1).

Current approaches toward medical treatment of UAB aim at providing additional stimulation of bladder muscarinic receptors. This can be done by a direct stimulation of muscarinic receptors by agonists such as bethanechol or carbachol. Alternatively, it can be done by inhibiting acetylcholinesterase, the enzyme inactivating the endogenous agonist acetylcholine. Common cholinesterase inhibitors

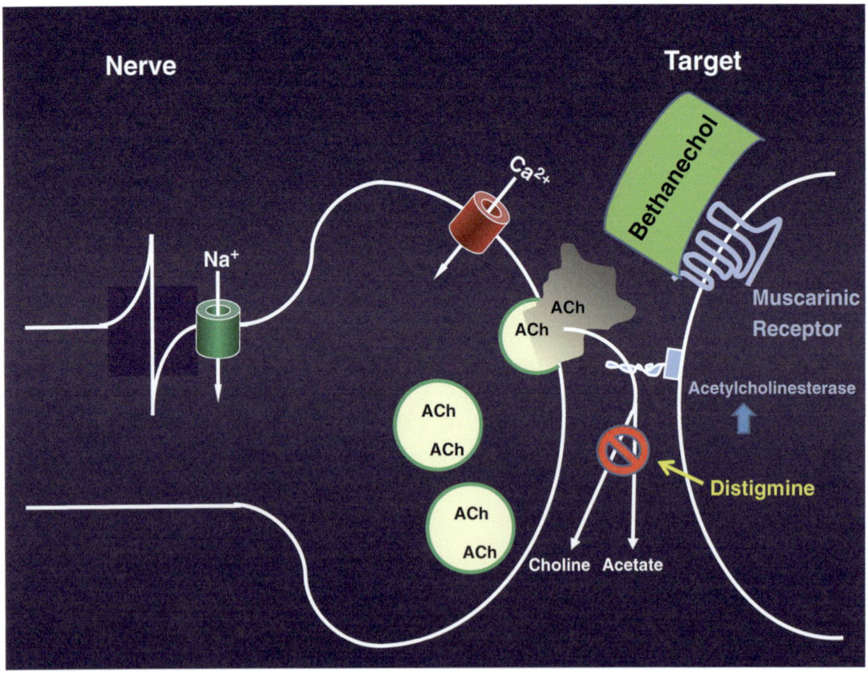

Fig. 6.1 Direct (bethanechol) and indirect (distigmine) agonist treatment of underactive bladder

include distigmine, pyridostigmine, and neostigmine (Tyagi et al. 2014). The latter approach depends on the presence of at least some endogenous acetylcholine, the effects of which can be amplified by inhibiting its breakdown by the cholinesterase inhibitor.

The most attractive feature of the use of direct muscarinic receptor agonists is that it does not require the presence of endogenous acetylcholine to be effective. One should remember that in order for muscarinic stimulation or cholinesterase inhibition to have a chance to work, it depends on some degree of preserved responsiveness to acetylcholine in the bladder wall.

Muscarinic Mechanisms

There are five bladder muscarinic receptor subtypes based on molecular cloning and four different receptor subtypes based on pharmacology (M_1 to M_5) (Yoshimura and Chancellor 2011; Yamaguchi et al. 1996). Ligand receptor binding studies revealed that M_2 receptors predominate but it is mostly M_3 receptors that mediate cholinergic contractions in the urinary bladder. Muscarinic receptors are also located on the bladder on cholinergic nerve terminals prejunctionally (Yoshimura and Chancellor 2011; Somogyi and de Groat 1992).

M_1 prejunctional receptor activation will facilitate acetylcholine release. whereas activation of M_2 receptors inhibits the release (Somogyi and de Groat 1992; Braverman, Kohn et al. 1998). It has been proposed that inhibitory M_2–M_4 receptors are preferentially activated by auto-feedback mechanisms during short periods of low-frequency nerve activity and thereby suppress cholinergic transmission during urine storage (Somogyi and de Groat 1992). M_1 receptors are activated during more prolonged high-frequency nerve firing that would occur during voiding. M1 receptors participate in an amplification mechanism to promote complete bladder emptying (Somogyi et al. 1996; Tyagi et al. 2014). The ability to modulate neurotransmission in the bladder through the selective activation and inhibition of specific presynaptic receptors may lead to novel forms of pharmacologic therapy for UAB.

Clinical Results of Muscarinic Agents for UAB

Available data show little beneficial effect of parasympathomimetic agents in treating or preventing UAB (Barendrecht et al. 2007; Krishnamoorthy and Kekre 2009). The main reason why these agents are approved by regulatory agencies in many countries for treating UAB is that such registration was typically obtained many years ago prior to requirement of randomized clinical trials.

Table 6.1 lists the randomized clinical trials on the use of muscarinic agents to treat UAB. The table is a modification and update of the excellent work by Barendrecht et al. (2007) who published a systematic review of randomized clinical

Table 6.1 Current drug treatment of underactive bladder

Treatment	Indication	Patients #	Endpoint	Did drug help	Results	Evidence level	Reference
Bethanechol 50 mg × 3 oral from 3 days after surgery, vs. no treatment	Prophylaxis of detrusor hypotonia after radical hysterectomy	40	Hospital stay, catheter treatment, rate of cystitis, and residual urine	Yes	Hospital stay 18.6 vs. 15.5 days; catheter treatment 13.3 vs. 9.6 days; rate of cystitis 25.0 vs. 18.8 %; residual urine <50 mL after 13 vs. 8 days for no treatment vs. bethanechol; all differences $p<0.01$	2b	Kemp et al. (1997)
Bethanechol 25, 50 or 100 mg × 1 oral vs. placebo 60 min before urodynamic investigation	Women with persistent high residual urine but no sign of neurological disease or outlet obstruction	48	Urodynamic parameters	No	No significant difference between groups for voided volume, residual volume, % residual volume, mean flow rate, and intravesical pressure	2b	Barrett (1981)
Bethanechol 15 mg every 4 h (6 doses) vs. no treatment	Prevention of acute urinary retention postpartum	1,796	Catheterization and residual volume	No	No significant difference between both groups	2b	Fleming (1957)

Bethanechol 25 mg × 1 oral vs. placebo for 2 weeks in cross-over design	Treatment of underactive bladder	16	Urodynamic parameters	Yes	Significant reduction of residual urine and increase in max urinary flow vs. placebo ($p<0.02$ and <0.03), detrusor pressure tended to increase	1b	Riedl et al. (2002)
Bethanechol 4 × 50 mg daily oral + intravesical PGE_2 × 1/week vs. placebo for 6 weeks	Treatment of underactive bladder	19	Residual urine volume	Inconclusive	Relative to baseline statistically significant reduction with active treatment but not with placebo, but effect size judges as "limited therapeutic effect" by investigator	1b	Hindley et al. (2004)

(continued)

Table 6.1 (continued)

Treatment	Indication	Patients #	Endpoint	Did drug help	Results	Evidence level	Reference
Bethanechol 20 mg tid vs. placebo	Prevention of underactive bladder after radical hysterectomy	62	Rate of urethral catheter removal at 1 week post surgery	Yes	67.7 % in treatment group vs. 38.7 % in placebo group had catheter removal at 1 week postoperatively ($p=0.04$). Residual urine volume and infection at 1 month were similar between groups	2b	Manchana and Prasartsakulchi (2011)
Cholinesterase inhibitor							
Distigmine 0.5 mg i.m. × 1 for 4 days vs. placebo	Treatment of acute urinary retention after prostatectomy	93	Flow rates and re-catheterization rate	No	No significant difference between groups	2b	Shah et al. (1983)
Combination therapy							
Carbachol/diazepam 2 mg each vs. alfuzosin 2.5 mg vs. placebo, all 1 × oral	Treatment of acute urinary retention after general surgery	249	Voiding within 2 h after medication	No	No significant difference between groups	2b	Burger et al. (1997)
Bethanechol 10 mg × 1 s.c. vs. midazolam vs. combination vs. placebo	Treatment of acute urinary retention after anorectal surgery	132	Incidence of catheterization	Yes	0 vs. 69 % responders for placebo and bethanechol ($p=0.05$) irrespective of other treatments	2b	Gottesman et al. (1989)

Bethanechol 20 mg × 3 or distigmine 5 mg × 3 oral vs. urapidil 30 mg × 2 vs. combined for 4 weeks	Treatment of underactive bladder	119	Urinary flow rate, post-void residual volume, and symptom scores	No	No significant effect of cholinergic agonists vs. baseline	2b	Yamanishi et al. (2004)
Distigmine 5 mg × 1 oral vs. phenoxybenzamine 10 mg × 2 oral vs. intravesical $PGF_2\alpha$ 7.5 mg vs. placebo from 1 day after surgery	Prevention of acute urinary retention after vaginal surgery for genital prolapse	100	Residual urine volume	No	Statistically significant increase of residual urine for distigmine vs. placebo	2b	Savona-Ventura et al. (1991)
Bethanechol 30 mg/day, cisapride (5HT4) receptor agonist 30 mg/day, both and placebo	Prevention of underactive bladder after radical hysterectomy	79	Urodynamic parameters	Yes	After 30 days, bethanechol and cisapride decreased bladder capacity at first desire to void, increased maximum flow rate and higher detrusor pressure at maximum flow, with lower post-void residual volumes	2b	Madeiro et al. (2006)

Adopted and updated from Barendrecht et al. (2007)

trials on muscarinic agents to treat UAB. The study was independently evaluated by two investigators and scored for its technical quality and evidence level, according to the Oxford Centre for Evidence-Based Medicine (2001).

A number of the studies involved one sex whereas others have reported both sexes. Studies have used placebo (Savona-Ventura et al. 1991; Gottesman et al. 1989; Burger et al. 1997; Shah et al. 1983; Barrett 1981; Hindley et al. 2004; Riedl et al. 2002), no treatment (Kemp et al. 1997; Fleming 1957), or other active treatments (Yamanishi et al. 2004) as control and involved a wide range of number of patients from less than 20 to almost 2,000. There was considerable heterogeneity in treatment methods and in some cases the muscarinic agonist was administered as part of a combined treatment (Burger et al. 1997; Hindley et al. 2004; Yamanishi et al. 2004). The dose, route of administration, and duration of treatment differed among studies. The efficacy of treatment was also assessed heterogeneously with clinical and/or urodynamic endpoints.

Some of the studies included patients with urodynamically confirmed detrusor underactivity (Hindley et al. 2004; Yamanishi et al. 2004; Riedl et al. 2002) and in neurologically normal women with elevated residual urine volume (Barrett 1981). Studies were reported for settings including postpartum women (Fleming 1957) and in patients after general surgery (Burger et al. 1997), prostatectomy (Shah et al. 1983), radical hysterectomy (Kemp et al. 1997), vaginal prolapse surgery (Savona-Ventura et al. 1991), or anorectal surgery (Gottesman et al. 1989).

Madeiro et al. (2006) evaluated the effects of bethanechol and cisapride, a drug that acts on serotonin 5-HT$_4$ receptor agonist and indirectly as a parasympathomimetic, on urodynamic parameters in patients undergoing radical hysterectomy. Stimulation of the serotonin receptors has been shown to increase acetylcholine release in the enteric nervous system. Medication was administered postoperatively for 30 days and urodynamics repeated. Results of study indicated that post-radical hysterectomy, bethanechol and cisapride correlated with decreased bladder capacity, a higher maximum flow rate and higher detrusor pressure at maximum flow and lower post-void residual volumes. The authors concluded that early use of bethanechol and cisapride results in improved detrusor function after radical hysterectomies.

Manchana and Prasartsakulchi (2011) reported a placebo-controlled randomized study between bethanechol 20 mg tid and placebo for the prevention of UAB after radical hysterectomy (31 subjects in each group). The subject received treatment on third to seventh postoperative days. The primary end point was the rate of urethral catheter removal at 1 week postoperatively. If PVR was more than 30 % of voided volume, the urethral catheter was reinserted, and medication would be continued but not for more than 1 month. Twenty-one patients (68 %) in the treatment group and 12 patients (39 %) in the control group had the urethral catheter removed at 1 week postoperatively ($p=0.04$). Median duration of urethral catheterization was shorter in the treatment group (7 and 14 days, $p=0.03$). However, the PVR and the incidence of urinary tract infection at 1 month postoperatively were not significantly different. Nine patients (29 %) in the treatment group had adverse events such as nausea, abdominal distension, and abdominal cramping versus 1 patient in the control group. The authors concluded that bethanechol chloride decreases the duration of urethral catheterization in patients who underwent radical hysterectomy with manageable adverse events.

Reasons for Poor Response

Combined studies involved in the meta-analysis by Barendrecht et al. (2007) had over 2,700 patients. The heterogeneity of patient populations, treatments, and assessments of treatment efficacy made the formal meta-analysis difficult. However, the data suggests that discrepancies among studies were unrelated to treatment versus preventive strategies, gender, or study size. Possible reasons why parasympathomimetic may not work well for UAB include (Hegde 2006; Yoshimura and Chancellor 2011):

- Underactive bladder may represent an *unresponsiveness* of the detrusor toward neurostimulation. Therefore, agents directly acting on detrusor smooth muscle contractility may be necessary. But such drugs are not yet available.
- Current parasympathomimetic agents are *under dosed* to be effective on the detrusor. The reasons for under dosing include side effects such as nausea, vomiting, flushing, diarrhea, gastrointestinal cramps, bronchospasms, salivation, sweating, headache, and difficulty with visual accommodation. Rare but deadly side effects include acute circulatory failure and cardiac arrest. Bladder-specific parasympathomimetic agents need to be developed.

Optimizing Distigmine Treatment

In a recent study by Tomoe (2014), 11 women with detrusor underactivity and without bladder outlet obstruction diagnosed on the basis of an urodynamic study were randomly divided into two groups. One group took distigmine bromide 5 mg orally 30 min before the morning meal (preprandial administration group; $n=6$) and the other group that took distigmine 5 mg orally 30 min after the morning meal (postprandial administration group; $n=5$). Plasma distigmine concentrations were assessed before and 4 weeks after the start of administration. In addition, quality of life questionnaires were assessed before and 4 weeks after treatment (Tomoe 2014). The plasma distigmine bromide concentration was 2.4 times higher in the preprandial administration group than in the postprandial administration group. Uroflowmetry in the patients with detrusor activity showed a tendency for flow rate and post-void residual urine volume to improve in both the preprandial group and the postprandial group. Conversely, patients with no detrusor activity showed no significant urodynamic improvement.

Quality of life indices significantly improved from before distigmine treatment to after the 4-week period of treatment; however, there were no significant differences between preprandial or postprandial administration. Tomoe (2014) concluded that distigmine might not be effective in the absence of detrusor contractility but may be beneficial in cases where there is some remaining detrusor activity. In addition, pre meal administration may be the optimal time to prescribe distigmine for UAB.

Conclusion

Current peer-reviewed medical literature shows little evidence to support the use of muscarinic receptor agonists in the treatment of UAB. The minor reported beneficial effect of parasympathomimetic drugs in some studies needs to be weighed against the risk of frequent mild and rare serious side effects. Parasympathomimetics are not routinely recommended in preventing or treating UAB.

References

Abrams P, Cardozo L, Fall M, Griffiths D, Rosier P, Ulmsten U, van Kerrebroeck P, Victor A, Wein A (2002) The standardisation of terminology of lower urinary tract function: report from the Standardisation Sub-committee of the International Continence Society. Neurourol Urodyn 21:167–178

Barendrecht MM, Oelke M, Laguna MP, Michel MC (2007) Is the use of parasympathomimetics for treating an underactive urinary bladder evidence-based? BJU Int 99:749–752

Barrett DM (1981) The effect of oral bethanechol chloride on voiding in female patients with excessive residual urine: a randomized double-blind study. J Urol 126:640–642

Braverman AS, Kohn IJ et al (1998) Prejunctional M1 facilitatory and M2 inhibitory muscarinic receptors mediate rat bladder contractility. Am J Physiol 274(2 Pt 2):R517–R523

Burger DH, Kappetein AP, Boutkan H, Breslau PJ (1997) Prevention of urinary retention after general surgery: a controlled trial of carbachol/diazepam versus alfuzosine. J Am Coll Surg 185:234–236

Chancellor MB, Diokno A (2014) CURE-UAB: shedding light on the underactive bladder syndrome. Int Urol Nephrol 46(Suppl 1):S1–S46

Fleming AR (1957) The use of urecholine in the prevention of postpartum urinary retention; final report. Am J Obstet Gynecol 74:569–571

Gottesman L, Milsom JW, Mazier WP (1989) The use of anxiolytic and parasympathomimetic agents in the treatment of postoperative urinary retention following anorectal surgery. A prospective, randomized, double-blind study. Dis Colon Rectum 32:867–870

Hegde SS (2006) Muscarinic receptors in the bladder: from basic research to therapeutics. Br J Pharmacol 147(Suppl 2):S80–S87

Hindley RG, Brierly RD, Thomas PJ (2004) Prostaglandin E2 and bethanechol in combination for treating detrusor underactivity. BJU Int 93:89–92

Kemp B, Kitschke HJ, Goetz M, Heyl W (1997) Prophylaxis and treatment of bladder dysfunction after Wertheim–Meigs operation: the positive effect of early postoperative detrusor stimulation using the cholinergic drug betanecholchloride. Int Urogynecol J Pelvic Floor Dysfunct 8:138–141

Krishnamoorthy S, Kekre NS (2009) Detrusor underactivity: to tone or not to tone the bladder? Indian J Urol 25:407–408

Madeiro AP, Rufino AC, Sartori MG, Baracat EC, Lima GR, Girão MJ (2006) The effects of bethanechol and cisapride on urodynamic parameters in patients undergoing radical hysterectomy for cervical cancer. A randomized, double-blind, placebo-controlled study. Int Urogynecol J Pelvic Floor Dysfunct 17:248–252

Manchana T, Prasartsakulchi C (2011) Bethanechol chloride for the prevention of bladder dysfunction after radical hysterectomy in gynecologic cancer patients: a randomized controlled trial study. Int J Gynecol Cancer 21:730–736

Osman NI, Chapple CR, Abrams P, Dmochowski R, Haab F, Nitti V, Koelbl H, van Kerrebroeck P, Wein AJ (2014) Detrusor underactivity and the underactive bladder: a new clinical entity? A review of current terminology, definitions, epidemiology, aetiology, and diagnosis. Eur Urol 65:389–398

Oxford Centre for Evidence-Based Medicine: Levels of evidence and grades of recommendation (2001) Available at: http://www.cebm.net/levels_of_evidence.asp. Accessed Nov 2006

Riedl CR, Daha LK, Knoll M, Pflueger H (2002) Bethanechol in the restitution of the acontractile detrusor: a prospective, randomized, double blind, placebo-controlled study. Neurourol Urodyn 21:376

Savona-Ventura C, Grech ES, Saliba I (1991) Pharmacological measures to prevent post-operative urinary retention; a prospective randomized study. Eur J Obstet Gynecol Reprod Biol 41:225–229

Shah PJ, Abrams PH, Choa RG et al (1983) Distigmine bromide and post-prostatectomy voiding. Br J Urol 55:229–232

Smith PP (2010) Aging and the underactive detrusor: a failure of activity or activation? Neurourol Urodyn 29:408–412

Smith PP, Tyagi P, Kuchel GA et al (2014) Advanced therapeutic directions to treat the underactive bladder. Int Urol Nephrol 46(Suppl 1):S35

Somogyi GT, de Groat WC (1992) Evidence for inhibitory nicotinic and facilitatory muscarinic receptors in cholinergic nerve terminals of the rat urinary bladder. J Auton Nerv Syst 37:S89–S97

Somogyi GT, Tanowitz M et al (1996) M1 muscarinic receptor facilitation of ACh and noradrenaline release in the rat urinary bladder is mediated by protein kinase C. J Physiol 496:245–254

Tomoe H (2014) Assessment of the usefulness and optimal method of administration of distigmine bromide for the treatment of voiding dysfunction due to underactive detrusor. Paper presented at the AUGS/IUGA Scientific Meeting. Washington, DC. 22–26 July 2014

Tyagi P, Smith PP, Kuchel GA et al (2014) Pathophysiology and animal modeling of underactive bladder. Int Urol Nephrol 46(Suppl 1):S11

Yamaguchi O, Shishido K et al (1996) Evaluation of mRNAs encoding muscarinic receptor subtypes in human detrusor muscle. J Urol 156:1208–1213

Yamanishi T, Yasuda K, Kamai T et al (2004) Combination of a cholinergic drug and an α-blocker is more effective than monotherapy for the treatment of voiding difficulty in patients with underactive detrusor. Int J Urol 11:88–96

Yoshimura N, Chancellor MB (2011) Physiology and pharmacology of the bladder and urethra. In: Wein AJ, Kavoussi LR, Novick AC, Partin AW, Peters CA, editors. Campbells urology. 10th edn Elsevier, Philadelphia, PA, USA

Chapter 7
Novel Drugs for Underactive Bladder

Pradeep Tyagi and Mahendra Pratap Kashyap

Need for Novel Drugs

The International Continence Society (ICS) defines UAB as a detrusor contraction of inadequate strength and/or duration resulting in prolonged bladder emptying and/or a failure to achieve complete bladder emptying in the absence of urethral obstruction (Abrams et al. 2002). A multifactorial etiology is implicated (Tyagi et al. 2014) including aging for idiopathic UAB, neurogenic UAB as a consequence of Parkinson disease, multiple sclerosis, spinal cord injury or cauda equina (e.g., herniated disc, pelvic fractures), infection (e.g., AIDS, herpes zoster infection), and myogenic UAB secondary to diabetes mellitus or bladder outlet obstruction.

Medical management of UAB does not always achieve satisfactory results and it remains an undertreated and underreported condition. Despite the enormous amount of new biologic insights, very few drugs with mechanism of action other than direct and indirect muscarinic agonists have passed as yet the proof-of-concept stage. Research and development of novel therapeutic options for UAB is therefore an area of active interest (Smith et al. 2014b). Although the exact etiology of UAB is unknown, pharmacological therapy has been targeted to both the central and peripheral nervous system. In order to understand the pharmacology guiding the enterprise of drug discovery for this ailment, it is important to describe the potential sites available for action by novel drugs. Complete bladder emptying during voluntarily initiated voiding relies on intact afferent transmission from the bladder to brain, which then activate the efferent outflow for coordinating the contraction and relaxation of the bladder and sphincter, respectively. During voiding, the pontine micturition reflex center stimulates the sacral parasympathetic nucleus to increase

P. Tyagi, PhD (✉) • M.P. Kashyap, PhD
Department of Urology, University of Pittsburgh School of Medicine, Pittsburgh, PA, USA
e-mail: tyagpradeep@gmail.com

M.B. Chancellor, A.C. Diokno (eds.), *The Underactive Bladder*,
DOI 10.1007/978-3-319-23687-2_7

parasympathetic activity. This results in bladder contraction via activation of post-synaptic muscarinic receptors (M2/3) and relaxation of both urethral and prostatic smooth muscle by nitric oxide (NO) release (Tyagi et al. 2014). A defect at any link in the chain (from urothelium to nerve to detrusor smooth muscle) can ultimately lead to prolonged bladder emptying that characterizes UAB (Tyagi et al. 2014). Molecular pathways participating at each stage of micturition reflex can be potential drug targets for UAB.

Novel Drugs

A number of promising new drugs that target key molecular pathways (Fig. 7.1) (Table 7.1) involved in micturition control at the levels of the urothelium, detrusor muscle, peripheral and central nervous systems are being considered for treatment of UAB (Smith et al. 2014b). Preferred drug candidates either increase the afferent activity or the detrusor contractile force while decreasing the outflow resistance. Molecular targets in the periphery include muscarinic, prostaglandin receptors, neurotrophins, potassium, pannexin, and transient receptor potential (TRP) and hyperpolarization-activated cyclic nucleotide-gated (HCN) channels. Potential targets in the CNS include dopamine, serotonin (5-HT), and opioid neurotransmission. In the standard pharmacotherapy for UAB, bethanechol mimics the acetylcholine action, which is the primary excitatory neurotransmitter involved in bladder (detrusor) contraction and emptying. Therefore, bethanechol can address the deficits in both afferent and efferent neurotransmission, but its clinical utility is limited by the lack of receptor selectivity and cholinergic side effects of sialorrhea, nausea, abdominal distension, and abdominal cramping (Manchana and Prasartsakulchai 2011), vision, and, potentially, cardiovascular and CNS effects. Further preclinical and clinical studies are therefore needed to meet the unmet medical need.

Drugs Targeting Urothelium Signaling

The sensory side of the micturition reflex (Smith et al. 2012) is a potential therapeutic target for UAB. Mechanoreceptive afferents residing in the bladder wall not only convey the state of bladder fullness during storage phase but also convey the magnitude of spontaneous (non-voiding) and voiding detrusor contractions (Meng et al. 2008). Several reports have suggested that reduced release of various substances, including adenosine triphosphate (ATP) (Munoz et al. 2011), prostaglandins, and acetylcholine (ACh), from bladder urothelium could contribute to decreased bladder sensation and cause a deficit in afferent input from the bladder(Smith et al. 2012). In addition, attenuated contractile stimulus (acetylcholine and ATP) can also lead to

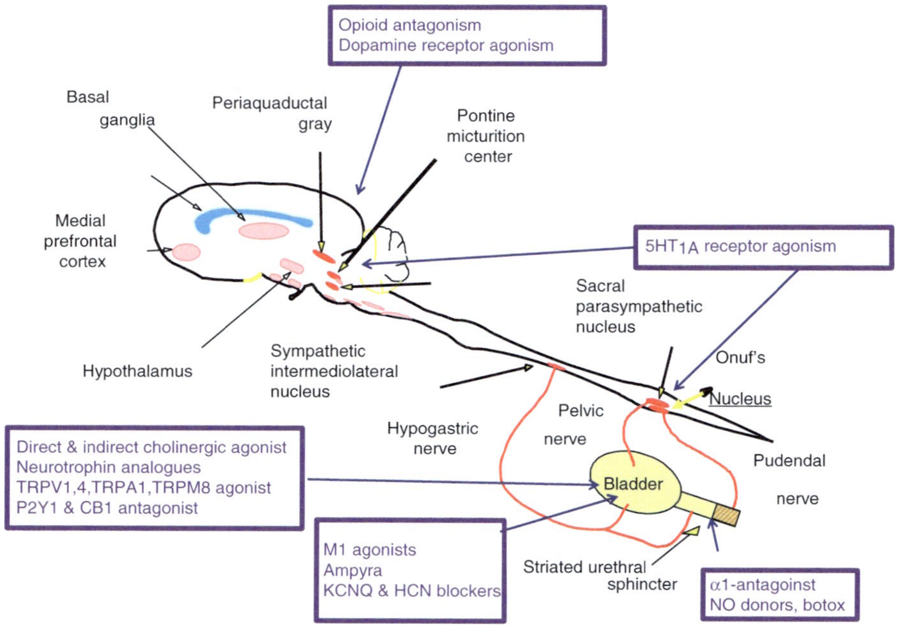

Fig. 7.1 Potential new drugs for UAB target key molecular pathways involved in micturition control at the levels of the urothelium, detrusor muscle autonomic and afferent pathways, spinal cord, and brain. Various drug classes are included in *purple boxes* with *arrows* indicating sites of action

Table 7.1 Novel drugs for underactive bladder

Drugs
Drugs targeting urothelium signaling
Acetylcholine
Improve bladder emptying by indirect acting agonists
Neurotrophin mimetics
Neurite growth enhancer
Prostaglandins
Agents that activate pannexin channels
Agents that sensitize afferent nerve endings
TRPV1 and TRPV4 agonists
TRPA1 agonists
Transient receptor potential melastatin 8 (TRPM8) channel agonists
Cannabinoid receptor antagonists
Drugs improving muscle function for myogenic UAB
By facilitating nerve-evoked contraction
M_1 muscarinic agonists
N-Type high-voltage-activated Ca(2+) channels (HVACCs) agonists
By facilitating spontaneous contraction
Potassium channels
Hyperpolarization-activated cyclic nucleotide-gated (HCN) channels
Centrally acting drugs for neurogenic UAB
Drugs acting on dopamine pathway
Drugs acting on serotonin pathway
Drugs acting on opioid pathway
Drugs that decrease urethral resistance

decreased detrusor contractility. Therefore, drugs that target urothelium can improve the defective initiation of afferent signals and enhance detrusor contractility.

Acetylcholine

Bladder urothelium possesses a nonneuronal cholinergic system and high density of muscarinic receptors. Impaired afferent signaling(Smith et al. 2014a) due to either reduced acetylcholine release from urothelium or due to changes in the sensitivity and coupling of the suburothelial interstitial cell network is offered as an explanation for UAB phenotype. Agents can either directly mimic the release of acetylcholine in the bladder or act indirectly by inhibiting the metabolism of acetylcholine. Acetylcholine released from parasympathetic nerves together with ATP (Burnstock 2013) at the detrusor neuromuscular synapse mediates detrusor contraction. ATP exerts activation of excitatory purinergic $P2X_1$ receptors on the detrusor smooth muscle, and inhibitory action on $P2Y_1$ receptors in cholinergic nerve endings controls the acetylcholine release.

Improve Bladder Emptying by Indirect Acting Agonists

Considering the adverse effect profile of direct acting agonists of acetylcholine, namely, bethanechol, there is a definite incentive for enhancing the action of acetylcholine through indirect means. Distigmine inhibits the enzyme, acetylcholinesterase, and thereby increases the pharmacodynamic half-life of endogenously released ACh. Three times daily treatment of distigmine 5 mg for 4 weeks was recently tested in 27 UAB patients (Bougas et al. 2004). In the phase II trial on UAB patients, distigmine was generally well tolerated by UAB patients. Pressure flow studies were conducted before the initiation of distigmine and at follow-up. Distigmine obviated the need for intermittent self-catheterization in 11 patients and PVR was significantly reduced. Treated patients also showed slight increase in maximum flow rate and detrusor pressure at maximum flow. Apart from cholinesterase inhibition for UAB, drugs that downregulate the expression of acetylcholinesterase can be another alternative option. Antagonists for P2Y1 receptor are known to block the ATP-mediated increase of cholinesterase activity with aging (Choi et al. 2003).

Neurotrophin Mimetics

A common trait shared by voiding dysfunctions such as UAB, irrespective of their origin, is dysregulation in synthesis and secretion of neurotrophins (Kim et al. 2005; Nirmal et al. 2014; Wang et al. 2015). Four neurotrophins have been identified in mammalian cells: most notably nerve growth factor (NGF), brain-derived neurotrophic factor (BDNF), neurotrophin-4/5 (NT-4/5). These target tissue-derived neurotrophins exert their effects upon binding to their high-affinity receptors abundantly expressed in the bladder (Girard et al. 2011) and neuronal circuits regulating micturition function (Garraway et al. 2011). Studies have demonstrated that constitutive expression of NGF and BDNF from urothelium and detrusor smooth muscle cells can promote neuronal survival and maturation (Elmariah et al. 2004; Gonzalez et al. 1999). BDNF interacts with serotoninergic and cholinergic transmission as serotonin reuptake inhibitors increase BDNF levels (Song et al. 2014), and BDNF is known to increase the cholinergic transmission through a presynaptic mechanism (Slonimsky et al. 2003). In a recent study, exogenous expression of BDNF was shown to upregulate the expression of cholinergic genes in the bladder (Kashyap et al. 2014b, 2015).

It is known that NGF activates the cell-surface transmembrane glycoprotein TrkA receptor, whereas BDNF acts via high-affinity receptor tropomyosin-related kinase B (TrkB). TrkB receptor is co-expressed with acetylcholine receptors along the postsynaptic membrane of the neuromuscular junction, and expression is innervation dependent (Funakoshi et al. 1995; Pitts et al. 2006). TrkB signaling was demonstrated to be a key regulator of neuromuscular function as blockade of TrkB signaling (Kulakowski et al. 2011) attenuated the neuromuscular transmission and fragmented postsynaptic acetylcholine receptors. Drugs mimicking BDNF action can therefore be potential drugs for increasing the cholinergic transmission in the bladder of UAB patients.

Neurite Growth Enhancer

Studies on animal models of neuropathy showed that TAC-302 a cyclohexenoic-long fatty alcohol derivative was able to enhance the outgrowth of neurites. Chronic oral administration of TAC-302 improved the voiding in diabetic bladder dysfunction with dose-dependent reduction in residual urine volume and increased voided volume in UAB secondary to streptozotocin (STZ)-induced diabetes (Takahisa et al. 2013; Yoshizawaa et al. 2012).

Prostaglandins

Prostaglandins, namely, PGE2, are synthesized by cyclooxygenase-1 (COX-1) and COX-2 in the bladder, which is released during bladder stretch and believed to be responsible for the spontaneous detrusor contractions (Fry et al. 2004). Instillation of PGE2 was able to reduce the voiding interval in UAB secondary to STZ-induced diabetes mellitus (Nirmal et al. 2014). In similar studies on UAB induced by lumbar canal stenosis (LCS), PGE2 infusion increased the frequency of small-amplitude phasic contractions during the filling phase of cystometry under urethane anesthesia performed 4 weeks after LCS (Fig. 7.2), whereas

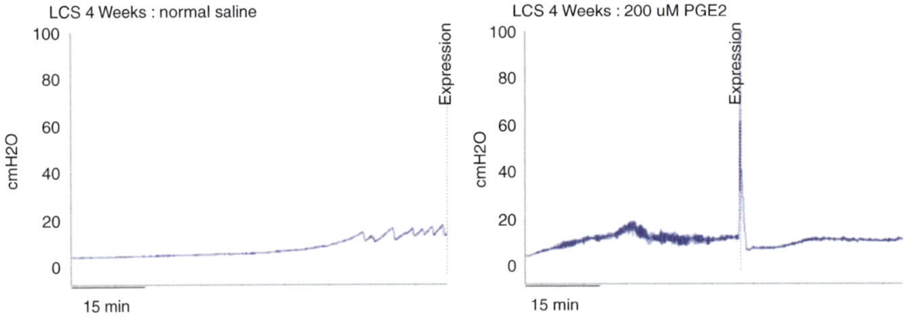

Fig. 7.2 The effect of PGE2 instillation on basal tone of the bladder in rat model of neurogenic UAB induced by lumbar canal stenosis. Bladder infusion of PGE2 in the concentration (200 uM) induced small-amplitude phasic contractions during the filling phase of cystometry under urethane anesthesia performed 4 weeks after LCS procedure (*right panel*). Saline-treated LCS rats at the same time point showed the acontractile phenotype with the absence of phasic contractions (*left panel*)

saline-treated group remained acontractile (Wang et al. 2015). Intravenous injection of sulprostone, a prostaglandin E receptor 3 (EP3) agonist at 2 weeks, reproduced the cystometric changes observed following intravesical PGE2 in 4-week old LCS rats under urethane anesthesia (Wang et al. 2015). In a clinical study, once-weekly intravesical PGE2 (1.5 mg in 20 mL 0.9 % saline) was combined with bethanechol 50 mg four times daily for a total of 6-week therapy of 17 male and 2 female UAB patients (Hindley et al. 2004). Combined therapy only showed limited therapeutic effect over placebo, where majority of the patients included in the trial were reliant on clean intermittent self-catheterization with PVR consistently >300 mL. Overall, studies support PGE2 analogues and EP1 receptor as potential drugs and drug target for UAB, respectively.

Agents That Activate Pannexin Channels

It is known that the bladder response to purinergic agents increases with age, whereas the response to cholinergic agents decreases with age (Yoshida et al. 2004). These age-dependent biochemical changes support the rationale of developing drugs acting on purinergic pathway for age-associated disorders such as UAB. A recent study showed that in response to distension, ATP is released through pannexin channels into the lumen (Beckel et al. 2015). Considering that aging is associated with loss of responsiveness to bladder filing (Smith et al. 2012), it is suggested that pannexin functionality is reduced with aging. Drugs that activate pannexin channels such as ATP diphosphohydrolase (apyrase) can be potential drugs for UAB.

Agents That Sensitize Afferent Nerve Endings

Bladder and urethral afferent dysfunction seen in UAB associated with diabetes (Lee et al. 2009) is associated with destruction of capsaicin-sensitive fibers in the bladder and urethra (Yang et al. 2010). Age-related decline in bladder sensation is also related to the sparse to moderate densities of TRPV1 immunoreactive nerves in the suburothelium and sparse fibers in the muscle layers. The capsaicin-sensitive afferents in the bladder are known to contain several peptides. These include tachykinins (such as substance P and neurokinin A and B), vasoactive intestinal polypeptide, and calcitonin gene-related peptide. Agents mimicking the action of these peptides can be potential drugs for UAB. Activation of transient receptor potential (TRP) channels on afferent nerves in the bladder induces the release of neurokinins, which increase detrusor contractility. Several partial or complete agonist of TRP channels TRPV1. TRPV4, TRPA1 and TRPM8 are potential drug candidates for UAB.

Transient Receptor Potential Vanilloid 1 (TRPV1) and TRPV4 Agonists

TRPV1 and TRPV4 are molecular transducers of hot temperature into neuronal signal. GSK 1016790A is a TRPV4 agonist and its intravesical instillation transiently decreased bladder capacity and voided volume (Aizawa et al. 2012). TRPV4 stimulation in the urothelium is considered to facilitate the micturition reflex by activation of the mechanosensitive, capsaicin-insensitive C-fibers of the primary bladder afferents. Extravesical application of piperine, a TRPV1 agonist to rat bladder, increased afferent input and detrusor contractility (Gevaert et al. 2007). Overall, studies support use of TRPV4 and TRPV1 agonists as a potential therapeutic approach for UAB.

Transient Receptor Potential Ankyrin 1 (TRPA1) Agonists

A recent study demonstrated that TRPV1 immunoreactivity in unmyelinated nerve fibers within the urothelium, suburothelial space, and muscle layer of the bladder is co-localized with TRPA1 immunoreactivity (Streng et al. 2008). Activation of TRPA1 by allyl isothiocyanate increased the micturition frequency and reduced the voided volume in rat. Findings support agonism of TRPA1 as a potential approach for improving afferent deficit in UAB.

Transient Receptor Potential Melastatin 8 (TRPM8) Channel Agonists

TRPM8 is a molecular thermal sensor for translating cold temperature into neuronal activity (Lei et al. 2013). It is recognized that cold temperature elicits urgency response in individuals with voiding dysfunction. Since sensory endings in the skin are responsible for perception of thermal cues, their stimulation can be harnessed to improve clinical outcomes. Spraying of menthol that activates TRPM8 decreased the voiding interval, micturition volume, and bladder capacity of rats (Lei et al. 2013), suggesting that topical activation of TRPM8 can be used to improve bladder emptying in UAB patients.

Cannabinoid Receptor Antagonists

In contrast to agonism of TRP channels, antagonism of cannabinoid receptors is a potential therapeutic approach for increasing afferent input from the bladder and reducing bladder capacity (Dmitrieva and Berkley 2002) in UAB patients.

Cannabinoid receptors were suggested to be responsible for the pathogenesis of UAB associated with diabetes (Li et al. 2013), and activity of bladder afferents was reduced following activation of CB1 receptors in mouse bladder (Walczak et al. 2009). Based on available research, we postulate that CB1 antagonist, rimonabant (Pataky et al. 2013), is a potential candidate for repositioning in UAB.

Drugs Improving Muscle Function for Myogenic UAB

The underlying pathobiology for myogenic UAB is considered to be either abnormal detrusor muscle contractility or secondary to bladder outlet obstruction. Decreased detrusor contractility can result from a lack of contractile stimulus from acetylcholine and ATP or a lack of tissue responsiveness to contractile stimuli due to irreversible changes in the bladder wall that are described as sarcopenia (loss of muscle tissue, increased collagen deposition) (Tyagi et al. 2014). The lack of tissue responsiveness to contractile stimuli may be due to altered excitation–contraction coupling mechanisms contributed by changes in the properties and density of calcium and potassium channels, gap junctions, and receptors in detrusor smooth muscles. It is considered that stimulus intensity of efferent nerve-evoked bladder contraction relies on afferent input (Zeng et al. 2012), which in turn is dependent on the strength of spontaneous detrusor contractions detected during storage phase. In fact, patients with mixed UAB (coexistence of both neurogenic and myogenic phenotype) are considered to have attenuated spontaneous detrusor contractions that reduce the afferent input (Andersson 2010), which ultimately causes insufficiency in nerve-evoked detrusor contractility. Therefore, drugs can address myogenic UAB by facilitating nerve-evoked contraction and/or by facilitating spontaneous contractions in UAB with acontractile bladder phenotype.

Drugs That Facilitate Nerve-Evoked Contraction

It is established that activation of muscarinic receptors in the bladder is responsible for normal voiding, and a subtype of muscarinic receptor can be pharmacologically manipulated for attenuating the prolonged bladder emptying of UAB. Presynaptic M1 muscarinic receptors on parasympathetic nerve terminals are involved in an auto-facilitatory mechanism that markedly enhances acetylcholine release (Somogyi and de Groat 1999). The facilitatory muscarinic mechanism is dependent upon a protein kinase A (Oliveira and Correia-de-Sa 2005)-mediated second messenger pathway and influx of extracellular Ca^{2+} into the parasympathetic nerve terminals via N-type Ca^{2+} channels. Both M1 receptors and N-type Ca^{2+} channels are suitable drug targets for UAB.

M_1 Muscarinic Agonists

Recent studies reported upregulation of M1 receptor subtype in an animal model of UAB induced by prolonged ischemia (Zhao et al. 2015), which suggests there is compensatory upregulation of receptors that can enhance the release of acetylcholine from nerves innervating the UAB. Presynaptic M1 receptors can facilitate the release of acetylcholine from nerves and thereby facilitate afferent signaling and voiding contraction (Witsell et al. 2012). Application of M1 agonist, cevimeline increased the spontaneous contractions of isolated guinea pig bladder strips (Arisawa et al. 2002). Intravenous administration of cevimeline (0.3 mg/kg or higher) in rats increased the non-voiding contractions, suggesting that the release of various substances, including acetylcholine (ACh) and ATP (Munoz et al. 2011), from bladder urothelium and efferent nerves in the bladder was increased. Oral dosing of cevimeline in rats at 30 mg/kg increased the urine volume, pH, and urinary excretion of Na^+ and Cl^- ions. Xanomeline [3(3-hexyloxy-1,2,5-thiadiazol-4-yl)-1,2,5,6-tetrahydro-1-methylpyridine] (Shannon et al. 1994) is another M1 agonist available as a drug candidate for UAB.

N-Type High-Voltage-Activated Ca(2+) Channels (HVACCs) Agonists

Since N-type HVACC are involved in facilitating the release of ACh from parasympathetic nerve terminals in the bladder, drugs that activate these channels can be potential agents for UAB. 4-Aminopyridine (4-AP) sold as Ampyra is known to directly stimulate presynaptic N-type VGCC at the concentration of 0.5 mM and blocks Kv1 family channels at 1 mM concentration (Wu et al. 2009). Ampyra and similar drug fampridine (Cardenas et al. 2014) can potentiate the release of neurotransmitters from both sensory and motor nerve terminals and improve neuromuscular function in patients with spinal cord injury, myasthenia gravis, or multiple sclerosis (Wu et al. 2009). The effect of Ampyra on improving bladder emptying was tested much earlier by Maggi et al., in urethane-anesthetized rats (Maggi et al. 1988). Ampyra potentiated nerve-evoked bladder contractions, and intravenous injection in the dose ranging from 0.15 to 2 mg/kg i.v. produced a dose-dependent potentiation of voiding frequency and activation of high-amplitude, hexamethonium-sensitive rhythmic bladder contractions.

Drugs That Facilitate Spontaneous Contraction

Spontaneous contractile activity of the urinary bladder (Turner and Brading 1997) is considered to underlie the basal tone that allows the bladder to maintain an optimum shape as it expands to accommodate increasing volumes of urine. In addition, spontaneous contractions (Fry et al. 2004) are known to facilitate the generation of bladder sensation and afferent activity (Andersson 2010). Several tools have been used to investigate the origin of spontaneous activity in the bladder, which have noted that Ca^{2+} wave in the propagation of spontaneous activity arise in the suburothelial layer of interstitial cells and then spreads to the detrusor layer (Kanai et al. 2007). Interstitial cells are considered pacemaker cells that activate the periodic spontaneous inward currents (pacemaker currents) responsible for the origin of Ca^{2+} waves.

Several reports suggest that attenuated spontaneous activity of the bladder contributes to the UAB phenotype (Wang et al. 2015; Nirmal et al. 2014) by reducing the intensity of afferent input from the bladder. Incidentally, acontractile bladder that is devoid of spontaneous activity is frequently observed in iatrogenic UAB patients (Drossaerts et al. 2015; Mitchell et al. 2014). Therefore, drugs that can selectively augment the dormant spontaneous contractions in the bladder will be preferable agents for UAB as they can improve the afferent input from the bladder. Several channel isoforms selectively expressed in the bladder can be leveraged to increase spontaneous activity in UAB.

Potassium Channels

Several types of potassium currents have been characterized in the bladder, but the subtype of K_v is considered to play an important role in spontaneous activity by regulating the resting membrane potential of smooth muscles and for repolarizing the action potential (Petkov 2012). Other types include BK channels that control action potential duration and the resting membrane potential, whereas SK currents underlie after-hyperpolarizations (Thorneloe and Nelson 2003). KCNQ (K_v7) currents are outwardly rectifying, voltage-dependent K^+ currents that activate at potentials positive to −60 mV with little inactivation (Gribkoff 2008; Gu et al. 2005). Five genes encoding the KCNQ family of ion channel proteins have been identified, each encoding a different KCNQ α-subunit (1–5). KCNQ are considered important in the regulation of smooth muscle contractility and tone (Anderson et al. 2013). KCNQ subtypes 1–5 are functionally expressed in detrusor smooth muscle as KCNQ channel inhibitors XE991, linopirdine, or chromanol 293B increased the amplitude of tetrodotoxin TTX-insensitive myogenic spontaneous contractions (Anderson et al. 2013). KCNQ inhibition by XE991 depolarized the cell membrane and evoked transient depolarizations in quiescent cells. XE991 also increased the frequency of Ca^{2+}-oscillations in detrusor smooth muscles of guinea pig bladder (Anderson et al. 2013). On the other hand, spontaneous activity was inhibited by the KCNQ channel activators flupirtine or meclofenamic acid (Anderson et al. 2013), and, in a separate study, another KCNQ activator, retigabine, decreased the capsaicin-induced bladder overactivity in a freely moving, conscious rat (Streng et al. 2004). Taken together, blockade of KCNQ locally in the bladder is a potential approach for UAB.

Hyperpolarization-Activated Cyclic Nucleotide-Gated (HCN) Channels

HCN channels (Cuttle et al. 2001; Greenwood and Prestwich 2002) belong to a family of nonselective cationic channels that conduct Na^+ and K^+ current and are activated by hyperpolarization in neurons and smooth muscles. HCN channels are comprised of four subtypes encoded by four genes (HCN1-4), which form the structural component of a voltage-gated inwardly rectifying I*h* current, which restores the resting membrane potential (Cuttle et al. 2001; Greenwood and Prestwich 2002). HCN channels are directly activated by direct binding of intracellular cyclic adenosine monophosphate (cAMP) inside the cells (Cuttle et al. 2001; Greenwood and Prestwich 2002). Expression of HCN channels has been recently reported in the rat and human bladder (He et al. 2012; Xue et al. 2012). Furthermore, the adenylate cyclase responsible for generating cAMP in the bladder smooth muscle, urothelium, and interstitial cells can be theoretically modulated by activation of M2 muscarinic receptor and β3 adrenoceptor, which raises the possibility of using bladder-selective M2 agonist or β3 adrenoceptor antagonists for modulating the kinetics of HCN channel.

Direct inhibition of HCN channels in the bladder with ZD7288 was shown to augment the spontaneous activity of the bladder (Green et al. 1996; Kashyap et al. 2015). Conversely, agents that activate HCN channels (Postea and Biel 2011; Albertson et al. 2011), such as lamotrigine and gabapentin, attenuate spontaneous activity of rat bladder (Kashyap et al. 2014a). We found that cumulative application of ZD7288 dose dependently increased the tetrodotoxin -insensitive phasic contractions of rat bladder (Fig. 7.3) as reported earlier by Green et al. (1996). In vitro studies suggested that a direct action of ZD7288 on HCN channels expressed by detrusor smooth muscles or interstitial cells is responsible for the increased spontaneous activity.

It is known that mechanosensitive Aδ bladder neurons play an important role in the control of normal voiding (de Groat and Yoshimura 2006), and localized blockade of HCN channels expressed in Aδ bladder neurons (Masuda et al. 2006) following intrathecal injection of ZD7288 (1 μg) blocked the voiding in normal rat. In a separate study, chronic administration of HCN channel activator, lamotrigine (20 mg/kg) (Loutochin et al. 2012), caused a urodynamic improvement in spinal cord-injured rat model. Apparently different subtypes of HCN channels are expressed in different tissue, such that expression of HCN 4 subtype (HCN4) is predominant in the bladder and HCN2 predominate in the heart (Kuwabara et al. 2013). There are also species differences in the bladder with predominant expression of HCN1 in rodents and HCN4 in human bladder (He et al. 2012; Xue et al. 2012). Based on available data, it is postulated that basal levels of intracellular cAMP constitutively activate the HCN channels, and therefore, agents that cannot penetrate the blood–brain barrier and are excreted unchanged in urine would be preferable to selectively block HCN4 channels in the bladder for augmenting spontaneous activity in the bladder of UAB patients without any cardiac effects. In contrast, selective activation of HCN channels expressed in bladder afferent neurons would be an alternative approach for increasing spontaneous activity in the bladder.

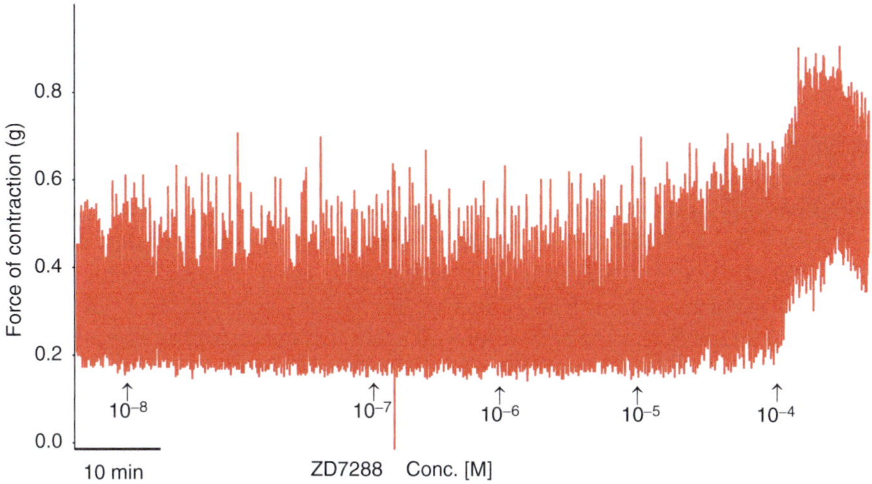

Fig. 7.3 The effect of HCN channel blocker ZD7288 on spontaneous activity of rat bladder. Cumulative application of ZD7288 dose dependently increased the tetrodotoxin-insensitive phasic contractions in bladder strips from healthy rats. Spontaneous contractility was measured in the presence of tetrodotoxin 1 μM

Centrally Acting Drugs for Neurogenic UAB

The potential targets for managing neurogenic UAB exist in the molecular pathways involved in spinal and supraspinal control of voiding reflex at the levels of autonomic and afferent pathways, spinal cord, and brain (Tyagi et al. 2014). Supraspinal control of the voiding reflex is dependent upon the normal relay of afferent input to the bladder as any deficit correlates with reduced activation in the insula and dorsal anterior cingulate cortex in the brain of older adults (Tadic et al. 2013). Therefore, efficient afferent signaling is integral for an efficient efferent outflow to the bladder, and neurogenic UAB can impact upon the key processes of perception and integration of afferent input from the bladder.

Drugs Acting on Dopamine Pathway

Age-related decline of dopamine binding has been reported in brain areas involved in cognition, and there is a tremendous overlap among regions involved in cognition and those involved in interpretation of afferent input from the bladder (MacDonald et al. 2012). Therefore, drugs that augment dopamine signaling can be potential drugs for neurogenic UAB. It is known that D1 receptors tonically inhibit and D2 facilitate micturition reflex, because D2-selective agonists and D1-selective antagonists produce a reduction of the bladder capacity in conscious rat (Brusa et al. 2006). Studies on subcutaneous administration of apomorphine (a nonselective dopamine receptor agonist) 0.01–0.5 mg/kg in rodents found that it raises intravesical pressure through its biphasic action on the dopamine receptors, which is characterized by initial increase in afferent activity followed by a decrease (Uchiyama et al. 2009). Apomorphine increases the afferent activity and stimulates central micturition center. These pharmacodynamic characteristics of apomorphine suggest that D2-selective agonists can be potential agents for increasing afferent input and involuntary detrusor contraction threshold (reflex volume) (Brusa et al. 2006) in UAB patients. Apomorphine can be absorbed sublingually, which suggest that an on-demand therapy for bladder emptying is a possibility. Metoclopramide is another FDA-approved agent that can modulate dopaminergic pathways in UAB.

Drugs Acting on Serotonin Pathway

Drugs acting on serotonin pathway can increase the afferent input from bladder and urethra which in turn determines the force and duration of detrusor contraction. It is known that urethral afferents responding to urine flow in the urethra potentiate the detrusor contraction and bladder emptying (Torrens and Morrison 1987; de Groat et al. 1993; Jung et al. 1999). These reflexes require the integrative action of neuronal populations at multiple levels of the nervous system involving serotoninergic transmission (Song et al. 2014). In a recent study, supraspinal micturition reflex in rats with bilateral avulsion injury of the L5–S2 ventral roots was elicited by agonists for the $5HT_{1A}$ receptor, 8-hydroxy-2-(di-n-propylamino)-tetralin (8OH-DPAT) (Chang and Havton 2013). The voiding efficiency of rats exhibiting UAB phenotype was increased by 20 %, and there was an evidence of coordinated contraction of the bladder and activation of the external urethral sphincter.

Drugs Acting on Opioid Pathway

Pharmacologic experiments revealed that endorphins are inhibitory transmitters in the spinal and supraspinal control of micturition reflex. Agents inhibiting the opioid action have been used to reverse opioid-induced urinary retention. Blood–brain barrier non-permeant analogues of naloxone, namely, methylnaltrexone, are effective in reversing opioid-induced constipation in patients, but not effective in reversing urinary retention (Rosow et al. 2007). The effect of quaternary amine, methylnaltrexone, suggests that volitional control over micturition involve endogenous opioids as the neurotransmitter in polysynaptic pathways mediating the coordination between the urinary bladder and the urethra.

Drugs That Decrease Urethral Resistance

Bladder emptying is facilitated by non-cholinergic/non-adrenergic nitric oxide (NO) release onto the internal urethral sphincter resulting in a relaxation of the urethral outlet and by removal of excitatory inputs to the urethra (Takeda et al. 2010). Therefore, drugs that reduce the urethral resistance can improve bladder emptying with deficient detrusor contractility by reducing the back pressure from urethral resistance. Clinical use of α_1 adrenoceptor antagonists in UAB patients was able to improve the bladder emptying by reversing obstruction and increasing PVR (Yamanishi et al. 2004; Chang et al. 2008). A drug approved for angina, isosorbide dinitrate, has been reported to decrease urethral pressures in spinal cord injury (Mamas et al. 2001; Reitz et al. 2004) as urethral relaxation is mediated by NO. Chemodenervation of the urethra and rhabdosphincter with botulinum toxin has also been tried to reduce urethral resistance (Kuo 2003).

Conclusions

The future for the development of new modalities for the UAB treatment looks promising as several different therapeutic pathways are being explored in preclinical studies. Future prospective therapies are aimed at novel targets with novel mechanisms of action, including M1 receptor agonist, N-type HVACC agonist, KCNQ and HCN channel blockers, serotonin, and dopamine signaling modulators. Among other investigational therapies, purinergic receptor agonism, TRP channel agonism, cannabinoid receptor antagonism, neurotrophin mimetics, and neurokinin receptor agonists are of considerable interest. There is great hope that just as drugs for OAB and ED better define the disease condition in the general population, an effective drug capable of reducing PVR will also help in better definition and management of UAB.

References

Abrams P, Cardozo L, Fall M, Griffiths D, Rosier P, Ulmsten U, van Kerrebroeck P, Victor A, Wein A, Standardisation Sub-committee of the International Continence S (2002) The standardisation of terminology of lower urinary tract function: report from the Standardisation Sub-committee of the International Continence Society. Neurourol Urodyn 21:167–178

Aizawa N, Wyndaele JJ, Homma Y, Igawa Y (2012) Effects of TRPV4 cation channel activation on the primary bladder afferent activities of the rat. Neurourol Urodyn 31(1):148–55. doi:10.1002/nau.21212

Albertson AJ, Yang J, Hablitz JJ (2011) Decreased hyperpolarization-activated currents in layer 5 pyramidal neurons enhances excitability in focal cortical dysplasia. J Neurophys 106(5): 2189–2200. doi:10.1152/jn.00164.2011

Anderson UA, Carson C, Johnston L, Joshi S, Gurney AM, McCloskey KD (2013) Functional expression of KCNQ (Kv7) channels in guinea pig bladder smooth muscle and their contribution to spontaneous activity. Br J Pharmacol 169(6):1290–1304. doi:10.1111/bph.12210

Andersson KE (2010) Detrusor myocyte activity and afferent signaling. Neurourol Urodyn 29(1):97–106. 2009/12/22 edn. doi:10.1002/nau.20784.

Arisawa H, Fukui K, Imai E, Fujise N, Masunaga H (2002) General pharmacological profile of the novel muscarinic receptor agonist SNI-2011, a drug for xerostomia in Sjogren's syndrome. 4th communication: effects on gastrointestinal, urinary and reproductive systems and other effects. Arzneimittelforschung 52(4):225–232. doi:10.1055/s-0031-1299885

Beckel JM, Daugherty SL, Tyagi P, Wolf-Johnston AS, Birder LA, Mitchell CH, de Groat WC (2015) Pannexin 1 channels mediate the release of ATP into the lumen of the rat urinary bladder. J Physiol 593(8):1857–1871. doi:10.1113/jphysiol.2014.283119

Bougas DA, Mitsogiannis IC, Mitropoulos DN, Kollaitis GC, Serafetinides EN, Giannopoulos AM (2004) Clinical efficacy of distigmine bromide in the treatment of patients with underactive detrusor. Int Urol Nephrol 36(4):507–512

Brusa L, Petta F, Pisani A, Miano R, Stanzione P, Moschella V, Galati S, Finazzi Agro E (2006) Central acute D2 stimulation worsens bladder function in patients with mild Parkinson's disease. J Urol 175(1):202–206. doi:10.1016/S0022-5347(05)00058-3

Burnstock G (2013) Purinergic signalling in the lower urinary tract. Acta Physiol 207(1):40–52. doi:10.1111/apha.12012

Cardenas DD, Ditunno JF, Graziani V, McLain AB, Lammertse DP, Potter PJ, Alexander MS, Cohen R, Blight AR (2014) Two phase 3, multicenter, randomized, placebo-controlled clinical trials of fampridine-SR for treatment of spasticity in chronic spinal cord injury. Spinal Cord 52(1):70–76. doi:10.1038/sc.2013.137

Chang HH, Havton LA (2013) Serotonergic 5-HT(1A) receptor agonist (8-OH-DPAT) ameliorates impaired micturition reflexes in a chronic ventral root avulsion model of incomplete cauda equina/conus medullaris injury. Exp Neurol 239:210–217. doi:10.1016/j.expneurol.2012.10.015

Chang SJ, Chiang IN, Yu HJ (2008) The effectiveness of tamsulosin in treating women with voiding difficulty. Int J Urol Off J Jpn Urol Assoc 15(11):981–985. doi:10.1111/j.1442-2042.2008.02134.x

Choi RC, Siow NL, Cheng AW, Ling KK, Tung EK, Simon J, Barnard EA, Tsim KW (2003) ATP acts via P2Y1 receptors to stimulate acetylcholinesterase and acetylcholine receptor expression: transduction and transcription control. J Neurosc Off J Soc Neurosci 23(11):4445–4456

Cuttle MF, Rusznak Z, Wong AY, Owens S, Forsythe ID (2001) Modulation of a presynaptic hyperpolarization-activated cationic current (I(h)) at an excitatory synaptic terminal in the rat auditory brainstem. J Physiol 534(Pt 3):733–744, 2001/08/03 edn

de Groat WC, Booth AM, Yoshimura N (1993) Neurophysiology of micturition and its modification in animal models of human disease, vol 1. Harwood Academic Publishers, London 227–90

de Groat WC, Yoshimura N (2006) Mechanisms underlying the recovery of lower urinary tract function following spinal cord injury. Prog Brain Res 152:59–84

Dmitrieva N, Berkley KJ (2002) Contrasting effects of WIN 55212–2 on motility of the rat bladder and uterus. J Neurosci Off J Soc Neurosci 22(16):7147–7153. doi: jneurosci.org/content/22/16/7147

Drossaerts J, Rademakers K, van Koeveringe G, Van Kerrebroeck P (2015) The value of urodynamic tools to guide patient selection in sacral neuromodulation. World J Urol. doi:10.1007/s00345-015-1479-6 epub

Elmariah SB, Crumling MA, Parsons TD, Balice-Gordon RJ (2004) Postsynaptic TrkB-mediated signaling modulates excitatory and inhibitory neurotransmitter receptor clustering at hippocampal synapses. J Neurosci Off J Soc Neurosci 24(10):2380–2393. doi:10.1523/JNEUROSCI.4112-03.2004

Fry CH, Sui GP, Severs NJ, Wu C (2004) Spontaneous activity and electrical coupling in human detrusor smooth muscle: implications for detrusor overactivity? Urology 63(3 Suppl 1):3–10. 2004/03/12 edn. doi:10.1016/j.urology.2003.11.005

Funakoshi H, Belluardo N, Arenas E, Yamamoto Y, Casabona A, Persson H, Ibanez CF (1995) Muscle-derived neurotrophin-4 as an activity-dependent trophic signal for adult motor neurons. Science 268(5216):1495–1499

Garraway SM, Turtle JD, Huie JR, Lee KH, Hook MA, Woller SA, Grau JW (2011) Intermittent noxious stimulation following spinal cord contusion injury impairs locomotor recovery and reduces spinal brain-derived neurotrophic factor-tropomyosin-receptor kinase signaling in adult rats. Neuroscience 199:86–102. 2011/10/27 edn. doi:10.1016/j.neuroscience.2011.10.007

Gevaert T, Vandepitte J, Hutchings G, Vriens J, Nilius B, De Ridder D (2007) TRPV1 is involved in stretch-evoked contractile changes in the rat autonomous bladder model: a study with piperine, a new TRPV1 agonist. Neurourol Urodyn 26(3):440–450. doi:10.1002/nau.20343

Girard BM, Malley SE, Vizzard MA (2011) Neurotrophin/receptor expression in urinary bladder of mice with overexpression of NGF in urothelium. Am J Physiol Renal Physiol 300(2): F345–355. 2010/11/05 edn. doi:10.1152/ajprenal.00515.2010

Gonzalez M, Ruggiero FP, Chang Q, Shi YJ, Rich MM, Kraner S, Balice-Gordon RJ (1999) Disruption of Trkb-mediated signaling induces disassembly of postsynaptic receptor clusters at neuromuscular junctions. Neuron 24(3):567–583

Green ME, Edwards G, Kirkup AJ, Miller M, Weston AH (1996) Pharmacological characterization of the inwardly-rectifying current in the smooth muscle cells of the rat bladder. Br J Pharmacol 119(8):1509–1518. 1996/12/01 edn

Greenwood IA, Prestwich SA (2002) Characteristics of hyperpolarization-activated cation currents in portal vein smooth muscle cells. Am J Physiol Cell Physiol 282(4):C744–753. 2002/03/07 edn. doi:10.1152/ajpcell.00393.2001

Gribkoff VK (2008) The therapeutic potential of neuronal K V 7 (KCNQ) channel modulators: an update. Exp Opin Ther Targets 12(5):565–581. doi:10.1517/14728222.12.5.565

Gu N, Vervaeke K, Hu H, Storm JF (2005) Kv7/KCNQ/M and HCN/h, but not KCa2/SK channels, contribute to the somatic medium after-hyperpolarization and excitability control in CA1 hippocampal pyramidal cells. J Physiol 566(Pt 3):689–715. 2005/05/14 edn. doi:10.1113/jphysiol.2005.086835

He P, Deng J, Zhong X, Zhou Z, Song B, Li L (2012) Identification of a hyperpolarization-activated cyclic nucleotide-gated channel and its subtypes in the urinary bladder of the rat. Urology 79(6):1411 e7–13. doi:10.1016/j.urology.2012.01.037

Hindley RG, Brierly RD, Thomas PJ (2004) Prostaglandin E2 and bethanechol in combination for treating detrusor underactivity. BJU Int 93(1):89–92

Jung SY, Fraser MO, Ozawa H, Yokoyama O, Yoshiyama M, De Groat WC, Chancellor MB (1999) Urethral afferent nerve activity affects the micturition reflex; implication for the relationship between stress incontinence and detrusor instability. J Urol 162. S0022-5347(05)68742-3 [pii]. doi:10.1097/00005392-199907000-00069

Kanai A, Roppolo J, Ikeda Y, Zabbarova I, Tai C, Birder L, Griffiths D, de Groat W, Fry C (2007) Origin of spontaneous activity in neonatal and adult rat bladders and its enhancement by stretch and muscarinic agonists. Am J Physiol Renal Physiol 292(3):F1065–1072. doi:10.1152/ajprenal.00229.2006

Kashyap M, Yoshimura N, Smith P, Chancellor M, Tyagi P (2015) Characterization of the role of HCN channels in β3-adrenoceptor mediated rat bladder relaxation. Bladder 2(2):15–23. doi:10.14440/bladder.2015.44

Kashyap M, Yoshimura N, de Groat WC, Tyagi P (2014) Exogenous overexpression of Brain Derived Neurotrophic Factor (BDNF) in rat bladder evokes bladder overactivity. J Urol 191(4):4

Kashyap MP, Pore S, De Groat WC, Chermansky C, Yoshimura N, Tyagi P (2015) BDNF overexpression alters the phenotype of cholinergic neurons in rat bladder. J Urol 193(4):1108

Kim JC, Park EY, Hong SH, Seo SI, Park YH, Hwang TK (2005) Changes of urinary nerve growth factor and prostaglandins in male patients with overactive bladder symptom. Int J Urol Off J Jpn Urol Assoc 12(10):875–880. doi:10.1111/j.1442-2042.2005.01140.x

Kulakowski SA, Parker SD, Personius KE (2011) Reduced TrkB expression results in precocious age-like changes in neuromuscular structure, neurotransmission, and muscle function. J Appl Physiol 111(3):844–852. doi:10.1152/japplphysiol.00070.2011

Kuo HC (2003) Effect of botulinum a toxin in the treatment of voiding dysfunction due to detrusor underactivity. Urology 61(3):550–554. 2003/03/18 edn. doi:science/article/pii/S0090429502025414

Kuwabara Y, Kuwahara K, Takano M, Kinoshita H, Arai Y, Yasuno S, Nakagawa Y, Igata S, Usami S, Minami T, Yamada Y, Nakao K, Yamada C, Shibata J, Nishikimi T, Ueshima K, Nakao K (2013) Increased expression of HCN channels in the ventricular myocardium contributes to enhanced arrhythmicity in mouse failing hearts. J Am Heart Assoc 2(3):e000150. doi:10.1161/JAHA.113.000150

Lee WC, Wu HP, Tai TY, Yu HJ, Chiang PH (2009) Investigation of urodynamic characteristics and bladder sensory function in the early stages of diabetic bladder dysfunction in women with type 2 diabetes. J Urol 181(1):198–203. doi:10.1016/j.juro.2008.09.021

Lei Z, Ishizuka O, Imamura T, Noguchi W, Yamagishi T, Yokoyama H, Kurizaki Y, Sudha GS, Hosoda T, Nishizawa O, Andersson KE (2013) Functional roles of transient receptor potential melastatin 8 (TRPM8) channels in the cold stress-induced detrusor overactivity pathways in conscious rats. Neurourol Urodyn 32(5):500–504. doi:10.1002/nau.22325

Li Y, Sun Y, Zhang Z, Feng X, Meng H, Li S, Zhu Y, Chen S, Wang Y, Wang J, Zhang D, Jiang X, Li N, Shi B (2013) Cannabinoid receptors 1 and 2 are associated with bladder dysfunction in an experimental diabetic rat model. BJU Int 112(2):E143–150. doi:10.1111/bju.12172

Loutochin O, Afraa TA, Campeau L, Mahfouz W, Elzayat E, Corcos J (2012) Effect of the anticonvulsant medications Pregabalin and Lamotrigine on Urodynamic parameters in an animal model of neurogenic detrusor overactivity. Neurourol Urodyn 31(7):1197–1202. 2012/04/05 edn. doi:10.1002/nau.21214

MacDonald SW, Karlsson S, Rieckmann A, Nyberg L, Backman L (2012) Aging-related increases in behavioral variability: relations to losses of dopamine D1 receptors. J Neurosci Off J Soc Neurosci 32(24):8186–8191. doi:10.1523/JNEUROSCI.5474-11.2012

Maggi CA, Santicioli P, Borsini F, Giuliani S, Conte B, Lecci A, Meli A (1988) The effect of 4-aminopyridine on micturition reflex in normal or capsaicin-desensitized rats. Brain Res 449(1–2):61–70

Mamas MA, Reynard JM, Brading AF (2001) Augmentation of nitric oxide to treat detrusor-external sphincter dyssynergia in spinal cord injury. Lancet 357(9272):1964–1967

Manchana T, Prasartsakulchai C (2011) Bethanechol chloride for the prevention of bladder dysfunction after radical hysterectomy in gynecologic cancer patients: a randomized controlled trial study. Int J Gynecol Cancer Off J Int Gynecol Cancer Soc 21(4):730–736. doi:10.1111/IGC.0b013e3181f7d6de

Masuda N, Hayashi Y, Matsuyoshi H, Chancellor MB, de Groat WC, Yoshimura N (2006) Characterization of hyperpolarization-activated current (Ih) in dorsal root ganglion neurons innervating rat urinary bladder. Brain Res 1096(1):40–52. 2006/06/13 edn. doi:10.1016/j.brainres.2006.04.085

Meng E, Young JS, Brading AF (2008) Spontaneous activity of mouse detrusor smooth muscle and the effects of the urothelium. Neurourol Urodyn 27(1):79–87. 2007/05/10 edn. doi:10.1002/nau.20456

Mitchell CR, Mynderse LA, Lightner DJ, Husmann DA, Krambeck AE (2014) Efficacy of holmium laser enucleation of the prostate in patients with non-neurogenic impaired bladder contractility: results of a prospective trial. Urology 83(2):428–432. doi:10.1016/j.urology.2013.09.035

Munoz A, Smith CP, Boone TB, Somogyi GT (2011) Overactive and underactive bladder dysfunction is reflected by alterations in urothelial ATP and NO release. Neurochem Int 58(3):295–300. doi:10.1016/j.neuint.2010.12.002

Nirmal J, Tyagi P, Chuang YC, Lee WC, Yoshimura N, Huang CC, Rajaganapathy B, Chancellor MB (2014) Functional and molecular characterization of hyposensitive underactive bladder tissue and urine in streptozotocin-induced diabetic rat. PloS One 9(7):e102644. doi:10.1371/journal.pone.0102644

Oliveira L, Correia-de-Sa P (2005) Protein kinase A and Ca(v)1 (L-Type) channels are common targets to facilitatory adenosine A2A and muscarinic M1 receptors on rat motoneurons. Neurosignals 14(5):262–272. doi:10.1159/000088642

Pataky Z, Gasteyger C, Ziegler O, Rissanen A, Hanotin C, Golay A (2013) Efficacy of rimonabant in obese patients with binge eating disorder. Exp Clin Endocrinol Diabetes Off J German Soc Endocrinol German Diabetes Assoc 121(1):20–26. doi:10.1055/s-0032-1329957

Petkov GV (2012) Role of potassium ion channels in detrusor smooth muscle function and dysfunction. Nat Rev Urol 9(1):30–40. doi:10.1038/nrurol.2011.194

Pitts EV, Potluri S, Hess DM, Balice-Gordon RJ (2006) Neurotrophin and Trk-mediated signaling in the neuromuscular system. Int Anesthesiol Clin 44(2):21–76.

Postea O, Biel M (2011) Exploring HCN channels as novel drug targets. Nat Rev Drug Discov 10(12):903–914. 2011/11/19 edn. doi:10.1038/nrd3576

Reitz A, Knapp PA, Muntener M, Schurch B (2004) Oral nitric oxide donors: a new pharmacological approach to detrusor-sphincter dyssynergia in spinal cord injured patients? Eur Urol 45(4):516–520. 2004/03/26 edn. doi:10.1016/j.eururo.2003.11.006. S030228380300575X [pii]

Rosow CE, Gomery P, Chen TY, Stefanovich P, Stambler N, Israel R (2007) Reversal of opioid-induced bladder dysfunction by intravenous naloxone and methylnaltrexone. Clin Pharmacol Ther 82(1):48–53. doi:10.1038/sj.clpt.6100164

Shannon HE, Bymaster FP, Calligaro DO, Greenwood B, Mitch CH, Sawyer BD, Ward JS, Wong DT, Olesen PH, Sheardown MJ, Swedberg MD, Suzdak PD, Sauerberg P (1994) Xanomeline: a novel muscarinic receptor agonist with functional selectivity for M1 receptors. J Pharmacol Exp Ther 269(1):271–281

Slonimsky JD, Yang B, Hinterneder JM, Nokes EB, Birren SJ (2003) BDNF and CNTF regulate cholinergic properties of sympathetic neurons through independent mechanisms. Mol Cell Neurosci 23(4):648–660. 2003/08/23 edn

Smith PP, Chalmers DJ, Feinn RS (2014a) Does defective volume sensation contribute to detrusor underactivity? Neurourol Urodyn. doi:10.1002/nau.22653 epub.

Smith PP, DeAngelis A, Kuchel GA (2012) Detrusor expulsive strength is preserved, but responsiveness to bladder filling and urinary sensitivity is diminished in the aging mouse. Am J Physiol Regul Integr Comp Physiol 302(5):R577–586. doi:10.1152/ajpregu.00508.2011

Smith PP, Tyagi P, Kuchel GA, Pore S, Chermansky C, Chancellor M, Yoshimura N, Levanovich P (2014b) Advanced therapeutic directions to treat the underactive bladder. Int Urol Nephrol 46(Suppl 1):S35–44 doi:10.1007/s11255-014-0809-8

Somogyi GT, de Groat WC (1999) Function, signal transduction mechanisms and plasticity of presynaptic muscarinic receptors in the urinary bladder. Life Sci 64(6–7):411–418

Song QX, Chermansky CJ, Birder LA, Li L, Damaser MS (2014) Brain-derived neurotrophic factor in urinary continence and incontinence. Nat Rev Urol 11(10):579–588. doi:10.1038/nrurol.2014.244

Streng T, Axelsson HE, Hedlund P, Andersson DA, Jordt SE, Bevan S, Andersson KE, Hogestatt ED, Zygmunt PM (2008) Distribution and function of the hydrogen sulfide-sensitive TRPA1 ion channel in rat urinary bladder. Eur Urol 53(2):391–399. doi:10.1016/j.eururo.2007.10.024

Streng T, Christoph T, Andersson KE (2004) Urodynamic effects of the K+ channel (KCNQ) opener retigabine in freely moving, conscious rats. J Urol 172(5 Pt 1):2054–2058

Tadic SD, Tannenbaum C, Resnick NM, Griffiths D (2013) Brain responses to bladder filling in older women without urgency incontinence. Neurourol Urodyn 32(5):435–440. doi:10.1002/nau.22320

Takahisa N, Yoshida S, Hakozaki A, Orimoto N, Sasaki E, Hayashi Y (2013) Therapeutic effect of Tac-302, a novel neurite outgrowth enhancer, on voiding dysfunction in rats with STZ-induced diabetes J Urol 189(4):e49

Takeda M, Araki I, Mochizuki T, Nakagomi H, Kobayashi H, Sawada N, Zakohji H (2010) The forefront for novel therapeutic agents based on the pathophysiology of lower urinary tract dysfunction: pathophysiology of voiding dysfunction and pharmacological therapy. J Pharmacol Sci 112(2):121–127

Thorneloe KS, Nelson MT (2003) Properties and molecular basis of the mouse urinary bladder voltage-gated K+ current. J Physiol 549(Pt 1):65–74. doi:10.1113/jphysiol.2003.039859

Torrens M, Morrison JFB (1987) The physiology of the lower urinary tract. Springer, London

Turner WH, Brading AF (1997) Smooth muscle of the bladder in the normal and the diseased state: pathophysiology, diagnosis and treatment. Pharmacol Ther 75(2):77–110

Tyagi P, Smith PP, Kuchel GA, de Groat WC, Birder LA, Chermansky CJ, Adam RM, Tse V, Chancellor MB, Yoshimura N (2014) Pathophysiology and animal modeling of underactive bladder. Int Urol Nephrol 46(Suppl 1) S11–S21. doi:10.1007/s11255-014-0808-9

Uchiyama T, Sakakibara R, Yoshiyama M, Yamamoto T, Ito T, Liu Z, Yamaguchi C, Awa Y, Yano HM, Yanagisawa M, Yamanishi T, Hattori T, Kuwabara S (2009) Biphasic effect of apomorphine, an anti-parkinsonian drug, on bladder function in rats. Neuroscience 162(4):1333–1338. doi:10.1016/j.neuroscience.2009.06.001

Walczak JS, Price TJ, Cervero F (2009) Cannabinoid CB1 receptors are expressed in the mouse urinary bladder and their activation modulates afferent bladder activity. Neuroscience 159(3):1154–1163. doi:10.1016/j.neuroscience.2009.01.050

Wang HJ, Tyagi P, Chuang YC, Yoshimura N, Huang CC, Chancellor MB (2015) Pharmacologic and molecular characterization of underactive bladder induced by lumbar canal stenosis. Urology 85(6):1284–90. doi:10.1016/j.urology.2015.01.017

Witsell DL, Stinnett S, Chambers MS (2012) Effectiveness of cevimeline to improve oral health in patients with postradiation xerostomia. Head Neck 34(8):1136–1142. doi:10.1002/hed.21894

Wu ZZ, Li DP, Chen SR, Pan HL (2009) Aminopyridines potentiate synaptic and neuromuscular transmission by targeting the voltage-activated calcium channel beta subunit. J Biol Chem 284(52):36453–36461. doi:10.1074/jbc.M109.075523

Xue L, Li Y, Han X, Yao L, Yuan J, Qin W, Liu F, Wang H (2012) Investigation of hyperpolarization-activated cyclic nucleotide-gated channels in interstitial cells of Cajal of human bladder. Urology 80(1):e213–228. doi:10.1016/j.urology.2012.04.005

Yamanishi T, Yasuda K, Kamai T, Tsujii T, Sakakibara R, Uchiyama T, Yoshida K (2004) Combination of a cholinergic drug and an alpha-blocker is more effective than monotherapy for the treatment of voiding difficulty in patients with underactive detrusor. Int J Urol 11(2):88–96

Yang Z, Dolber PC, Fraser MO (2010) Differential vulnerabilities of urethral afferents in diabetes and discovery of a novel urethra-to-urethra reflex. Am J Physiol Renal Physiol 298(1):F118–124. doi:10.1152/ajprenal.00281.2009

Yoshida M, Miyamae K, Iwashita H, Otani M, Inadome A (2004) Management of detrusor dysfunction in the elderly: changes in acetylcholine and adenosine triphosphate release during aging. Urology 63(3 Suppl 1):17–23. doi:10.1016/j.urology.2003.11.003

Yoshizawaa T, Hayashi Y, Yoshida A, Ito Y, Yamada S, Takahashia S (2012) Therapeutic effects of the cyclohexenone derivative Tac-302 on the bladder dysfunction in Streptozotocin (Stz)-induced diabetic rats. J Urol 187(4):e43.

Zeng J, Pan C, Jiang C, Lindstrom S (2012) Cause of residual urine in bladder outlet obstruction: an experimental study in the rat. J Urol 188(3):1027–1032. doi:10.1016/j.juro.2012.04.101

Zhao Z, Yang J, Thurmond P, Azadzoi K (2015) Prolonged ischemia mediates overactive bladder transition to underactive bladder. J Urol 193(4):e76.

Chapter 8
Neuromodulation Treatment of Underactive Bladder

Michael B. Chancellor

Introduction

Table 8.1 lists the neuromodulatory methods to treat underactive bladder (UAB) that will be discussed in this chapter. Sacral nerve stimulation (SNS) is a minimally invasive technique which requires subcutaneous implantation of the electrode and pulse generator. Direct sacral nerve stimulation is typically done by the Brindley device. More investigational techniques of neuromodulation include bidirectional pudendal nerve stimulation and blockade as described by Tai, nerve reroute (the Xiao procedure), and direct electrode stimulation of the detrusor wall and indirect intravesical catheter-based electrostimulation (Chancellor and Diokno 2014).

Sacral Nerve Stimulation

The sacral nerve stimulation (SNS) device (InterStim, Medtronic, Minneapolis, MN) has approval from the US Food and Drug Administration for the indications of refractory urge incontinence, refractory urgency, and frequency, and approved indications include urinary urge incontinence, urgency–frequency, nonobstructive urinary retention, and fecal incontinence. As a minimally invasive urologic procedure, it has demonstrated long-term efficacy and safety.

Electrical stimulation of the sacral nerve can paradoxically inhibit urge incontinence in overactive bladder-wet patients and yet restore spontaneous urination in

M.B. Chancellor, MD
Department of Urology, Aikens Research Center, Oakland University William Beaumont School of Medicine, Rochester, MI, USA

Neurourology Program, Beaumont Health System, Royal Oak, MI, USA
e-mail: Michael.Chancellor@beaumont.edu

M.B. Chancellor, A.C. Diokno (eds.), *The Underactive Bladder*,
DOI 10.1007/978-3-319-23687-2_8

Table 8.1 Neuromodulatory approaches to treat underactive bladder

Sacral nerve stimulation (SNS)
(Interstim, Medtronic, Minneapolis, MN, USA)
Direct stimulation to the sacral nerve roots; the Brindley device
(Finetech Medical, Hertfordshire, UK)
Pudendal nerve interruption or blockade; Tai procedure
Nerve reroute: Xiao procedure
Create artificial "skin–central nervous system–bladder" reflex pathway
Direct bladder wall electrode placement and stimulation
Transurethral intravesical stimulation

underactive bladder patients with idiopathic urinary retention. The effects of sacral neuromodulation depend on electrical stimulation of the afferent axons in the spinal roots that in turn modulate voiding and continence reflex pathways in the central nervous system (Leng and Chancellor 2005). The stimulation effect is afferent mediated because the intensities of stimulation do not activate movements of striated muscles.

How does neuromodulation treat nonobstructive urinary retention? I believe that SNS activates the somatic afferent inputs that modulate sensory processing and micturition reflex pathways in the sacral spinal cord (Yoshimura and Chancellor 2011). In cases of UAB and dysfunctional voiding, SNS can inhibit the aberrant guarding reflexes.

Micturition Reflexes and Nerve Pathways

Most visceral organs such as the blood vessels, heart, and gastrointestinal tract receive a tonic autonomic regulation and are "turned on" most of the time. The urinary bladder is different because it is functionally "turned off" most of the time except for the six to eight times a day when a person voluntarily urinates.

The bladder is turned on in an "all-or-none" manner to eliminate urine (Fig. 8.1). The ability to "turn on," in switch-like fashion, to urinate is facilitated by positive feedback loops in the micturition reflex pathway. Amplification of bladder afferent activity can activate sufficient efferent excitatory signals to the bladder to initiate micturition. This positive feedback is effective for promoting sustained bladder contraction until the bladder is emptied (Yoshimura and Chancellor 2011).

Bladder afferent nerves send signals of bladder fullness and discomfort to the brain in order to initiate the micturition reflex (Yoshimura and de Groat 1997; de Groat 1997). The bladder afferent pathways are composed mostly of two types of axons: small myelinated A-delta fibers and unmyelinated C-fibers. A-delta fibers transmit signals mainly from mechanoreceptors that detect bladder fullness. The

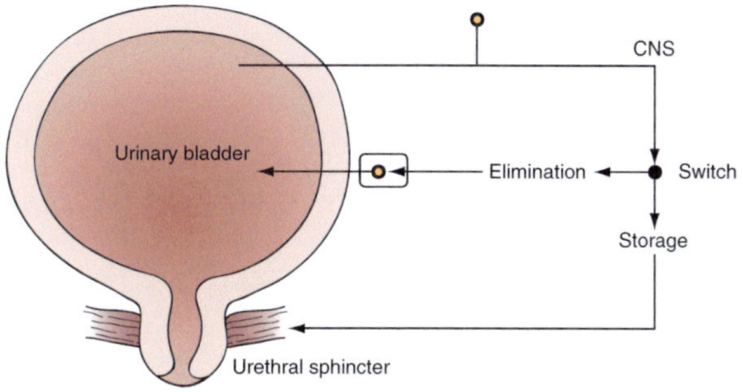

Fig. 8.1 Diagram illustrating the anatomy of the lower urinary tract and the "switch-like" function of the micturition reflex pathway. During urine storage, a low level of afferent activity activates efferent input to the urethral sphincter. A high level of afferent activity induced by bladder distention activates the switching circuit in the central nervous system (*CNS*), producing firing in the efferent pathways to the bladder, inhibition of the efferent outflow to the sphincter, and urine elimination. The guarding reflex prevents urinary incontinence. When there is a sudden increase in intravesical pressure, such as during a cough, the urinary sphincter contracts via the spinal guarding reflex to prevent urinary incontinence. The spinal guarding reflex is turned off by the brain to urinate (Permission from Yoshimura and Chancellor (2011))

C-fibers mainly detect noxious signals and initiate painful sensations. The bladder C-fiber nociceptors perform a similar function and signal the central nervous system during urinary tract infection, inflammation after radiation, or intravesical chemotherapy. C-fiber bladder afferents can also trigger voiding in abnormal conditions such as neurogenic detrusor overactivity (Yoshimura and de Groat 1997).

Guarding Reflexes

The urethra and urinary sphincter are on a "turned-on" state except for short periods when we urinate and voluntarily relax our sphincter muscle. There is an important bladder to urethral reflex that is mediated by sympathetic efferent pathways to the urethra. This excitatory reflex promotes urethral smooth muscle contraction during the bladder storage phase and thus is called the guarding reflex (de Groat et al. 1997).

The guarding reflex is not activated during micturition, but rather, when bladder pressure is momentarily increased during events such as a sneeze or cough. A second guarding reflex is triggered and amplified by bladder afferent signaling, which then synapses with sacral interneurons that in turn activate urethral external sphincter efferent neurons via the pudendal nerve (Shaker and Hassouna 1998; Yoshimura and Chancellor 2011). The activation of pudendal urethral efferent pathways contracts the external urinary sphincter and prevents stress urinary incontinence (Fig. 8.2).

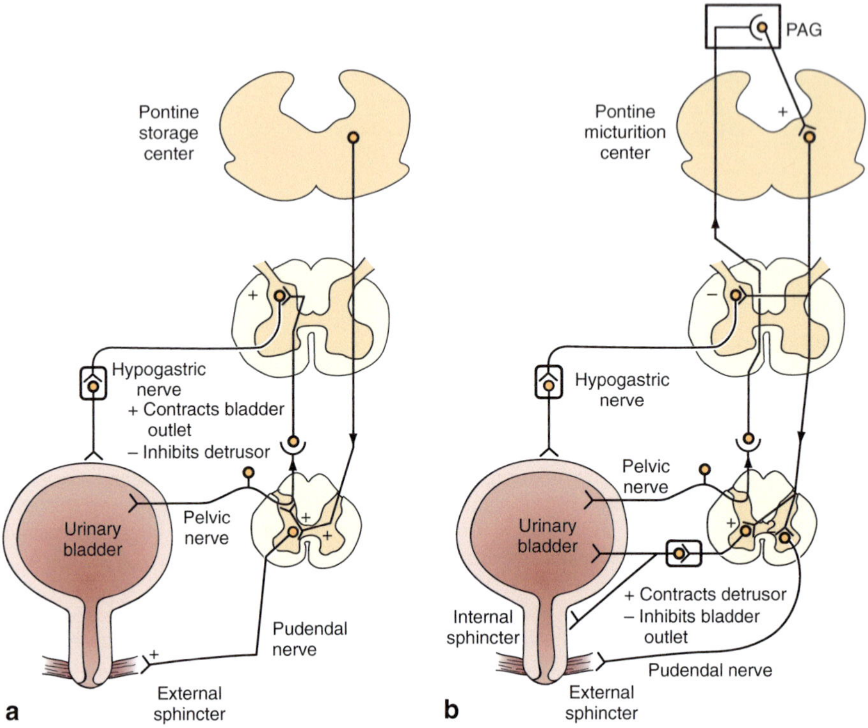

Fig. 8.2 Mechanism of storage and voiding reflexes. (**a**) Storage reflexes. During the storage of urine, distention of the bladder produces low-level bladder afferent firing. Afferent firing in turn stimulates the sympathetic outflow to the bladder outlet (base and urethra) and pudendal outflow to the external urethral sphincter. These responses occur by spinal reflex pathways and represent "guarding reflexes," which promote continence. Sympathetic firing also inhibits detrusor muscle and transmission in bladder ganglia. (**b**) Voiding reflexes. At the initiation of micturition, intense vesical afferent activity activates the brainstem micturition center, which inhibits the spinal guarding reflexes (sympathetic and pudendal outflow to the urethra). The pontine micturition center also stimulates the parasympathetic outflow to the bladder and internal sphincter smooth muscle. Maintenance of the voiding reflex is through ascending afferent input from the spinal cord, which may pass through the periaqueductal gray matter (PAG) before reaching the pontine micturition center (Permission from Yoshimura and Chancellor (2011))

Rationale for Neuromodulation to Facilitate Voiding

Brain pathways are necessary to turn off sphincter and urethral guarding reflexes to allow efficient bladder emptying. Thus, spinal cord injury produces bladder–external sphincter dyssynergia and inefficient bladder emptying by eliminating the brain mechanisms. This may also occur after more subtle neurologic lesions in patients with idiopathic urinary retention. Before the development of brain control of micturition, at least in animals, the stimulation of somatic afferent pathways passing through the pudendal nerve from the perineum can initiate efficient voiding by activating bladder efferent pathways and turning off the excitatory pathways to the urethral outlet (de Groat 1997). Sacral nerve stimulation may elicit similar responses in patients with urinary retention and turn off excitatory outflow to the urethral outlet and promote bladder emptying. Because sphincter activity can generate afferent input to the spinal cord that can in turn inhibit reflex bladder activity, an additional benefit of suppressing sphincter reflexes would be a facilitation of bladder activity.

The voiding and guarding reflexes discussed are activated at different and opposite times. When we urinate, the voiding reflex is turned on and the guarding reflex is turned off. When we are sleeping, the voiding reflex is turned off while the guarding reflex is turned on. Anatomically the neuronal wiring of the voiding and guarding reflexes is located in close proximity to each other in the S2–S4 levels of the human spinal cord (Table 8.2). For patients with UAB, neuromodulation's benefit is believed to activate the pudendal nerve afferents originating from the pelvic organs into the spinal cord and restore the inhibited voiding reflexes by suppressing exaggerated guarding reflexes (Leng and Chancellor 2005; Yoshimura and Chancellor 2011) (Fig. 8.3). In patients with overactive bladder, pudendal afferents may activate the afferent limb of inhibitory reflexes that promote bladder storage. This blocks input to the pontine micturition center, thereby restricting involuntary detrusor contractions without interfering with normal voiding patterns. In patients with fecal incontinence, the pudendal afferent somatic fibers are believed to be working by inhibiting colonic propulsive activity and activating the internal anal sphincter.

Sacral Stimulation Techniques

Current approved indications for sacral neuromodulation include urinary urge incontinence, urgency–frequency, nonobstructive urinary retention, and fecal incontinence (Noblett and Cadish 2014). SNS involves a two-stage procedure. The initial phase is considered the test stimulation period where the patient is allowed to evaluate whether the therapy is effective. There are two techniques that exist to perform the test stimulation.

Table 8.2 Sacral 2, 3, and 4 nerve root stimulation reflex responses

Nerve root	Sensation	Pelvic floor	Ipsilateral leg
S2	"Pulling" sensation of vagina or penis	Anal sphincter contraction	Lateral leg rotation, contraction of foot and toes
S3	"Pulling" in rectum, variable sensations in labia, tip of penis, or scrotum	"Bellows" response of pelvic floor, bladder, and urethral sphincter contraction	Great toe plantar flexion
S4	"Pulling" in rectum	"Bellows" response of pelvic floor	Usually none

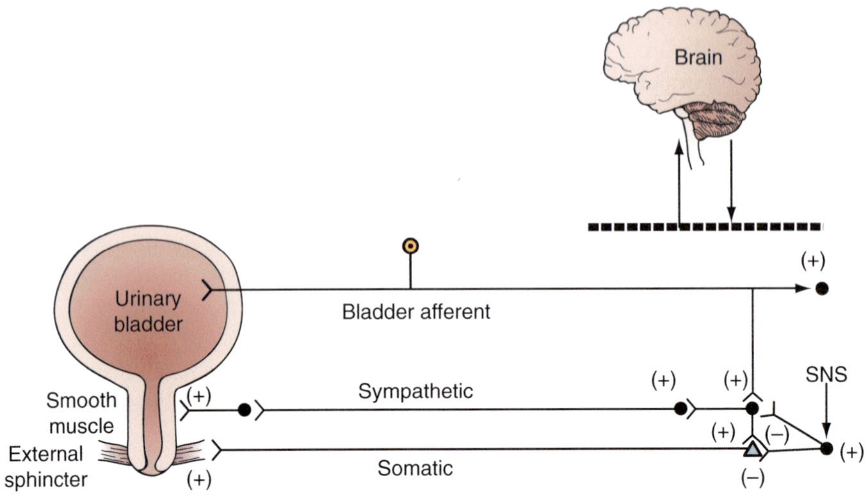

Fig. 8.3 When there is a sudden increase in intravesical pressure, such as during a cough, the urinary sphincter contracts by means of the spinal guarding reflex to prevent urinary incontinence (guarding reflex). The spinal guarding reflexes can be turned off by the brain for urination. In cases of neurologic diseases or pelvic floor overactivity, the brain cannot turn off the guarding reflex, and retention can occur. The sacral nerve stimulation (*SNS*) restores voluntary micturition in cases of voiding dysfunction and urinary retention but inhibits the guarding reflex (Permission from Yoshimura and Chancellor (2011))

Percutaneous Nerve Evaluation (PNE)

Percutaneous nerve evaluation (PNE) involves placing a temporary wire electrode through the S3 sacral foramen under local anesthesia. This can be done with or without fluoroscopic guidance. The wire is connected to an external generator worn for a trial period of 3–7 days (Fig. 8.4). Those with at least 50 % improvement in symptoms during the test phase are candidates for permanent implant of the lead and implantable pulse generator (IPG). The advantage of the PNE is that it is a minimally invasive office procedure requiring only local anesthesia. The disadvantage is that the wire is not securely anchored in place and the lead can migrate away from the proper position with patient's daily activity.

Staged Implant

The second option is a staged implant introduced by Spinelli et al. (2003). This procedure involves the placement of a quadripolar lead wire next to a sacral nerve root using a self-anchoring lead, and the patient undergoes a test phase for 7–14 days. The advantage of this technique is that it allows for a longer trial period with minimal risk of lead migration. During the second stage, the previously placed tined lead remains in place and is connected to an implanted IPG. The disadvantage of the staged implant is that it requires two visits to the operating room and may be more costly (Figs. 8.5 and 8.6).

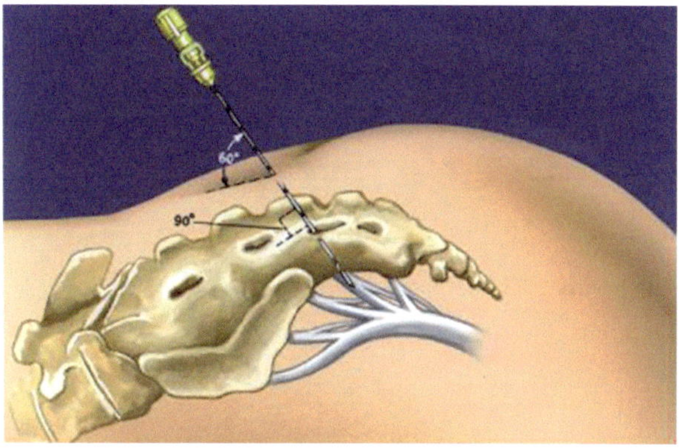

Fig. 8.4 Percutaneous nerve stimulation with optimal placement of the needle at approximately 60° angle into the medial and superior portion of the S3 foramen (With permission from Medtronic, Inc.)

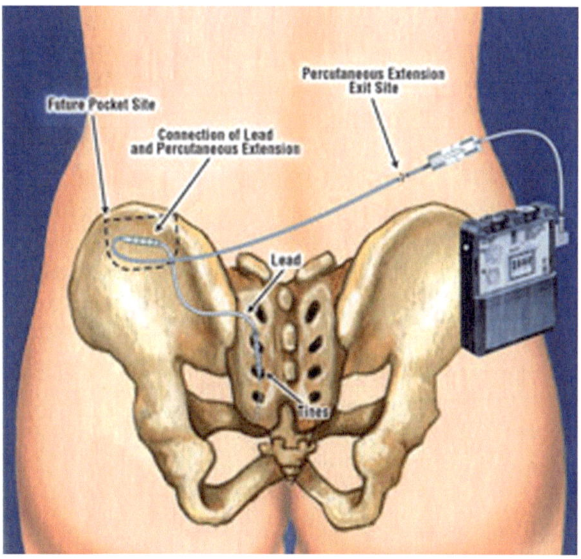

Fig. 8.5 During the trial period, the device consists of the chronic lead wire connected to the temporary wire extension (With permission from Medtronic, Inc.)

Sacral Neuromodulation Results

In a registry study from 1993 to 1997, a mixture of overactive bladder and UAB patients were evaluated with SNS. Thirty-one of the 51 UAB patients (61 %) were able to eliminate catheter use, and another 16 % had a 50 % reduction in catheter use. At 6 months with the stimulation off, the mean volume per catheterization increased back up to 264 ml (van Kerrebroeck et al. 2007). Aboseif and coworkers

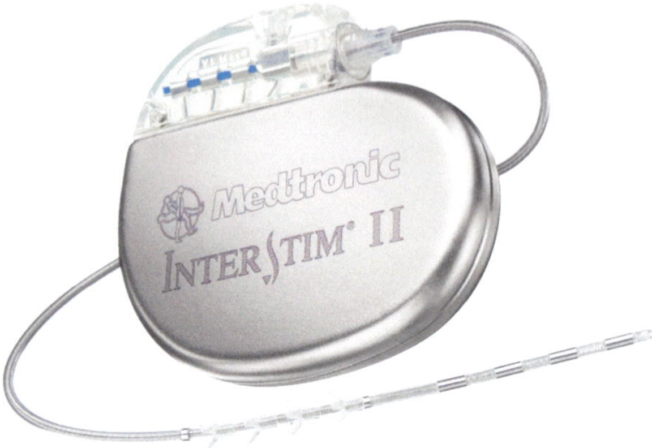

Fig. 8.6 Sacral nerve stimulation InterStim permanent implantable device components (With permission from Medtronic, Inc.)

(2002) evaluated the efficacy and change in quality of life in patients with idiopathic nonobstructive urinary retention. Thirty-two patients requiring intermittent catheterization underwent PNE. Permanent implants were placed in 20 patients (17 women) who showed more than 50 % improvement in symptoms. Eighteen patients (90 %) were subsequently able to void and no longer required catheterization; one patient required bilateral SNS implants. Average-voided volumes increased from 48 to 198 m. Post-void residual volume decreased from 315 to 60 ml. Eighteen patients (90 %) reported more than 50 % improvement in quality of life, although the questionnaire used in the study was not described.

A randomized multicenter trial to evaluate the efficacy of SNS for urinary retention was performed by Jonas et al. (2001). After a PNE for up to a week, 68 patients (38 % of those evaluated) with chronic urinary retention qualified for permanent implantation. Patients were randomly assigned to the treatment or control group, in which treatment was delayed for 6 months. Successful results were initially achieved in 83 % of patients who received the implant, with 69 % able to discontinue intermittent catheterization completely. At 18 months, 71 % of patients available for follow-up had sustained improvement. These results have been corroborated by later studies with longer follow-up (Datta et al. 2008; White et al. 2008).

Are there any predictors of success for SNS in UAB? Goh and Diokno (2007) reported their experience in patients who underwent SNS implantation for nonobstructive urinary retention. They found a significant difference in predicting success of test stimulation for patients with a preimplantation ability to void >50 ml versus non-voiders. Bertapelle et al. (2008) developed a urodynamic detrusor contractility test in urinary retention patients as an exclusion criteria for SNS. The take-home message appears to be that UAB patients with detrusor acontractility due to irreversible bladder myopathy and/or complete neurogenic lesions are not appropriate candidates for sacral neuromodulation (Fig. 8.7).

Onset of clinical improvement in patients with UAB may not be as rapid as in patients undergoing SNS for UAB. A longer PNE period and a permanent implant lead evaluation of 4 weeks or more have been suggested. It has also been proposed

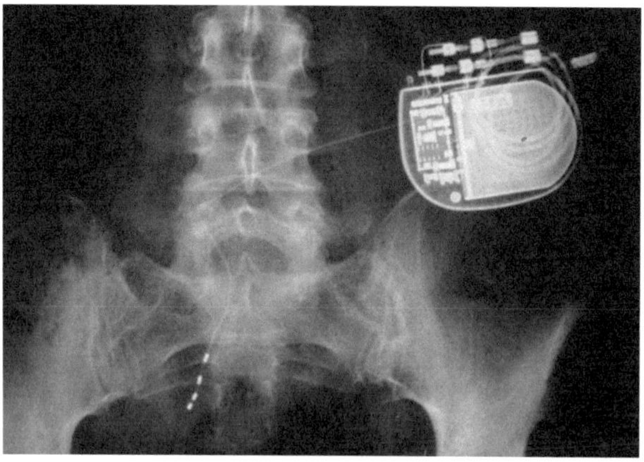

Fig. 8.7 X-ray of SNS implant

that for UAB, bilateral SNS should also be considered when an initial unilateral SNS trial has failed (Pham et al. 2008; van Kerrebroeck et al. 2005).

Pudendal Nerve Stimulation

The pudendal nerve is a peripheral branch of the sacral nerve roots, and stimulating the pudendal nerve allows for afferent stimulation to all three of the sacral nerve roots (S2–S4). Therefore, there is rationale for stimulating the more peripheral pudendal nerve instead of the S3 nerve. Stimulation of the more peripheral pudendal may decrease risk of discomfort in the thighs, calves, and feet. Peters et al. (2005) compared the effectiveness of sacral and pudendal nerve stimulation for voiding dysfunction in a prospective, single-blinded, randomized crossover trial of 30 patients (22 with urgency/frequency, five with urgency incontinence, and three with urinary retention). Twenty-four of the 30 patients (80 %) demonstrated a significant clinical response and had an implantable pulse generator placed. Sacral nerve stimulation resulted in 46 % improvement in symptoms, while pudendal nerve stimulation demonstrated 63 % improvement in symptoms.

SNS Summar

Sacral nerve neuromodulation holds promise for a large number of patients who suffer from a spectrum of lower urinary tract dysfunctions including a select subset of underactive bladder patients that may otherwise be refractory to conventional therapies. Neuromodulation therapy continues to advance, and the therapeutic indications are increasing. In the future, more patients with underactive bladder may benefit from this minimally invasive treatment option.

Brindley Device

Direct electrical stimulation to the sacral nerve roots to restore urination was developed approximately 30 years ago by Brindley (1994). Since then, the Brindley device has been used mainly in spinal cord-injured patients. Simultaneous bladder and striated sphincter stimulation is negated by performing a posterior sacral rhizotomy. The stimulation sequences and parameters are designed to lessen striated sphincter contraction during micturition, but complete sacral deafferentation is usually necessary except in patients with preserved genital sensation or reflex erections. An intact neural pathway between the bladder and sacral cord nuclei and a bladder that is capable of sustained contraction to adequately empty is required before considering the Brindley device in UAB patients.

Micturition, defecation, and erection programs are possible, with stimulus patterns tested and programmed specifically for each patient. Electrodes are applied intradurally to S2–S4 nerve roots (Finetech Medical, Hertfordshire, UK). Selective nerve roots may be activated independently through the programmer (Fig. 8.8). The detrusor is usually innervated primarily by S3 and to a smaller extent by S2 or S4. Rectal stimulation is by means of all three roots equally. Erectile stimulation is chiefly by S2 with a small contribution from S3 and none from S4.

The ventral sacral roots carry both parasympathetic fibers to the bladder and somatic fibers to the striated sphincter. Ventral root stimulation therefore occasionally results in detrusor–external sphincter dyssynergia. The current Brindley stimulator uses the principle of "poststimulus voiding" to minimize the sphincter

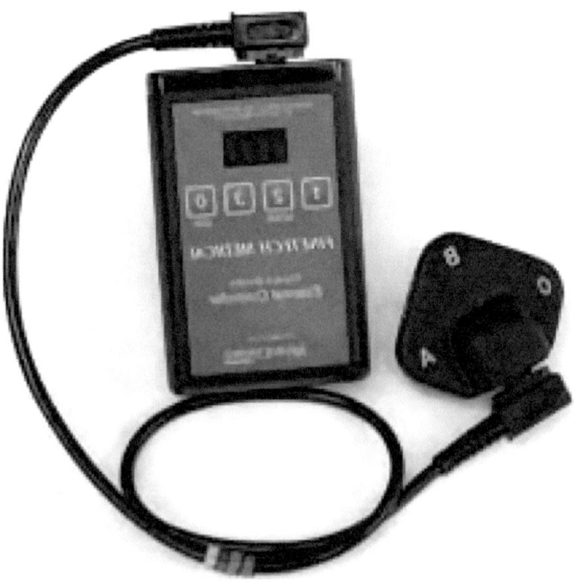

Fig. 8.8 Brindley device external components

dyssynergia (Jonas and Tanagho 1975). Relaxation time of the skeletal muscle external sphincter after a stimulus train is much shorter than the relaxation time of the smooth muscle detrusor. When interrupted pulse trains are used, voiding is achieved between the pulse trains because the detrusor contraction does not have time to relax and intravesical pressure is sustained.

Despite the advantage of requiring sacral rhizotomy, poststimulus voiding has several limitations: (1) When the stimulus parameters are not optimized, the voiding pressures can become too high, (2) Voiding occurs in spurts, and (3) Spasms and movement of the legs due to the close proximity of nerve fibers innervating the legs with that of the sacral roots.

Of the first 500 patients treated with this device, two patients were lost to follow-up, and 21 had died (Brindley 1994). Ninety-five reoperations were required for repair, six stimulators were removed with four infected, and two were awaiting repair. In 45 patients the stimulator was believed to be intact but not used for various reasons. In all others the stimulators were in use (411 for micturition and in most for defecation and in 13 for defecation alone), and the users were believed to be "pleased." Upper tract deterioration was reported in only 2 of 365 patients with full deafferentation and in 10 of 135 with incomplete or no deafferentation.

Van Kerrebroeck et al. (1997) reported the results of the Brindley device in 52 patients after screening 226 patients. Complete posterior sacral root rhizotomies were performed in all 52 patients. Thirty-seven of the patients had 6 months of follow-up; in these patients, complete daytime continence was achieved in 73 % and nighttime continence in 86 %. There were significant increases in bladder capacity and bladder compliance, and residual urine was reduced significantly. Complications included cerebrospinal fluid leaks, which resolved spontaneously in 23 patients, nerve damage that resolved in one patient, and one implant failure caused by a cable fracture, which was successfully repaired. Recent laparoscopic access and robotic techniques have minimized the invasiveness of this procedure and may have a role in the future in this select group of patients (Possover 2009).

Extradural stimulation has been used in the treatment of 19 patients with serious and refractory neuropathic voiding disorders (Tanagho and Schmidt 1988; Tanagho et al. 1989). After dorsal rhizotomy, a stimulator was implanted on the ventral component of S3 or S4 with selective peripheral neurotomy. In eight patients (42 %), complete success was achieved with continence, low-pressure storage, and low-residual voiding with electrical stimulation. Ten patients qualified as achieving partial success, regaining storage function and obtaining continence.

Brindley Device Summary

Electrical stimulation of the ventral sacral roots with ancillary techniques to reduce detrusor hyperactivity and obviate external sphincter dyssynergia has become an accepted treatment modality in selective spinal cord-injured patients in some countries, but the procedure is limited to centers of excellence in neurogenic bladder management. Prospective long-term comparative studies would be helpful for this remarkable technique.

Pudendal Nerve Interruption or Blockade (Tai Procedure)

Advances in neuromodulation, including the research by Tai and associates, may revolutionize neuromodulation to restore micturition for underactive bladder patients.

Relief of obstruction at the level of the striated sphincter may be achieved by pudendal neurectomy, but this method is seldom used because of high rate of impotence and may result in significant fecal and stress urinary incontinence. Tai et al. (2004) reported on the use of high-frequency electrical stimulation to provide a reversible pudendal nerve block in cats. The authors stated that the goal of this approach is to relax the external urethral sphincter only at the time of voiding, allowing normal function between voids to maintain continence (Fig. 8.9).

Inhibitory and excitatory stimulation frequencies of the pudendal–bladder reflexes: The pudendal nerve may have a dual mechanism depending on the frequency and continuity of stimulation. Tai et al. (2008) reported in anesthetized spinal cord-injured cats that at low frequency stimulation of the pudendal nerve inhibited bladder function and decreased bladder pressures, whereas, intermittent stimulation at 20 Hz improved the efficiency of the bladder to empty (Fig. 8.10). The development by Tai and associates of variable stimulation frequency neural prosthetic devices might be able to restore voluntary micturition function without rhizotomy.

Nerve Rerouting (Xiao Procedure) to Reestablish Micturition Reflex

One fascinating approach to surgically treat underactive bladder is not to directly increase detrusor contractility but rather through microscopic surgery to establish a new reflex pathway to initiate and maintain micturition (Xiao 2006). Xiao proposed to establish an artificial "skin–central nervous system (CNS)–bladder" reflex pathway to help spinal cord-injured patients to regain voluntary micturition. It is hoped that the motor axons of a somatic reflex arc may be able to regenerate into autonomic preganglionic nerves and thus reinnervate the bladder parasympathetic ganglion cells and transfer somatic reflex activity to the detrusor. This "skin–CNS–bladder" pathway is a somatic reflex arc with a modified efferent branch that transfers somatic motor impulses to the bladder and has been designed to allow patients to initiate voiding by scratching the skin (Fig. 8.11).

Preclinical work was first presented in rat studies where a crossover "skin–CNS–bladder" reflex pathway was established by intradural microanastomosis of the left

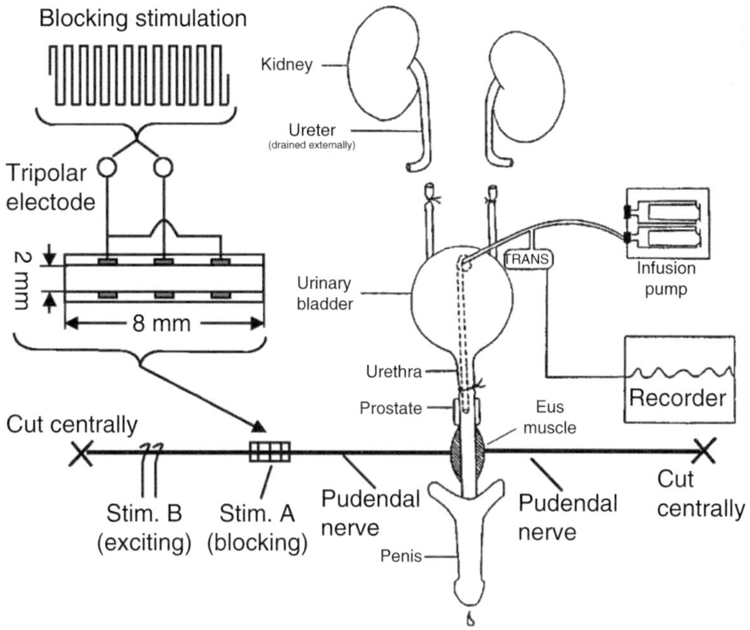

Fig. 8.9 Experimental setup of pudendal nerve block induced by high-frequency biphasic stimulation. *EUS* External urinary sphincter, *TRANS* Transducer (With Permission, Tai et al. (2008))

L4 ventral root to L6 ventral root, which innervated the bladder and external urethral sphincter in rats, while leaving the L4 dorsal root intact as a starter of micturition (Xiao et al. 1999). After axonal regeneration, 15 of the 24 rats with the new pathway underwent electrophysiological study. Single stimuli (0.3–3 mA, 0.02–0.2 ms duration) to the left L4 nerve resulted in evoked potentials (0.5–1 mV) recorded from the left L6 nerve distal to the anastomosis. Xiao et al. (1999) stated that bladder pressures increased to levels similar to controls with electrical stimulation and neural tracing study with horseradish peroxidase on six rats demonstrated that the somatic motor axons regenerated successfully into the pelvic nerve, and the bladder was reinnervated by the L4 somatic motor neurons. The bladder contraction could also be initiated by scratching the L4-related skin (Xiao 2006).

The first clinical trial of the Xiao procedure included 15 spinal cord-injured men with neurogenic detrusor overactivity and detrusor–external sphincter dyssynergia. The patients underwent hemi-laminectomy and ventral root microanastomosis, usually between the L5 and S2/S3 ventral roots. The L5 dorsal root was left intact as the trigger of micturition after axonal regeneration (Xiao et al. 2003). The trial in SCI patients was followed by a series of 20 spina bifida children with neurogenic bladder (Xiao et al. 2005), among whom 17 of 20 (85 %) demonstrated urodynamic improvements after surgery. Partial loss of L4 or L5 motor function, ranging from slight muscular weakness to visible foot drop, was reported in 5 of 20 patients (25 %).

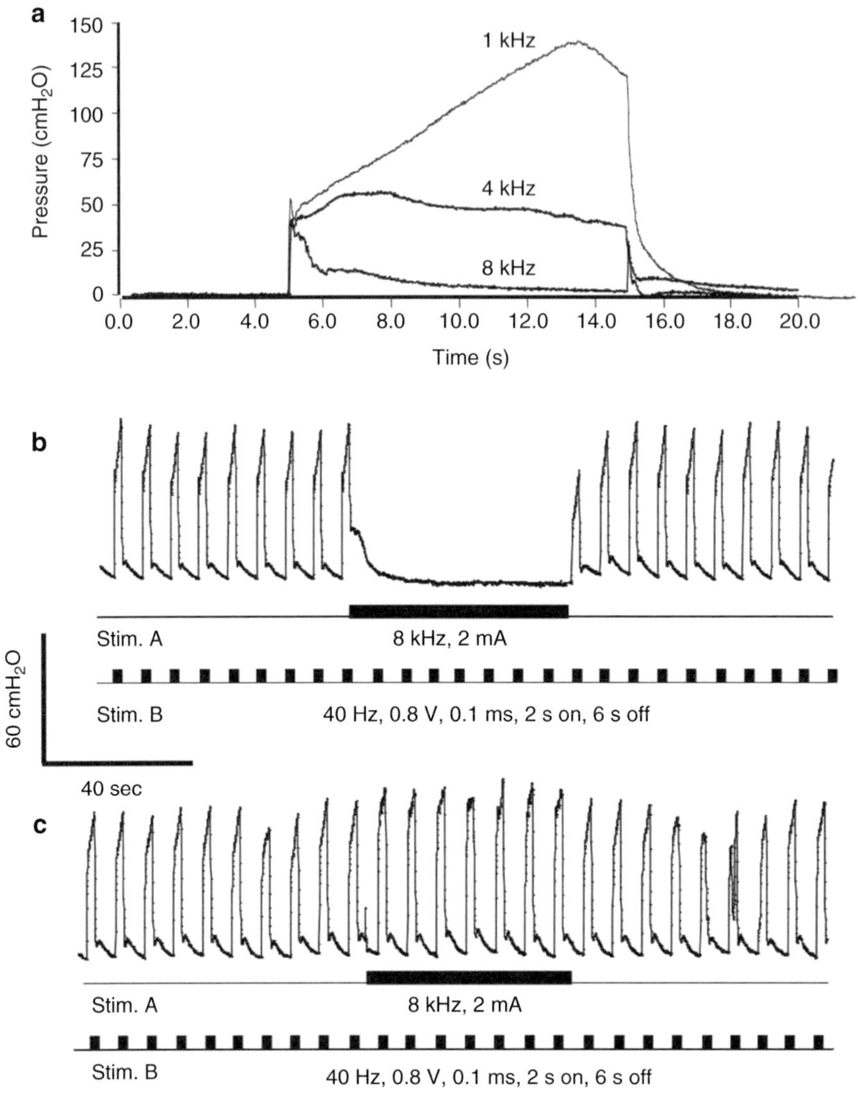

Fig. 8.10 Pudendal nerve block by biphasic high-frequency stimulation at 37 °C. (**a**) Urethral pressure induced by 10-s blocking stimulation A alone at 2 mA intensity. (**b**) Blocking stimulation A blocked urethral responses induced by stimulation B located centrally to stimulation A. *Horizontal bar* indicates stimulation duration (*ms*: milliseconds). (**c**) Blocking stimulation A failed to block urethral responses when stimulation B was moved to location distal to stimulation A (With Permission, Tai et al. (2008))

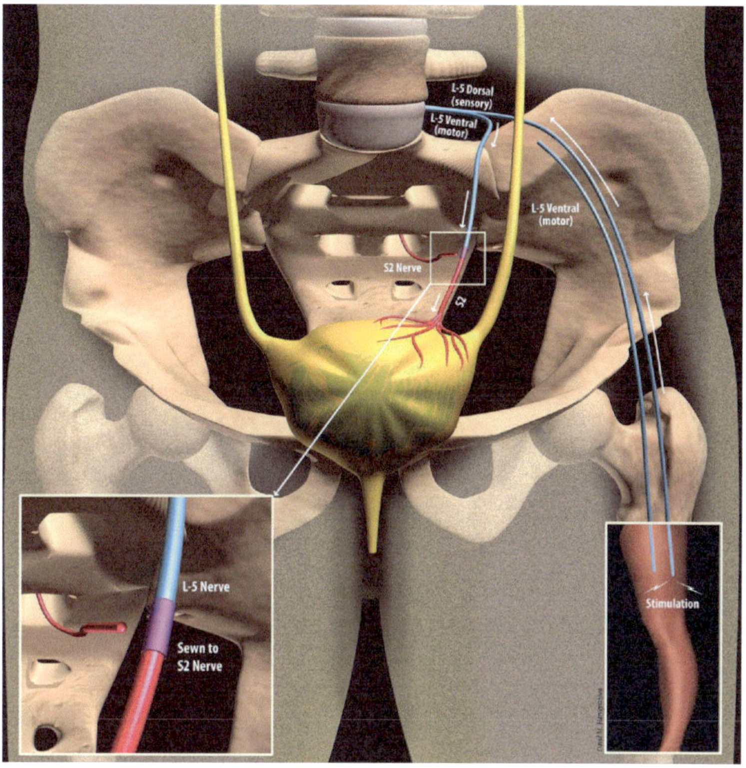

Fig. 8.11 Skin–CNS–bladder reflex reroute surgery as developed by Xiao. Left ventral lumbar (*L5*) to sacral (*S2*) nerve rerouting (With Permission Peters et al. (2010))

A more recent report of reroute operation to restore urination was by Peters et al. (2010) in nine spinal bifida patients with 1-year follow-up. At 1 year 7 patients (78 %) had an increase in bladder pressure with stimulation of the dermatome. Two patients were able to stop catheterization, and all safely stopped antimuscarinics. While no patient achieved total urinary continence, the majority did report improved bowel function. One patient was continent of stool at baseline, and four were continent at 1 year. Eight of nine patients (89 %) had variable weakness of lower extremity muscle groups at 1 month. One child had persistent foot drop, and the remainder returned to baseline by 12 months. The authors concluded longer follow-up and multi-institutional studies are needed to assess the risk/benefit ratio of this novel procedure.

Thüroff (2011) challenged the merit of reroute procedure stating that lumbar ventral spinal roots are mixed nerves with somatic and some autonomic outflow, and transection can result in irreversible lower extremity muscle weakness. Thüroff stated that "even if reinnervation of one sacral nerve is completely successful, this means that only one of eight sacral nerves innervating the bladder is activated on stimulation for micturition." He further noted that incontinence in spina bifida patients might be related to detrusor hyperreflexia, decreased sphincter innervation, low bladder compliance, or a combination of factors and questioned how all of these abnormalities may be controlled by reinnervation of a single sacral ventral spinal root.

Nerve Reroute Summary

The concept of nerve reroute is elegant and the dream of reestablishing voluntary micturition in the neurologically impaired patients noble. However, the Xiao procedure is currently investigational and should only be considered in regulatory approved studies.

Direct Bladder Electrical Stimulation

There was a time in neuromodulation development when direct electrical stimulation to the urinary bladder, performed by surgically implanting electrical leads in the detrusor wall, to facilitate emptying was championed, but clinical trials did not demonstrate efficacy, and the technique has largely been abandoned (Wein and Barrett 1988). Though there was some initial improvement, the device subsequently failed in almost all cases due to fibrosis, electrode malfunction, or bladder erosion. The spread of current to other pelvic organs often caused pain, spasticity, or defecation. There were reports of spasms of leg muscles and in men erection and ejaculation. The increase in intravesical pressure when the bladder is "turned on" was not coordinated with the sphincter being "turned off," and efficient bladder emptying did not occur.

Transurethral Electrical Stimulation

Intravesical electrotherapy is another technique that was popular for a number of years as a minimally invasive method to rehabilitate the neurogenic bladder and facilitate bladder emptying. The hypothesis was that transurethral electrical stimulation of the bladder can help bladder emptying by establishing conscious control of the initiation and completion of a micturition reflex (Fischer et al. 1993; Ebner et al. 1992). It was proposed that patients with incomplete central or peripheral nerve lesions, such as spina bifida, have some nerves connecting to the central nervous system preserved but are inadequate to empty the bladder. The hope was that transurethral electrical stimulation can be sufficient to activate mechanoreceptors in the bladder wall that can be amplified to reach a certain strength so that "vegetative afferentation" begins (Kaplan 2000). Sensory signals of sufficient magnitude can then travel to the brain and with repeated practice can reinforce efferent pathways that can lead to coordinated detrusor contractions of adequate magnitude to empty.

Procedure of Transurethral Electrical Stimulation

This technique involves direct intraluminal monopolar electrical stimulation with a special urethral catheter. Saline solution is used to allow current to spread throughout the bladder surface. Reinforcement is achieved by visual recording of detrusor contractions via stimulation of the catheter-based sensor. An intensive bladder training program has to be combined with transurethral electrical stimulation. Only patients with an incomplete spinal cord lesion, intact cortex, adequate residual bladder sensory receptors, and adequate detrusor contractility are candidates. Transurethral electrical stimulation is typically performed on a daily basis, lasting about 90 min, for several weeks to months.

Results of Transurethral Electrical Stimulation

Kaplan et al. (1989) reported outcome in 88 myelodysplastic children with 3–5 days a week stimulation session for a total of 15–30 sessions. Of 62 patients evaluated, 42 completed at least one series of treatment. "Success" was defined differently for infants than for older children. For infants, success implied a decrease in filling pressure, an increase in the quality of bladder contraction, and a decrease in residual urine. For older children, "success" implied a heightened awareness of detrusor contractions before and during a contraction, maintenance of low-pressure filling, effectively emptying detrusor contractions with low residual urine, and either a conscious urinary control or timely enough sensory input to allow clean intermittent catheterization for continence. Of children who initially had some detrusor contraction on initial evaluation, 80 % were said to have achieved some or all of the success parameters. Of those with no initial detrusor activity, 33 % achieved some success.

Enthusiasm for transurethral bladder stimulation subsequently diminished. Lyne and Bellinger (1993) reported the results of transurethral electrical stimulation treatment of 17 patients with neurologic dysfunction. Although all patients showed detrusor contraction after the many courses of stimulation, there was little clinical improvement in continence or increase in functional bladder capacity. Decter et al. (1994) reported a series of 25 patients with neurogenic voiding dysfunction where urodynamic showed a greater than 20 % increase in the age-adjusted bladder capacity in only 6 of 18 patients (33 %) with serial studies and clinically significant improvements in end-filling pressures in 5 (28 %). Even pioneers in the technique have dampened enthusiasm about the long-term success of transurethral electrical stimulation to attain the goal of volitional voiding (Kaplan 2000; Decter 2000).

Conclusions

Sacral nerve neuromodulation has been shown to help treat underactive bladder patients with nonobstructive urinary retention. Pudendal afferent input turns on voiding reflexes by suppressing the guarding reflex pathways. Pudendal afferent input to the sacral spinal cord can also turn off supraspinally mediated hyperactive voiding by blocking ascending sensory pathway inputs. Neuromodulation has proven to be safe and minimally invasive and holds great promise for future of underactive bladder therapeutics.

References

Aboseif S, Tamaddon K, Chalfin S et al (2002) Sacral neuromodulation in functional urinary retention: an effective way to restore voiding. BJU Int 90:662–665

Bertapelle P, Bodo G, Carone R (2008) Detrusor acontractility in urinary retention: detrusor contractility test as exclusion criteria for sacral neuromodulation. J Urol 180:215–216

Brindley GS (1994) The first 500 patients with sacral anterior root stimulator implants: general description. Paraplegia 32:795–805

Chancellor MB, Diokno A (2014) CURE-UAB: shedding light on the underactive bladder syndrome. Int Urol Nephrol 46(Suppl 1):S1

Datta SN, Chaliha C, Singh A et al (2008) Sacral neuromodulation for urinary retention: 10 year experience from one UK centre. BJU Int 101:192–196

Decter RM, Snyder P, Laudermilch C (1994) Transurethral electrical bladder stimulation: a follow-up report. J Urol 152:812–817

Decter RM (2000) Intravesical electrical stimulation of the bladder: con. Urology 56:5–8

de Groat WC (1997) Chapter 6. Central nervous system control of micturition. In: O'Donnell PD (ed) Urinary incontinence. Mosby Publisher, St. Louis, pp 33–47

de Groat WC, Araki I, Vizzard MA, Yoshiyama M, Yoshimura N, Sugaya K, Tai C, Roppolo JR (1997) Developmental and injury induced plasticity in the micturition reflex pathway. Behav Brain Res 92:127

Ebner A, Jiang C, Lindstrom S (1992) Intravesical electrical stimulation—an experimental analysis of the mechanism of action. J Urol 148:920–924

Fischer J, Madersbacher H, Zechberger J et al (1993) Sacral anterior root stimulation to promote micturition in transverse spinal cord lesions. Zentralbl Neurochir 54:77–79

Goh M, Diokno AC (2007) Sacral neuromodulation for nonobstructive urinary retention—is success predictable? J Urol 178:197–199

Jonas U, Fowler CJ, Chancellor MB et al (2001) Efficacy of sacral nerve stimulation for urinary retention: results 18 months after implantation. J Urol 165:15–19

Jonas U, Tanagho EA (1975) Studies on the feasibility of urinary bladder evacuation by direct spinal cord stimulation. II. Poststimulus voiding: a way to overcome outflow resistance. Invest Urol 13:151–153

Kaplan WE (2000) Intravesical electrical stimulation of the bladder: pro. Urology 56:2–4

Kaplan WE, Richards TW, Richards I (1989) Intravesical transurethral bladder stimulation to increase bladder capacity. J Urol 142:600–602

Leng WW, Chancellor MB (2005) How sacral nerve stimulation neuromodulation works. Urol Clin North Am 32:11–18

Lyne CJ, Bellinger MF (1993) Early experience with transurethral electrical bladder stimulation. J Urol 150:697–699

Noblett KL, Cadish LA (2014) Sacral nerve stimulation for the treatment of refractory voiding and bowel dysfunction. Am J Obst Gyn 210:99–106

Peters KM, Feber KM, Bennett RC (2005) Sacral versus pudendal nerve stimulation for voiding dysfunction: a prospective, single-blinded, randomized, crossover trial. Neurourol Urodyn 24:643–647

Peters KM, Girdler B, Turzewski C, Trock G, Feber K, Nantau W, Bush B, Gonzalez J, Cass E, de Benito J, Diokno A (2010) Outcomes of lumbar to sacral nerve rerouting for spina bifida. J Urol 184:702–708

Pham K, Guralnick ML, O'Connor RC (2008) Unilateral versus bilateral stage I neuromodulatory lead placement for the treatment of refractory voiding dysfunction. Neurourol Urodyn 27:779–781

Possover M (2009) The sacral LION procedure for recovery of bladder/rectum/sexual functions in paraplegic patients after explanation of a previous Finetech-Brindley controller. J Minim Invasive Gynecol 16:98–101

Spinelli M, Giardiello G, Arduini A, van den Hombergh U (2003) New percutaneous technique of sacral nerve stimulation has high initial success rate: preliminary results. Eur Urol 43:70–74

Shaker HS, Hassouna M (1998) Sacral root neuromodulation in idiopathic nonobstructive chronic urinary retention. J Urol 159:1476

Tai CF, Roppolo JR, de Groat WC (2004) Block of external urethral sphincter contraction by high frequency electrical stimulation of pudendal nerve. J Urol 172:2069–2072

Tai CF, Wang J, Chancellor MB, Roppolo JR, de Groat WC (2008) Influence of temperature on pudendal nerve block induced by high frequency biphasic electrical current. J Urol 180:1173–1178

Tanagho EA, Schmidt RA (1988) Electrical stimulation in the clinical management of the neurogenic bladder. J Urol 140:1331–1339

Tanagho EA, Schmidt RA, Orvis BR (1989) Neural stimulation for control of voiding dysfunction: a preliminary report in 22 patients with serious neuropathic voiding disorders. J Urol 142(2 Pt 1):340–346

Thüroff JW (2011) Re: outcomes of lumbar to sacral nerve rerouting for spina bifida. Eur Urol 59:173–175

van Kerrebroeck PE, van der Aa HE, Bosch JL et al (1997) Sacral rhizotomies and electrical bladder stimulation in spinal cord injury. I. Clinical and urodynamic analysis. Dutch Study Group on Sacral Anterior Root Stimulation. Eur Urol 31:263–271

van Kerrebroeck EV, Scheepens WA, de Bie RA, Weil EH (2005) European experience with bilateral sacral neuromodulation in patients with chronic lower urinary tract dysfunction. Urol Clin North Am 31:51–57

van Kerrebroeck PE, van Voskuilen AC, Heesakkers JP et al (2007) Results of sacral neuromodulation therapy for urinary voiding dysfunction: outcomes of a prospective, worldwide clinical study. J Urol 178:2029–2034

Wein AJ, Barrett DM (1988) Voiding function and dysfunction—a logical and practical approach. Year Book, Chicago

White WM, Dobmeyer-Dittrich C, Klein FA, Wallace LS (2008) Sacral nerve stimulation for treatment of refractory urinary retention: long-term efficacy and durability. Urology 71:71–74

Xiao C (2006) Reinnervation for neurogenic bladder: historic review and introduction of a somatic-autonomic reflex pathway procedure for patients with spinal cord injury or spina bifida. Eur Urol 49:22–29

Xiao CG, de Groat WC, Godec CJ, Dai C (1999) Xiao Q: "Skin-CNS-bladder" reflex pathway for micturition after spinal cord injury and its underlying mechanisms. J Urol 162(3 Pt 1):936–942

Xiao CG, Du MX, Dai C, Li B, Nitti VW et al (2003) An artificial somatic-central nervous system-autonomic reflex pathway for controllable micturition after spinal cord injury: preliminary results in 15 patients. J Urol 170:1237–1241

Xiao CG, Du MX, Li B, Liu Z, Chen M et al (2005) An artificial somatic-autonomic reflex pathway procedure for bladder control in children with spina bifida. J Urol 173:2112–2116

Yoshimura N, de Groat WS (1997) Neural control of the lower urinary tract. Int J Urol 4:111–125

Yoshimura N, Chancellor MB (2011) Physiology and pharmacology of the bladder and urethra. In: Wein AJ, Kavoussi LR, Novick AC, Partin AW, Peters CA (eds) Campbells urology, 10th edn Elsevier, Philadelphia, PA, USA

Chapter 9
Surgery for Underactive Bladder Treatment

Michael B. Chancellor

Surgery to Increase Bladder Emptying

Table 9.1 outlines the surgical options that have been advanced for the treatment of the underactive bladder (UAB). Section "Surgery to increase bladder emptying" will focus on bladder surgeries and section "Surgery to decrease outlet resistance" on surgical options is available to decrease urethral outlet resistance.

Cellular Therapy

I have been interested in the development of stem cells to treat bladder and urethral dysfunction since approximately 1997 (Yokoyama et al. 2000). Chancellor et al. (2000) demonstrated successful long-term survival of the injected muscle-derived stem cells in the bladder and urethra, with histochemical evidence that these muscle-derived stem cells can differentiate to smooth muscle. The technology has advanced further with urethral sphincter injection for the treatment of stress urinary incontinence (Carr et al. 2013) and it is currently in international phase 3 multicenter placebo-controlled double-blind studies.

M.B. Chancellor, MD
Department of Urology, Aikens Research Center, Oakland University William Beaumont School of Medicine, Rochester, MI, USA

Neurourology Program, Beaumont Health System, Royal Oak, MI, USA
e-mail: Michael.Chancellor@beaumont.edu

M.B. Chancellor, A.C. Diokno (eds.), *The Underactive Bladder*,
DOI 10.1007/978-3-319-23687-2_9

Table 9.1 Surgical methods for treating underactive bladder

I. Improve bladder emptying
Cellular therapy:
Intradetrusor application stem cells
Reduction cystoplasty:
Resection of bladder dome reduces capacity by up to 80 % in some cases
Bladder myoplasty:
Microneurovascular free transfer of autologous latissimus dorsi muscle
Bladder replacement:
Regenerative medicine with biodegradable bladder scaffold and cells seeding
II. Decrease outlet resistance
Incision of bladder neck and prostate
External sphincter defeating procedures:
Over dilation
Sphincterotomy
Urethral stent
Sphincter and pelvic floor botulinum toxin injection
Intraurethral prosthesis with a self-contained urinary pump (see Chap. 10)

Preclinical Results in Model of Underactive Bladder

Huard et al. (2002) demonstrated that muscle-derived stem cell (MDC) transplantation increased muscle contractility in the cryoinjury UAB model (Figs. 9.1 and 9.2):

- Demonstrated the feasibility and survival of MDC injection into the bladder wall
- Established improved detrusor contractility with MDC injection

Fig. 9.1 Physiological improvement of the injured bladder via muscle-derived cell implantation. Schematic representation of the cryoinjury model and location of the bladder strips (**a**). A representative contractile curve of bladder strips evoked by electrical stimulation (20 Hz 80 shocks) of control (**b**) and 30 s cryoinjured (**c**) rat bladders. Cryoinjured rat bladders with immediate saline and muscle-derived cells (pp6) injection both resulted in a significant (*P <0.05) decrease of contractile responses to electrical field stimulation when compared with the control bladder (**d**). However, the muscle-derived cells (pp6) injected at 1 week after cryoinjury in the rat bladder displayed a significant improvement in bladder contractility versus cryo+saline (1 week) injection (+P<0.05) for up to 80 % of the normal baseline level, which was not significantly different from the control group (**e**). The cryoinjured mouse bladder injected with muscle-derived cells (mc13) at 1 week after injury significantly improved bladder contractility in contrast to that observed with early plated myoblasts (pp1/pp2) (**f**). Compared with control; +compared with cryo+saline (With permission Huard et al. (2002))

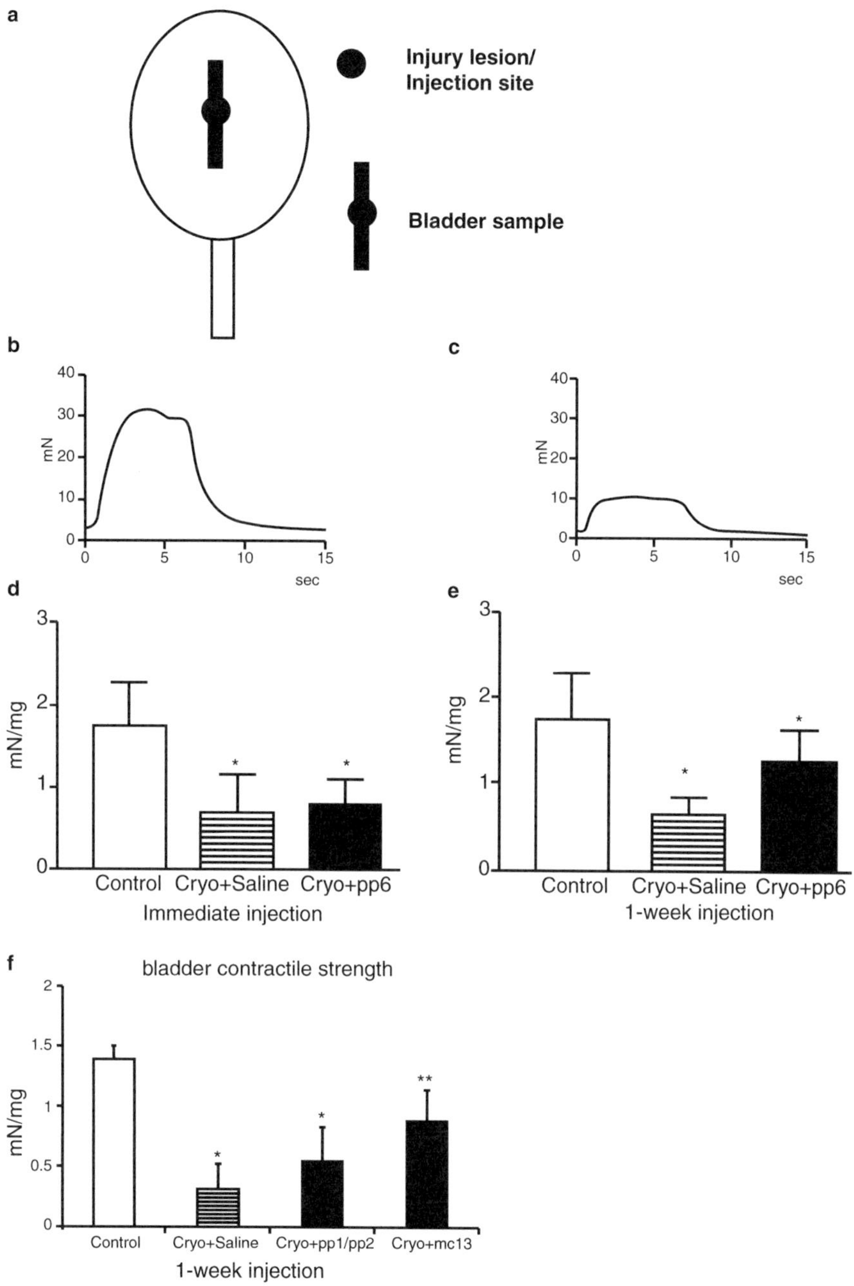
a
Injury lesion/
Injection site
Bladder sample
b
40
30
20
10
0
mN
0
5
10
15
sec
c
40
30
20
10
0
mN
0
5
10
15
sec
d
3
2
1
0
mN/mg
*
*
Control
Cryo+Saline
Cryo+pp6
Immediate injection
e
3
2
1
0
mN/mg
*
*
Control
Cryo+Saline
Cryo+pp6
1-week injection
f
bladder contractile strength
2
1.5
1
0.5
0
mN/mg
*
*
**
Control
Cryo+Saline
Cryo+pp1/pp2
Cryo+mc13
1-week injection

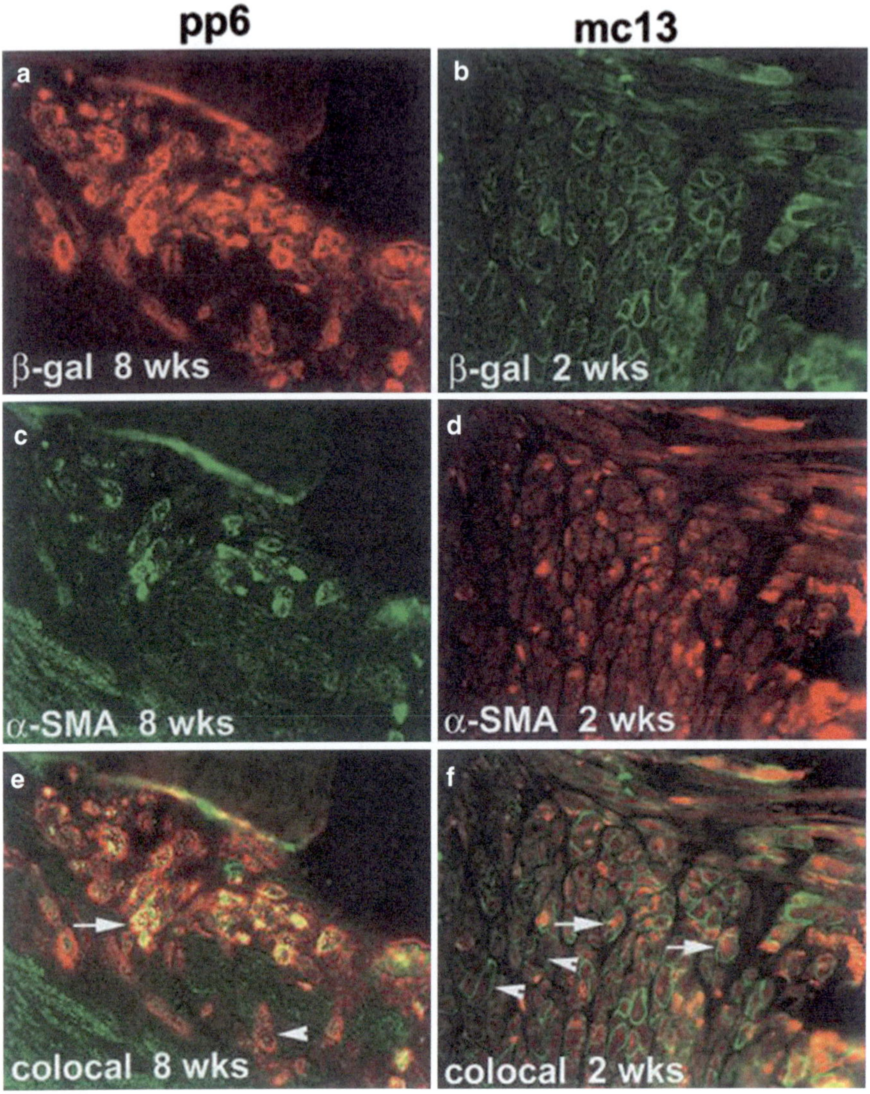

Fig. 9.2 Expression of alpha smooth muscle actin (a-SMA) in the injected muscle cells at the injected site. Bladders at 8 weeks (pp6) and 2 weeks (mc13) after injection were stained for b-galactosidase (**a**, **b**) and SMA (**c**, **d**). Although some of the cells expressing b-galactosidase did not colocalize with SMA (*arrowheads* **e**, **f**), many of the injected MDC expressed both markers (*arrows* **e**, **f**) showing their differentiation into the smooth muscle lineage. Magnification **a**–**f**,×200 (With Permission Huard et al. (2002))

- Revealed the maturity of the β-galactosidase-expressing myofibers in the injured bladder by demonstrating the presence of neuromuscular junctions based on the accumulation of AChRs in small segments of their membrane
- Supported MDC differentiating into a smooth muscle lineage when injected into the bladder wall

Peclinical data support that autologous MDC injections can be used as a nonallergenic agent to improve bladder contractility (Figs. 9.1 and 9.2) (Huard et al. 2002). Thus, cystoscopic injection of autologous muscle-derived stem cells, under local anesthesia in the outpatient clinic, may be a promising treatment strategy for patients with UAB.

Stem Cell Clinical Trials to Treat UAB

Due to the lack of medical treatment options available for persons with chronic UAB, approval was obtained from the FDA to treat a single patient with regenerative medicine stem cell therapy. The primary objective was to determine the safety of utilizing autologous muscle-derived cells (AMDC) to treat UAB. Additionally, the potential clinical efficacy of AMDC was evaluated.

In a 79-year-old man with chronic urinary retention despite having previously undergone two transurethral resections of the prostate (Levanovich et al. 2015), urodynamic studies demonstrated detrusor areflexia of over 800 ml. Alpha blockers and bethanechol have been tried on multiple occasions without benefit. The patient has been unable to void and has been performing clean intermittent catheterization 4–6 times daily for the past 5 years. The patient has had episodes of gross hematuria requiring bladder irrigation and recurrent febrile urinary tract infections requiring hospitalization.

Approximately 150 mg of the quadriceps femoris muscle was harvested under local anesthesia and the tissue was processed by Cook MyoSite (Pittsburgh, PA). The AMDC were isolated and expanded in culture over several weeks to a final concentration of approximately 250 million. Injections were performed utilizing a flexible cystoscope under direct visualization. The treatments were performed utilizing topical, local anesthesia. There were a total of 30 intradetrusor injections (0.5 ml per injection; 2 mm in depth) throughout the bladder.

No treatment-related adverse events or side effects were reported by the patient. Additionally, there were no complications during biopsy or injection, nor were there any cystoscopic abnormalities at 6 or 12 months. Global response assessment reported "moderate improvement" of UAB symptoms at 6 and 12 months. Reductions in first desire and strong urge to urinate, from 711 to 365 ml and 823 to 450 ml, respectively, were observed. A reduction in maximum cystometric capacity from 844 to 663 ml was noted as well. Using bladder diaries, the patient reported the ability to void a small volume of urine but has continued to require self-catheterization 1-year posttreatment.

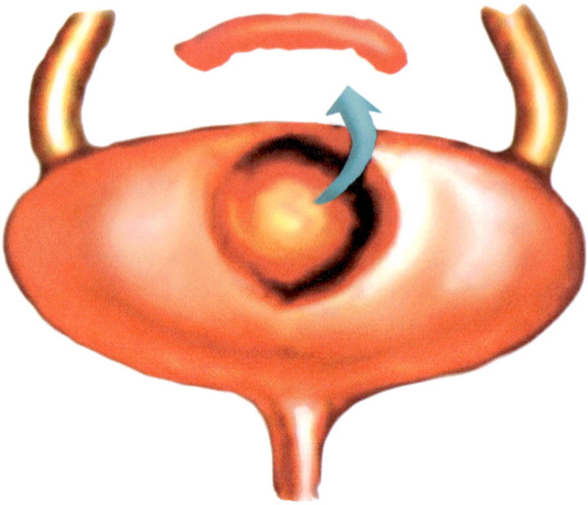

Fig. 9.3 Reduction cystoplasty whereby a segment of the bladder is excised and bladder capacity surgically reduced

The successful completion of this first report of cellular therapy to treat UAB with autologous muscle-derived stem cells has led to the FDA approval of an expanded phase 2 trial. The research study is currently underway and assesses the safety and efficacy of AMDC for UAB. In the future, cellular therapy may be a promising novel treatment for underactive bladder.

Reduction Cystoplasty

Partial cystectomy to reduce excess bladder capacity and potentially decrease the total work the detrusor must perform to adequately empty is conceptually attractive (Fig. 9.3). Over the years the technique of reduction cystoplasty has been intermittently advocated as treatment for excessively large UAB. However, the jury is still out on its efficacy over the long term as there is trend for the bladder to stretch out again over time.

How is reduction cystoplasty done? A number of techniques have been described, but most commonly, the most easily accessible portion of the bladder, the bladder dome is widely excised, and bladder closed together. Kinn (1985) reported on 10 patients with UAB and was successful in reducing the bladder capacity, reducing residual urine volume, and reducing frequency of urinary infection, but found no improvement of detrusor contractility after reduction cystoplasty. More encouraging results have been suggested in patients with retained hypocontractile detrusor function (Klarskov et al. 1988). Bukowski and Perlmutter (1994) reported on the long-term outcome of reduction cystoplasty in 11 boys with prune belly syndrome. They found that short-term reductions in bladder volume may have initially contributed to the decreased incidence of urinary infections, but bladder capacity and residual volumes tended to increase over time.

Reduction cystoplasty has not been proven to yield long-term success in UAB patients in controlled studies. Cost and benefit of reduction cystoplasty should be compared with the standard of care, clean intermittent catheterization. Reduction cystoplasty may be considered select patients with diminished detrusor contractility and an excessively large bladder capacity such as a bladder capacity that is 1 or 2 l or more. Perhaps combining reduction cystoplasty with implantation of stem cells may aid toward restoration of adequate bladder contractility after surgery.

Detrusor Myoplasty

Bladder myoplasty is a major surgical method for inducing micturition in UAB patients via augmentation of the bladder with a skeletal muscle wrap (Chancellor 1994; Chancellor et al. 1994a). The method comprises the steps of transecting a patient's rectus abdominis muscle, preserving the patient's inferior epigastric artery and 2–4 innervating intercostal nerves, wrapping the muscle around the patient's bladder, and attaching at least one electrical lead which is attached to a pulse generator similar to the one used for sacral neuromodulation (Fig. 9.4). Electrical stimulation from the signal generator to the bladder myoplasty can facilitate the emptying of the urinary bladder. Initial case report demonstrated encouraging result (Chancellor et al. 1994b), but due to the extensive surgery required, I decided to advance to intradetrusor injection of muscle-derived stem cells as a less invasive method to augment detrusor contractility.

Von Heyden et al. (1998) and Van Savage et al. (2000) reported early studies with electrically stimulated detrusor myoplasty in dogs. Von Heyden et al. (1998) described anastomosing the thoracodorsal nerve to the obturator nerve and the vascular supply to the external iliac vessels. The graft was then stimulated by electrodes connected to the anastomosed neural supply and with direct muscle stimulation. Van Savage et al. (2000) described detrusor myoplasty with rectus muscle with the addition of stimulation being achieved with electrodes inserted into the muscle near the nerve entrance. Initial positive results with acute stimulation generating bladder pressures adequate for bladder emptying but bladder emptying did not improve with chronic stimulation.

Stenzl et al. (1998) reported 3 UAB patients treated with a micro-neurovascular free transfer of autologous latissimus dorsi muscle. The main neural and vascular supply to the latissimus dorsi was anastomosed to the lowermost motor branch of the intercostal nerve and to the inferior epigastric vessels supplying the rectus abdominis muscle. The transferred muscle was wrapped around the bladder covering about 75 % of the mobilized bladder and leaving only the area of the trigone and the lateral pedicles uncovered. Patients were actively contracting the lower abdominal musculature when they want to urinate. Short-term follow-up revealed peak flow rates of 18–26 ml/s and residual urine volumes of 0–90 ml. Positive results were reported in a multicenter trial of latissimus dorsi detrusor myoplasty by Gakis et al. (2011) where 24 UAB patients were followed for 46 months (Fig. 9.5). Sixteen of 24 (67 %) regained spontaneous micturition without the need for intermittent catheterization while 3 were able to reduce the frequency of catheterization.

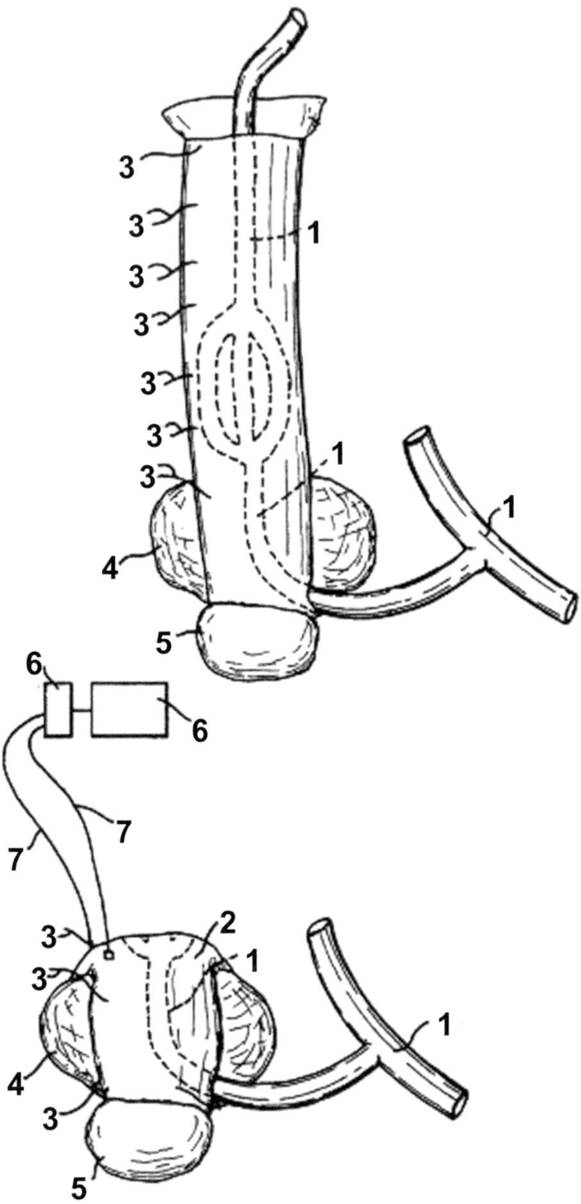

Fig. 9.4 Surgical technique of detrusor myoplasty. *Top* drawing is a diagram showing the human rectus abdominis muscle including innervation (*3*) and vascularization (*1*), the points of attachment of the rectus abdominis muscle to the pubic symphysis (*5*), and the bladder (*4*) before detrusor myoplasty. *Bottom* drawing is a diagram showing the points of attachment of the rectus abdominis muscle (*2*) and the bladder (*4*) wrapped with the rectus muscle after detrusor myoplasty. (*1*) Blood vessels of the rectus muscle; (*2*) rectus muscle; (*3*) nerves to the rectus muscle; (*4*) bladder; (*5*) pubic symphysis; (*6*) pulse generator; (*7*) wire that leads to detrusor myoplasty

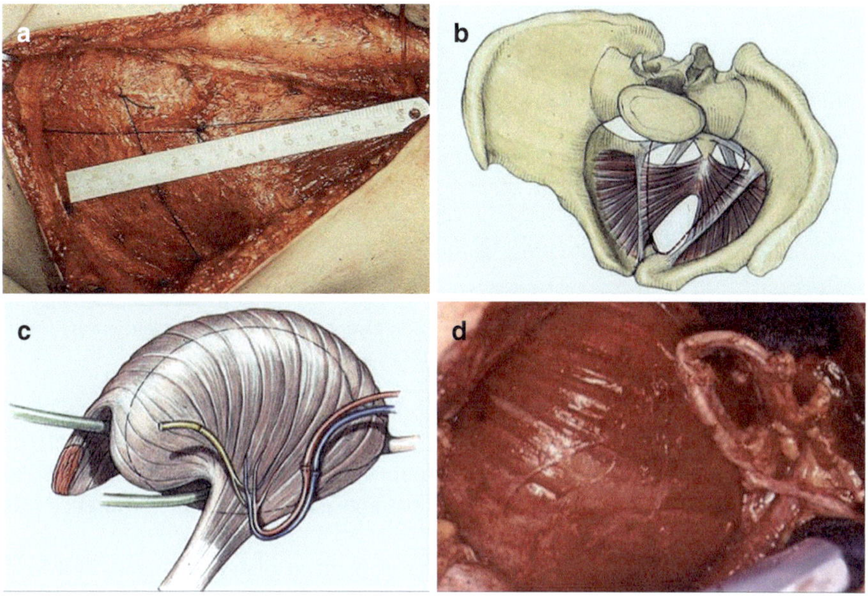

Fig. 9.5 (**a**) Latissimus dorsi muscle before harvesting. Sutures mark original length of muscle. (**b**) Fixation of latissimus dorsi muscle in pelvis (*broken line*). (**c**) Schematic drawing of position of muscle around bladder with neurovascular connections. (**d**) Final intraoperative aspect of muscle in pelvis with neurovascular connections (*right side*) (With permission Gakis et al. (2011))

Regenerative Medicine Bladder Replacement

The term "regenerative medicine" became popularized in the late 1990s, around the time when Atala pioneered bladder regeneration research and reported 7 children with myelomeningocele (4–19 years old) and high-pressure or poorly compliant bladders were treated with an engineered bladder to enhance vascularity (Fig. 9.6) (Atala et al. 2006). A bladder biopsy was obtained from each patient and urothelial and muscle cells were grown in culture. The expanded cells were then seeded on a collagen or collagen/polyglycolic acid-based biodegradable bladder-shaped scaffold. Approximately 7 weeks after the biopsy, the engineered bladder constructs were implanted. Serial follow-up evaluation was done with a mean follow-up of 46 months. Postoperatively, the mean bladder leak point pressure decreases at capacity, and the volume and compliance increase were greater in the composite engineered bladders with an omental wrap. No metabolic consequences were noted and renal function was preserved. No stones or mucus production occurred in the reconstructed bladders.

A subsequent industry sponsored FDA registry phase II trial (Joseph et al. 2014) in children with spina bifida requiring enterocystoplasty and did not report favorable results. Urothelial and smooth muscle cells were harvested via open bladder biopsy, grown in culture and seeded onto a biodegradable scaffold. Bladders were

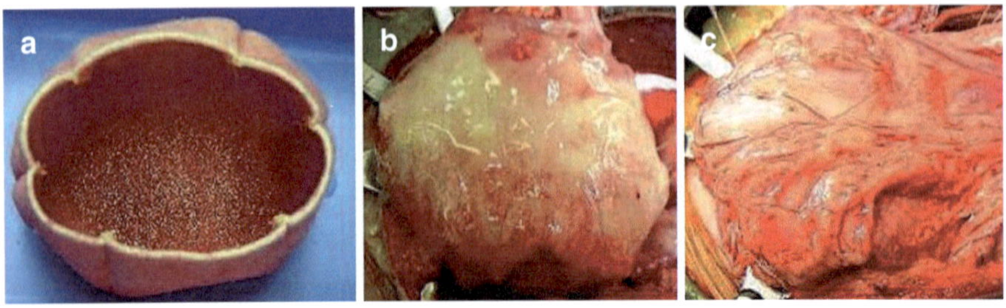

Fig. 9.6 Construction of engineered bladder scaffold seeded with cells (**a**) and engineered bladder anastamosed to native bladder with running 4-0 polyglycolic sutures (**b**). Implant covered with fibrin glue and omentum (**c**) (With permission Atala et al. (2006))

cycled postoperatively to promote regeneration. Although compliance improved in 4 of 11 patients at 12 months and in 5 of 11 patients at 36 months, the difference was not clinically or statistically significant.

There was no clinical or statistical improvement in bladder capacity at 12–36 months in any patient. Bowel obstruction and bladder rupture occurred in 4 patients (Joseph et al. 2014). The authors concluded that the procedure did not bladder capacity or compliance and was associated with serious adverse events.

During the last decade we have seen an expanding list of engineered tissues including tracheas, blood vessels, and urethras. More than 1,000 novel cell therapy trials are currently listed internationally (Li et al. 2014; Atala 2014). Although the field of regenerative medicine continues to expand and progress, challenges remain such as cost, patient selection, and regulatory and financial hurdles. Nonetheless, the future of regenerative medicine, stem cell transplantation, and tissue engineering is bright in the field of urology.

Surgical Assisting Detrusor Contractility Summary

- Management of poor detrusor contractility is limited and has few proven treatment options today.
- Clinical injection of muscle-derived stem cells into the underactive bladder has demonstrated proof of concept safety and signal of efficacy. Phase 2 FDA trial is ongoing.
- Reduction cystoplasty use remains debatable with only limited case series reported.
- Bladder myoplasty including augmentation of detrusor function with a skeletal muscle flap has been successfully performed in a few specialized centers but requires further study.
- Tissue engineering to regenerative the bladder is experimental but holds promise in the future.

Surgery to Decrease Outlet Resistance

Given the lack of effective pharmacologic agent and proven surgical methods that can reliably improve detrusor contractility, surgical treatment of UAB has historically focused attention on decreased outlet resistance to allow the UAB patient to have an easier time to void, even if detrusor contractility is diminished, by lower outlet resistance. Several approaches are presented based on the site of obstruction.

Bladder Neck and Prostate

The most common indication for transurethral resection or incision of the bladder neck is an anatomic or functional obstruction at the bladder neck or proximal urethra. Primary bladder neck obstruction is a video-urodynamically diagnosed condition, characterized by high-pressure, low-flow voiding, with radiographic evidence of obstruction at the bladder neck, without external sphincter or distal urethral obstruction (Padmanabhan and Nitti 2007). Common technique is either one or two incisions at the 5-o'clock and/or 7-o'clock positions with cystoscopic cautery or laser (Huckabay and Nitti 2005).

Surgical YV plasty of the bladder neck was reported historically for bladder neck obstruction, but with adoption of endoscopic bladder neck incision, surgical is now rarely performed. The most significant concern with bladder neck incision or resection is the development of retrograde ejaculation. There are a variety of surgical methods to treat benign prostatic obstruction that are well known to urologists. Specific surgical details are not central to the discussion in this chapter except the purpose of surgical treatment of the enlarged prostate is to relieve the obstruction to reduce afterload on an underactive bladder.

Striated Sphincter

Detrusor-external sphincter dyssynergia (DESD) is the most common cause of neurogenic sphincteric obstruction and is most often managed by intermittent catheterization. Avoidance of high intravesical pressure protects the upper tracts and decreases the risk for incontinence, infection, and stones (Chancellor and Rivas 1995) (Figs. 9.7 and 9.8). A number of sphincter defeating techniques are available.

Urethral Over dilation

Urethral over dilatation up to 40–50 Fr in women may achieve similar success as external sphincterotomy in men (Wang et al. 1989). But in women, over dilation is rarely performed because of the lack of a suitable external collecting device to

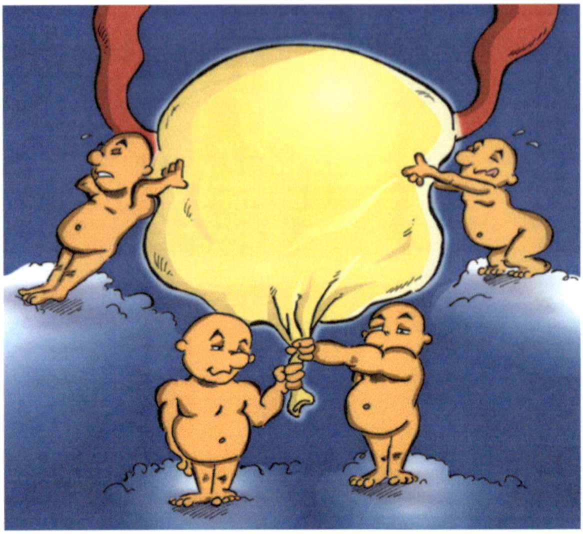

Fig. 9.7 Cartoon comically illustrating the simultaneous overactive and obstructive voiding pattern observed in patients with detrusor overactivity and detrusor-external sphincter dyssynergia (With permission, Chancellor and Smith (2011))

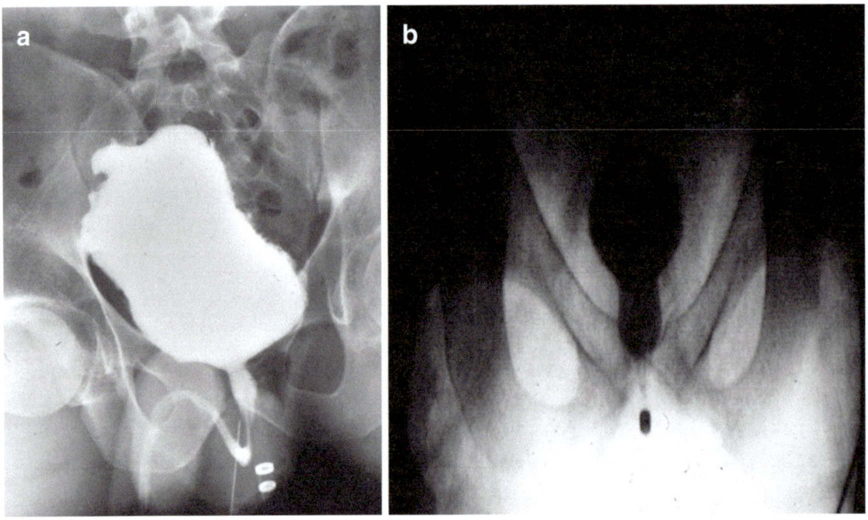

Fig. 9.8 (**a**) Voiding cystourethrogram image demonstrating detrusor-external sphincter dyssynergia in a male patient. Note the open bladder neck and prostatic urethral but abrupt cutoff of contrast at level of external urethral sphincter; (**b**) voiding cystourethrogram image of detrusor-external sphincter dyssynergia but in a female patient. Note the open bladder neck and proximal urethra but closure at the level of the external sphincter (With permission, Chancellor and Smith (2011))

manage the nearly total stress urinary incontinence when the sphincter is disrupted. Balloon dilatation of the external urethral sphincter was reported, but with either catheter or balloon, the benefit appears temporary and neither is commonly used today.

Surgical Sphincterotomy

Transurethral sphincterotomy has been used for over 50 years and yet it is still a controversial treatment with high complication rate of bleeding, erectile dysfunction, and failure rates in up to half of the patients. Sphincterotomy is performed by incision at the 12-o'clock position (Madersbacher and Scott 1975). Sphincterotomy can be performed using a knife electrode, resection with a loop electrode, or laser ablation. The incision extends from the level of the verumontanum at the proximal bulbous urethra. Visual controlled gradual deepening of the incision decreases risks of bleeding. A condom catheter is necessary postoperatively.

Failure rates following sphincterotomy have been reported to be as high as 50 % and the incidence of failure increases with time from the initial procedure (Yang and Mayo 1995). It requires considerable experience to completely transect the sphincter, and bleeding from the dorsal venous complex can be brisk. Therefore, failure is often due to incomplete resection and this leads to repeated treatments. Laser sphincterotomy is the current technique of choice by most experts for sphincter ablation and incision.

Urethral Stenting

Endourethral stents can be considered in selected patients with DESD. Stent placement can be as effective as conventional sphincterotomy and advantageous in regard to reduced hospital stay and reversibility. Continence is maintained by the competency of the bladder neck.

Chancellor and Rivas (1995) reported the initial multicenter North American data using the UroLume stent (American Medical Systems, Minnetonka, MN) in 153 patients at 15 centers. A significant decrease in detrusor leak pressure and residual urine volume was seen; however, 18 % of patients required more than one procedure to adequately open the sphincter, hyperplasia within the lumen was seen in 42 patients (33 %) at 3 months, and 10 devices were removed (7 for migration) and 7 were replaced. Bladder neck obstruction requiring treatment was seen in 13 patients (4 with α-blockers, 7 with incision, 2 with intermittent catheterization), and when removal was required (in 4), this was not a problem up to 12 months (Chancellor et al. 1999).

The reversibility of this procedure is attractive to some; however, stent removal, when necessary, may be difficult. Complications include obstruction by hyperplastic tissue ingrowth and migration of a stent across the membranous urethra has been adverse issues associated with stent management, thereby limiting its utility to a select group of patients.

Botulinum Toxin Injection in Sphincter and Pelvic Floor

The first clinical indication of botulinum toxin (BoNT) in urology was actually not for the overactive bladder but rather injection into the urethral sphincter in spinal cord-injured patients to treat DSD (Dykstra et al. 1988). Subsequent results include

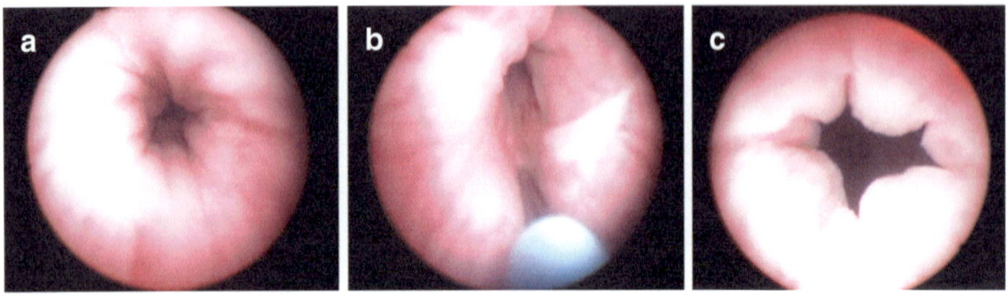

Fig. 9.9 Cystoscopic images of the male external urethral sphincter in a patient with detrusor-external sphincter dyssynergia. (**a**) Before injection, (**b**) during injection with botulinum toxin and (**c**) 1 month after injection (i.e., note lack of coaptation of urethral mucosa demonstrating relaxation of sphincter) (With permission, Chancellor and Smith (2011))

botulinum toxin usage in diverse groups with voiding dysfunction including the Fowler syndrome manifested by abnormal myotonus-like electromyographic activity in the striated urethral sphincter (Fowler et al. 1992).

Compared to external sphincterotomy or intraurethral stent placement, BoNT sphincter injection is attractive because the treatment is minimally invasive, is easy to perform, carries minimal morbidity, and is reversible (Chancellor and Smith 2011). The chemical denervation achieved by BoNT is temporary, which offers an advantage by giving male patient's the ability to determine if condom catheter is a reasonable bladder management option. In addition, this treatment option offers to the patient the hope of neurorecovery after SCI and the potential to walk again without a sphincter that is permanently damaged by sphincterotomy. BoNT also offers the opportunity to partially decrease urethral outlet resistance depending on the dosage chosen for moderate degrees of DESD in men and women with neurological diseases.

How to Do It

OnabotulinumtoxinA has been the most commonly used BoNT for the treatment of DESD and pelvic floor conditions. Other serotypes and brands of BoNT may also be effective but doses should be based on the specific toxin used. The following section on sphincteric application of botulinum toxin and details on techniques of toxin injection in the sphincter are adopted from Chap. 8 in the book "Botulinum Toxin in Urology" by Chancellor and Smith (2011, Springer Publishing).

Technique in Men: Male urethral sphincters are injected with a total of 200 U of onabotulinumtoxinA diluted in 4 ml of preservative free saline under local or general anesthesia using a rigid cystoscope loaded with an endoscopic injection needle (e.g., 25-gauge Cook® Williams Needle). BoNT is injected in equal aliquots at the 12, 3, 6, and 9 o'clock positions. It is recommended that the injection be directed deeper than urethral bulking agent injections to target the nerve terminals innervating the external (skeletal muscle) sphincter. Other methods described in the literature include perineal and/or transrectal ultrasound-guided external urethral sphincter injections (Fig. 9.9) (Chancellor and Smith 2011; Chen et al. 2010).

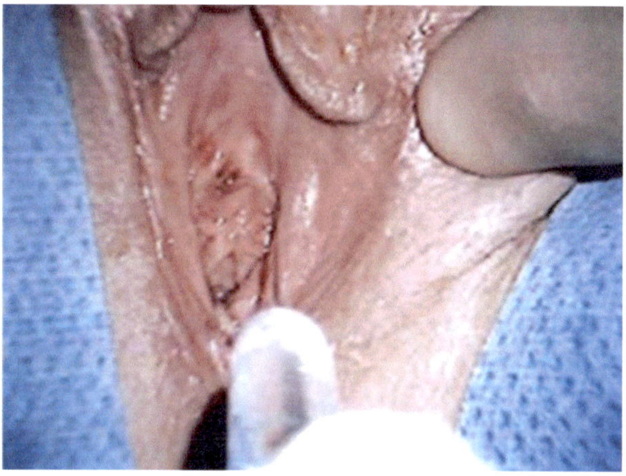

Fig. 9.10 Photograph displaying periurethral injection of the external urethral sphincter in the female (With permission, Chancellor and Smith (2011))

Technique in Women: A 22-gauge short spinal needle is inserted for 1.5 cm at the 3 o'clock and 9 o'clock positions 1 cm lateral to the urethral meatus in the periurethral folds. One ml of toxin (i.e. 50 U) is injected at each site (Fig. 9.10).

I typically use 100 U of onabotulinumtoxinA for patients with UAB who wish to void by abdominal straining as well as for patients with dysfunctional voiding or poor relaxation of the urethral sphincter. Medications for reduction of urethral resistance such as alpha blockers may be discontinued 1–2 weeks after the BoNT injections if the patient reports clinical improvement.

BoNT Sphincter Injection Results

Dykstra and associates reported the first use of BoNT to treat DESD in 1988. Eleven SCI patients with DESD were injected with 20 to 240 U of onabotulinumtoxinA into the external sphincter through the perineum or transurethrally with a cystoscope (Dykstra et al. 1988). After injection, ten patients were evaluated by electromyography and all showed signs of sphincter denervation. The maximal urethral pressures in the 7 patients in whom they were measured before and after treatment decreased an average of 27 cmH_2O after BoNT injection. Post-void residual urine volumes decreased by an average of 146 ml after toxin injection in 8 patients and autonomic dysreflexia decreased in 5 of 7 patients. The effects of BoNT sphincter injection lasted an average of 50 days.

About a dozen of peer-reviewed publications have investigated the use of BoNT to treat DESD in SCI and other neurological diseases including its use in pediatric patients (Schurch et al. 1996). Different toxin formulations, injection dosages, dilution protocols, cumulative dosages, injection frequencies, and injection approaches (cystoscopic vs. transperineal vs. transrectal) have been used in these studies which make comparisons between them difficult. However, most report clinical improvement in properly selected patients (Chancellor and Smith 2011). Chen and Kuo

Table 9.2 Sphincter botulinum toxin injection to improve bladder emptying results

Disease	Number patients	Significant improvement (%)	Moderate improvement (%)	No improvement (%)
Neurologically impaired patients				
1. DSD	29	8 (27.6 %)	15 (51.7 %)	6 (20.7 %)
2. Cauda equine lesion	8	5 (62.5 %)	1 (12.5 %)	2 (25 %)
3. Peripheral neuropathy	14	5 (35.7 %)	6 (42.9 %)	3 (21.4 %)
Patients without neurological diseases				
1. Dysfunctional voiding	20	6 (30 %)	14 (70 %)	0
2. Non-relaxing sphincter	10	8 (42.1 %)	7 (36.8 %)	4 (21.1 %)
3. Idiopathic UAB	13	8 (61.5 %)	4 (30.8 %)	1 (7.7 %)
Total	103	40 (38.8 %)	47 (45.7 %)	16 (15.5 %)

(2004) reported a 41 % reduction in intravesical pressures after BoNT sphincter injection. Smith et al. (2005) reported 52 patients with SCI, multiple sclerosis, and stroke with significant decreases in maximal voiding pressures and post-void residual urine volume after sphincter BoNT injection.

For DESD secondary to multiple sclerosis, a multicenter, placebo-controlled, randomized study by Gallien et al. (2005) used a single injection of 100 U of onabotulinumtoxinA via a transperineal approach and the authors reported a reduction in intravesical pressure by 21 % at 30 days (from 67 to 52 cmH_2O). However, treatment neither significantly reduced the post-void residual urine volume or maximal urethral pressures nor increased the maximal urinary flow rates. These results were less positive than findings reported in SCI patients. The differences in efficacy may represent differences in the pathophysiology of DESD between multiple sclerosis and SCI or differences in injection techniques (i.e., transperineal injection versus cystoscopic injection).

In a mixed series of 103 patients with voiding dysfunction, Kuo (2003) performed onabotulinumtoxinA urethral injections using either 50 U (n=48) or 100 U (n=55). Forty patients (i.e., 39 %) had an excellent result, forty-seven (46 %) had significant improvement, and sixteen (15 %) had treatment failure. Among the patients with an excellent result, UAB patients due to cauda equina lesion (63 %) or idiopathic cause (62 %) had the highest success rate, whereas those with DESD (28 %) had least improvement. The overall reported success rate was 85 %. Among the 45 patients presenting with urinary retention, indwelling catheters were removed or clean intermittent catheterization was discontinued in 39 (87 %) (Table 9.2).

Kuo (2007) evaluated the effects of BoNT urethral injection in 27 patients with idiopathic low detrusor contractility. Detrusor contractility recovered in 48 % of those treated. Patients with normal bladder sensation combined with poor relaxation or hyperactive urethral sphincter activity were most likely to respond to urethral injections with BoNT. In 38 % of patients, the therapeutic effect of restoring detrusor contractility lasted over 1 year. Kuo (2008) found that 61 % of 33 patients with neurogenic bladder treated with BoNT for their DESD were satisfied with their treatment. Their relatively low satisfaction rate was somewhat surprising especially given the fact that detrusor pressures and post-void residuals were reduced. The author found that the major reason for dissatisfaction was an increase in urgency and urge incontinence episodes.

Adverse Events

Complications of BoNT injection into the external sphincter are rare and usually self-limiting. Dykstra et al. (1988) injected 140 U of onabotulinumtoxinA at the first and 240 U at subsequent sessions in the external sphincter of five SCI patients with DESD. Three patients developed upper extremity weakness that caused difficulty in transferring for 2–3 weeks. This systemic adverse effect was documented by electromyography studies of the deltoid muscle in one of the patients. Appearance of new stress urinary incontinence and exacerbation of preexisting incontinence due to sphincter denervation by BoNT have also been reported. The use of sphincter BoNT is currently an off-label application of botulinum toxin.

Results for Bladder Neck Obstruction

Lim and Quek (2008) evaluated the effects of BoNT on voiding parameters in 8 men diagnosed by video urodynamic study and who had failed medical treatment. Eight patients with bladder-neck dyssynergia had 100 U of onabotulinumtoxinA injected transurethrally into the bladder neck and proximal prostatic urethra laterally (10 U/ml × 10 sites). At 6 weeks, 7 of 8 (88 %) patients had >50 % reduction of international prostate symptom scores from baseline. Six of 8 (75 %) patients had > 3 ml/s increase in peak urinary flow rate at 6 weeks. Micturition frequency decreased 46 % and quality of life component of the international prostate symptom scores improved by 47 %. Symptom relief lasted over 6 months and no patients reported any adverse effects or ejaculation dysfunction.

Botulinum Toxin Summary

The case for BoNT injection into the urinary sphincter and pelvic floor is based on a number of international trials but regulatory registry trials has not begun because of the small number of patients it can be used for versus the large patients with OAB. Despite promising positive results and high degree of safety with the use of sphincter BoNT injection to treat UAB, prospective randomized trials are necessary to fully evaluate the clinical effectiveness of this promising modality.

Surgical Decreasing Outlet Resistance Summary

- Transurethral incision of the bladder neck should be based on urodynamically confirmed anatomic or functional obstruction at the bladder neck. Most significant risk is the development of retrograde ejaculation.
- Urethral over dilatation may improve compliance and decrease outlet resistance but the result is short lasting.
- Early failure after sphincterotomy is often due to inadequate surgical technique, inadequate detrusor function, or obstruction at the level of the bladder neck or prostate. Late failure after sphincterotomy typically occurs with fibrosis.
- Urethral stenting offers a less invasive alternative to sphincterotomy with the advantage of being reversible. Complications include infection, migration, encrustation, and hyperplastic tissue overgrowth of the stent.
- Sphincter and pelvic floor injection of botulinum toxin is a simple procedure with multiple publication of successful outcome, but the treatment for UAB is an off-label use of the toxin.
- Intraurethral pump prosthesis with a self-contained urinary pump is a new development for the treatment of UAB (see Chap. 10).

References

Atala A (2014) Regenerative bladder augmentation using autologous tissue—when will we get there? J Urol 191:1204–1205

Atala A, Bauer SB, Soker S et al (2006) Tissue-engineered autologous bladders for patients needing cystoplasty. Lancet 367:1241

Bukowski TP, Perlmutter AD (1994) Reduction cystoplasty in the prune belly syndrome: a long-term follow up. J Urol 152:2113–2118

Carr LK, Robert M, Kultgen PL, Herschorn S, Birch C, Murphy M, Chancellor MB (2013) Autologous muscle derived cell therapy for stress urinary incontinence: a prospective, dose ranging study. J Urol 189:595–601

Chancellor MB (1994) Detrusor myoplasty and neuromuscular electrical stimulation of the urinary bladder. US Patent: 5,370,670, 6 Dec 1994

Chancellor MB, Rivas DA (1995) Current management of detrusor-sphincter dyssynergia. In: McGuire E (ed) Advances in urology. CV Mosby, St Louis, pp 291–324

Chancellor MB, Smith CP (2011) Botulinum toxin in urology. Springer, Berlin

Chancellor MB, Rivas DA, Acosta R, Erhard MJ, Moore J, Salzman SK (1994a) Detrusor-myoplasty, innervated rectus muscle transposition study, and functional effect on the spinal cord injury rat model. Neurol Urodyn 13:547–557

Chancellor MB, Rivas DA, Salzman SK (1994b) Lancet. Letter 343(8898):669

Chancellor MB, Bennett C, Simoneau AR et al (1999) Sphincteric stent versus external sphincterotomy in spinal cord injured men: prospective randomized multicenter trial. J Urol 161:1893–1898

Chancellor MB, Yokoyama T, Tirney S, Mattes CE, Yoshimura N, de Groat WC, Huard J (2000) Preliminary results of myoblast injection into the urethra and bladder wall: a possible method for the treatment of stress urinary incontinence and impaired detrusor contractility. Neuourol Urodyn 19:279–287

Chen YH, Kuo HC (2004) Botulinum A toxin treatment of urethral sphincter pseudodyssynergia in patients with cerebrovascular accidents or intracranial lesions. Urol Int 73:156–161

Chen SL, Bih LI, Chen GD, Huang YH, You YH, Lew HL (2010) Transrectal ultrasound-guided transperineal botulinum toxin a injection to the external urethral sphincter for treatment of detrusor external sphincter dyssynergia in patients with spinal cord injury. Arch Phys Med Rehabil 91:340–344

Dykstra DD, Sidi AA, Scott AB, Pagel JM, Goldish GD (1988) Effects of botulinum A toxin on detrusor-sphincter dyssynergia in spinal cord injury patients. J Urol 139:919–922

Fowler CJ, Betts C, Christmas T et al (1992) Botulinum toxin in the treatment of chronic urinary retention in women. Br J Urol 70:387–393

Gakis G, Ninkovic M, van Koeveringe GA, Raina S, Sturtz G, Rahnama'i MS, Sievert KD, Stenzl A (2011) Functional detrusor myoplasty for bladder acontractility: long-term results. J Urol 185:593–599

Gallien P, Reymann JM, Amarenco G, Nicolas B, de Seze M, Bellissant E (2005) Placebo controlled, randomised, double blind study of the effects of botulinum A toxin on detrusor sphincter dyssynergia in multiple sclerosis patients. J Neurol Neurosurg Psychiatry 76:1670–1676

Huard J, Pruchnic R, Yokoyama T, Smith CP, Qu Z, Kumon H, Yoshimura N, Somogyi G, de Groat WC, Chancellor MB (2002) Muscle based gene therapy and tissue for urological dysfunction. Gene Ther 9:1617–1626

Huckabay C, Nitti VW (2005) Diagnosis and treatment of primary bladder neck obstruction in men. Curr Urol Rep 6:271–275

Joseph DB, Borer JG, De Filippo RE et al (2014) Autologous cell seeded biodegradable scaffold for augmentation cystoplasty: phase II study in children and adolescents with spina bifida. J Urol 191:1389–1395

Kinn AC (1985) The lazy bladder-appraisal of surgical reduction. Scand J Urol Nephrol 19:93

Klarskov P, Holm-Bentzen M, Larsen S et al (1988) Partial cystectomy for the myogenous decompensated bladder with excessive residual urine. Scand J Urol Nephrol 22:251–256

Kuo HC (2003) Botulinum A toxin urethral injection for the treatment of lower urinary tract dysfunction. J Urol 170:1908–1912

Kuo HC (2007) Recovery of detrusor function after urethral botulinum A toxin injection in patients with idiopathic low detrusor contractility and voiding dysfunction. Urology 69:57–61

Kuo HC (2008) Satisfaction with urethral injection of botulinum toxin A for detrusor sphincter dyssynergia in patients with spinal cord lesion. Neurourol Urodyn 27:793–796

Levanovich PE, Diokno A, Hasenau DL, Lajiness M, Pruchnic R, Chancellor MB (2015) Intradetrusor injection of adult muscle-derived cells for the treatment of underactive bladder: pilot study. Int J Urol Nephrol 47:465–467. doi:10.1007/s11255-015-0924-1

Li MD, Atkins H, Bubela T (2014) The global land-scape of stem cell clinical trials. Regen Med 9:27

Lim SK, Quek PL (2008) Intraprostatic and bladder-neck injection of botulinum A toxin in treatment of males with bladder-neck dyssynergia: a pilot study. Eur Urol 53:620–625

Madersbacher H, Scott FB (1975) Twelve o'clock sphincterotomy. Urol Intern 30:75–81

Padmanabhan P, Nitti VW (2007) Primary bladder neck obstruction in men, women, and children. Curr Urol Rep 8:379–384

Schurch B, Hauri D, Rodic B et al (1996) Botulinum-A toxin as treatment of detrusor sphincter dyssynergia: a prospective study in 24 spinal cord injury patients. J Urol 155:1023–1029

Smith CP, Nishiguchi J, O'Leary M, Yoshimura N, Chancellor MB (2005) Single-institution experience in 110 patients with botulinum toxin A injection into bladder or urethra. Urology 65:37–41

Stenzl A, Ninkovic M, Kollé D et al (1998) Restoration of voluntary emptying of the bladder by transplantation of innervated free skeletal muscle. Lancet 351:1483–1485

Van Savage JG, Perez-Abadia GP, Palanca LG et al (2000) Electrically stimulated detrusor myoplasty. J Urol 164:969–972 von Heyden B, Anthon JP, Brock GB et al (1998) The latissimus dorsi bladder myoplasty to assist detrusor function. Urol Res 26:215–221

Wang SC, McGuire EJ, Bloom DA (1989) Urethral dilation in the management of urological complications of myelodysplasia. J Urol 142:1054–1055

Yang CC, Mayo ME (1995) External urethral sphincterotomy: long-term follow-up. Neurourol Urodyn 14:25–31

Yokoyama T, Huard J, Chancellor MB (2000) Myoblast therapy for stress incontinence and bladder dysfunction. World J Urol 18:56–61

Chapter 10
Advance Technology

Michael B. Chancellor

Intraurethral Valve-Pump

The inFlow Intraurethral Valve-Pump (Vesiflo, Redmond WA) is a nonsurgical urinary prosthesis intended to provide bladder drainage for women with underactive bladder. The term atonic bladder was used during the device's development and therefore part of the label and will be used in this chapter (Fig. 10.1). The inFlow mimics normal urination, providing an alternative to intermittent or indwelling urinary catheters. The inFlow is normally replaced monthly, but can be easily and safely removed at any time, even by patients.

The inFlow device with activator is indicated for use "in female patients 18 years of age or older who have incomplete bladder emptying due to impaired detrusor contractility of neurologic origin, and who are capable of operating it in accordance with instructions or who have trained caregivers. The device must be replaced every 29 days (or less)" (FDA 2014).

The FDA granted the approval based on non-clinical testing and a clinical trial that enrolled 273 women with impaired detrusor contractility using clean intermittent catheterization. Over half of the women stopped using the device as a result of discomfort and leakage of urine. The trial showed that 98 % of the 115 women that continued to use the inFlow device had comparable post-void residual urine volume with those who used the intermittent catheterization.

Adverse events associated with the device included asymptomatic bacteriuria, urinary tract infection, bladder inflammation, genital and urinary pain, blood in the urine (hematuria), urinary leakage around the device, urinary frequency/urgency,

M.B. Chancellor, MD
Department of Urology, Aikens Research Center, Oakland University William Beaumont School of Medicine, Rochester, MI, USA

Neurourology Program, Beaumont Health System, Royal Oak, MI, USA
e-mail: Michael.Chancellor@beaumont.edu

M.B. Chancellor, A.C. Diokno (eds.), *The Underactive Bladder*,
DOI 10.1007/978-3-319-23687-2_10

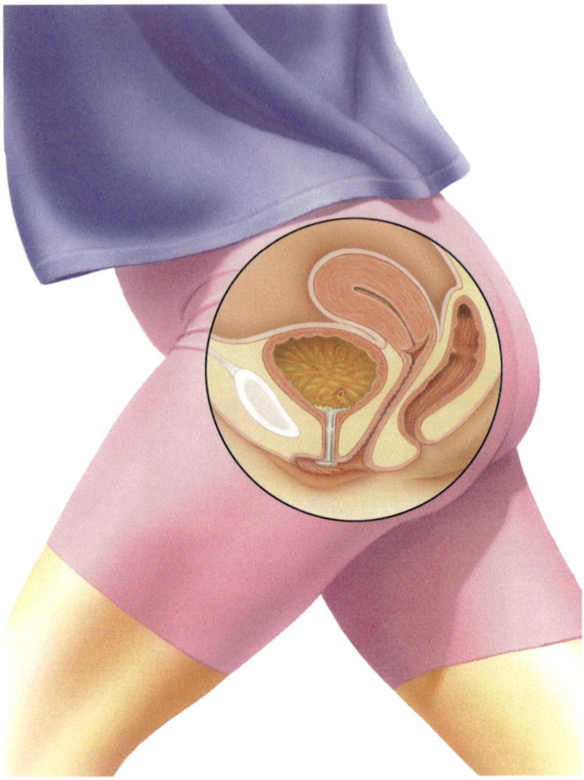

Fig. 10.1 The inFlow Intraurethral device in proper position in this drawing cross-sectional area of a woman's pelvis

bladder spasms, and vulvar, vaginal, and urethral disorders. It is noteworthy that urinary tract infection appeared to occur at a lower rate with the inFlow device as compared to clean intermittent catheterization. Among patients treated with the inFlow device, infection was stable and managed with antibiotics.

The inFlow has been sold outside the USA for a decade, mostly in Germany and Australia. Approximately 15,000 devices have been sold to date, amounting to over 1,000 women and years of use based on typical device use of 1 month each. No serious adverse events have been reported. In Germany, the inFlow is available and is reimbursed by the country's national health system.

Underactive Bladder, Atonic Bladder

Atonic bladder is a medical condition where patients are unable to spontaneously urinate due to insufficient detrusor muscle contraction. The inFlow device was developed to be an alternative to urinary catheters which are among the most commonly used medical devices. However, catheterization is associated with low quality of life, encrustation, stone formation, and recurrent urinary tract infections (UTIs).

Table 10.1 Bladder drainage options inFlow vs. catheterization

	Indwelling	Intermittent catheterization	inFlow
Allows bladder cycling		✓	✓
Allows use of toilet			✓
Easy to operate	✓		✓
Effectively empties bladder		✓	✓
Minimal UTI rate		✓	✓
Number of insertions/month	1	From 120 [×4/day] up to 240 [×8/day]	1

The present standard of care for UAB and atonic bladder is clean intermittent catheterization (CIC). If a woman cannot or will not use CIC, then she is likely to end up with a urethral or suprapubic catheter and urine drainage bag. The inFlow prosthetic device compensates for the inability of women with atonic bladder to generate bladder pressure by providing near complete evacuation of urine on demand. By allowing almost normal use of a toilet, the inFlow eliminates the need to catheterize multiple times daily and eliminates tubes/drainage bags, improving its users' self-image as well as their hygiene (Table 10.1).

Design

The inFlow device has four components: a sterilized, single-use urethral insert component with silicone shaft, fins, and flange; an introducer; an activator; and a sizing component. The device draws urine out to empty the bladder and blocks urine flow when continence is desired. A physician sizes the patient for an inFlow device and performs the initial insertion. After training, device insertion and removal can be performed by the patient or a caregiver. Each inserted component must be replaced at least once every 29 days.

To void, the user sits on a toilet, holds a remote control over the lower pelvic area, and presses a button. This magnetically activates the miniature internal pump, which drains the bladder at a normal flow rate. When the button is released, the valve is engaged, blocking further urine flow.

How the inFlow Works

The inFlow is a 3–7 cm long device in a silicone housing (shown on top with its disposable introducer and below after deployment). Nine sizes are available in order to account for variations in urethral length using a disposable introducer (Fig. 10.2).

Flexible "petals" open to hold the device at the bladder neck. Device sizing and initial insertion are performed by a physician. Thereafter, a new device is inserted every 29 days, typically by a caregiver or spouse. Insertion is similar to that for a

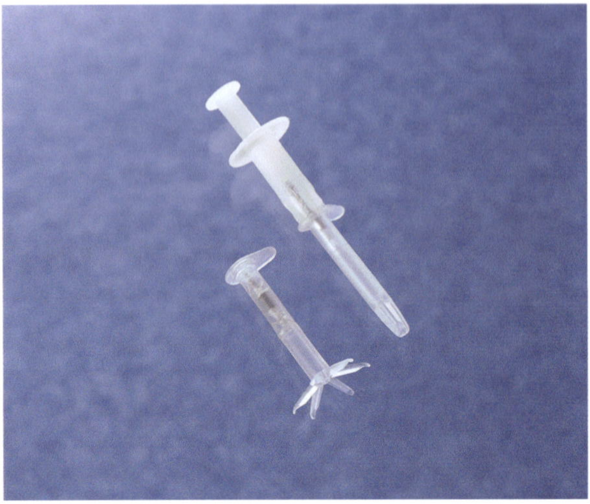

Fig. 10.2 InFlow device shown as supplied mounted on its disposable introducer (*top-right*) and without (*bottom-left*). The inflow device includes an internal value-pump mechanism

urinary catheter. The inserted device resides almost entirely in the urethra. To void, the patient sits on a toilet, holds a remote control over the lower pelvic area, and presses a button (right). This magnetically activates a miniature internal pump that spins at 10,000 rotations per minute (RPM) and drains the bladder at a normal flow rate. When the button is released, a valve is engaged, blocking further urine flow (Fig. 10.3).

Previous Experience with Intraurethral Prosthesis

Over a decade ago, Madjar et al. (1999) reported on 92 women, having the earlier version of the device for over 1 year and noted only that 3.9 % of subjects had a UTI in 357 months of device use and all resolved with oral antibiotics. Removal of the device within 2 weeks was required in 57 % of patients, mostly because of local discomfort and urinary leakage. In another 21 % of patients, the device was removed between 2 and 16 months after placement. Twenty-one patients (23 %) with the device still in place after more than 1 year were being followed.

Several investigator-initiated studies outside the USA have been published and included similar populations to the recent pivotal study (Chen et al. 2005; Nativ et al. 1997; Schurch et al. 1999). No serious or lasting adverse events were reported in any study. In a 1-year study of 20 atonic bladder patients, Lynch et al. (2003) reported 80 % improvement in quality of life and no negative tissue changes. This study also reported a high rate of device acceptance; only one patient discontinued device use for reasons related to the device. The mean flow rate was 10.7 ml/s (range 9–16 ml/s) and the post-void residual urine volume (PVR) 3 ml (range 0–17 ml). Two patients had a single UTI after the initial insertion of the InFlow and they responded to antibiotics. A higher rate of device acceptance can be achieved by providing pre-insertion patient education and post-insertion nursing support.

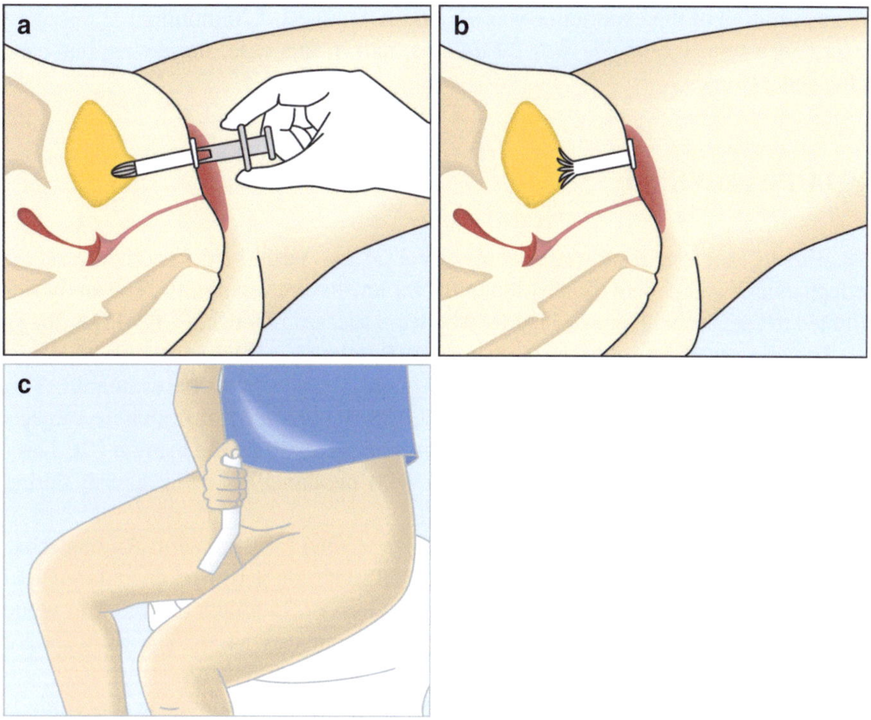

Fig. 10.3 Diagrams showing the inflow device (**a**) being inserted, (**b**) detached from the introducer, and (**c**) residing in situ within the urethra

In a study of 21 patients with voiding dysfunction who were followed for more than a year with a follow-up time of 12–44 months (mean 25 months), Madjar et al. (2000) reported "The new remote controlled intraurethral inFlow Catheter is useful for managing difficult voiding in women. The pump and valve assembly mimics normal urination by enabling a good stream of urine with complete bladder evacuation as well as continence between voids. The cost and incidence of symptomatic urinary tract infection are similar to those of clean intermittent catheterization. This device is safe and effective for women with difficult voiding."

In a study of 60 women with chronic urinary retention, median age of 62 years old (range 40–89 years old), Mazouni et al. (2004) found that the inFlow is effective in emptying the bladder, had few significant complications, and was a good solution for many users, but that a high percentage of subjects discontinued its use. The mean maximal peak flow measured after 1 month was 14 ml/s (range 7–18 ml/s). The post-void residual volume was 15 ml (range 0–40 ml). The incidence of urinary infection was 3 %. The abandonment of the prosthesis was noted in 50 % (30/60) of cases within the first 15 days after implantation. At the end of the procedure, 30 patients were using the In-Flow prosthesis with successful bladder emptying. The mean duration of the experience was 95 months (range 1–870 months). The longest experience with the device was 29 months, and in this case, the device has been changed 31 times.

FDA Phase 3 Study

An 18-site, single-arm crossover study ($n=273$) was performed to compare safety, effectiveness, and patient satisfaction of the inFlow device versus CIC. The study was limited to females with atonic bladder who were successfully using CIC (FDA 2013).

The primary endpoint of the study was PVR volume. All subjects with PVR data available for both baseline and treatment were considered to be evaluable. This resulted in a total of 115 evaluable subjects. 98 % (113/115) of evaluable subjects had a median inFlow treatment PVR that was no greater than the median CIC baseline PVR or both medians were <50 ml, with median PVR at each visit during inFlow treatment ranging from 10 to 20 ml.

Key secondary endpoint was quality of life (QOL) measurement. Among those subjects with both baseline and treatment QOL data, on a 100-point scale, patient scores for the Wagner I-QOL increased by a mean of 25 points ($p<0.0001$) while using the inFlow. The median percent improvement was 54 %. The results were both statistically and clinically significant.

Safety was monitored throughout the study. The UTI experience in this study is based on 417 patient-month cumulative exposure in 157 patients. Thus, the UTI rate observed is a representative and robust estimate of what might be expected in clinical use and the finding of equivalence is notable in that no indwelling bladder drainage device has been shown to have the same UTI rate as intermittent catheters. No serious or long-lasting adverse events associated with inFlow use were reported in the pivotal trial. As an indwelling device, it was anticipated that adverse events associated with inFlow use may be more frequent and severe than those for CIC, which contacts subjects for only minutes per day. There were no significant differences in event rates between the CIC baseline and inFlow treatment periods, however, except for hematuria, genitourinary pain, bladder inflammation, and urinary incontinence. All hematuria events were of mild or moderate severity and none required treatment or device removal. All bladder inflammation events were mild in severity. All genitourinary pain and incontinence events were mild to moderate in severity. Device awareness/discomfort increased during inFlow treatment, and although all cases were mild in severity, this caused numerous subjects to discontinue device use.

Conclusions

The US FDA approved in 2015 the inFlow Intraurethral Valve-Pump, a replaceable urinary prosthesis for use in adult women who cannot contract the muscles necessary to push urine out of the bladder. To void, the user sits on a toilet, holds a remote control over the lower pelvic area, and presses a button. This magnetically activates the miniature internal pump, which drains the bladder at a normal flow rate. When the button is released, the valve is engaged, blocking further urine flow. The approval of the InFlow is an important step toward advancing technology development and adoption for the treatment of underactive bladder.

References

Chen TYH, Ponsot Y, Carmel M, Bouffard N, Kennelly MJ, Tu LM (2005) Multi-centre study of intraurethral valve-pump catheter in women with a hypotonic or acontractile bladder. Eur Urol 48:628–633

FDA (2013) De novo classification request for inflow intraurethral valve-pump and activator. DEN130044, 25 Oct 2013

FDA (2014) http://www.fda.gov/NewsEvents/Newsroom/PressAnnouncements/ucm418835.htm

Lynch WJ, Testa GA, Bell D (2003) A study to determine subjective and objective benefits of a remote- controlled intra-urethral device for the management of female acontractile bladder. Br J Urol 92:960–963

Madjar S, Sabo E, Halachmi S, Wald M, Issaq E, Moskovitz B, Beyar M, Nativ O (1999) A remote controlled intraurethral insert for artificial voiding – a new concept for treating women with voiding dysfunction. J Urol 161:895–898

Madjar S, Halachmi S, Wald M, Issaq E, Moskovitz B, Beyar M, Nativ O (2000) Long-term follow-up of the inFlow™ intraurethral insert for the treatment of women with voiding dysfunction. Eur Urol 38:161–166

Mazouni C, Karsenty G, Bladou F, Serment G (2004) Urethral device in women with chronic urinary retention: an alternative to self-catheterization? Eur J Obstet Gynecol Reprod Biol 115:80–84

Nativ O, Moskovitz B, Issaq E, Condrea A, Kastin A, Halachmi S, Burbara J, Madjar S, Beyar M (1997) A new intraurethral sphincter prosthesis with a self-contained urinary pump. ASAIO J 43:197–203

Schurch S, Suter S, Dubs M (1999) Intraurethral sphincter prosthesis to treat hyporeflexic bladders in women – does it work? Br J Urol 84:789–794

Chapter 11
Diabetes and Other Neurogenic Underactive Bladder Conditions

En Meng and Yao-Chi Chuang

Introduction

Diabetes, a chronic metabolic condition, is a rising health concern across the world with significant medical and health economic issues. According to the International Diabetes Federation (IDF), the North American Region has a prevalence of diabetes of 8 % in the adult population (Allgot et al. 2003). Using Taiwan National Health Insurance claims data, Chang et al. reported that the prevalence of type 2 diabetes among those aged over 20 years was 7 % in Taiwan (Chang et al. 2010). Worldwide, it is estimated that 382 million people (prevalence 8 %) had diabetes in 2013 and is expected to rise to 592 million by 2035 (Guariguata et al. 2014).

Urological complications are always a concern in those affected by DM (both types I and II). It has been estimated that more than a quarter of diabetic patients will develop costly and debilitating urological complications, e.g., infections, overactive bladder (OAB), loss of bladder sensation, retention of urine, and underactive bladder (UAB) (Chancellor and Blaivas 1995; Yoshimura et al. 2005). Diabetic bladder dysfunction is a complex phenomenon and involves different pathophysiology and functional manifestations of the bladder (Daneshgari et al. 2009). Diabetic bladder dysfunction was earlier described as diabetic cystopathy with characteristics that included incomplete emptying, diminished contractility, and decreased sensation of bladder fullness (Yoshimura et al. 2005), which are also characteristics of UAB with a reported prevalence ranging from 25 to 87 % (Frimodt-Moller 1980).

E. Meng, MD, DPhil
Division of Urology, Department of Surgery, Tri-Service General Hospital, Taipei, Taiwan

National Defense Medical Center, Taipei, Taiwan

Y.-C. Chuang, MD (✉)
Department of Urology, Kaohsiung Chang Gung Memorial Hospital, Chang Gung University College of Medicine, Kaohsiung, Taiwan
e-mail: chuang82@ms26.hinet.net

M.B. Chancellor, A.C. Diokno (eds.), *The Underactive Bladder*,
DOI 10.1007/978-3-319-23687-2_11

Many elderly diabetic patients have concomitant lesions, such as benign prostatic enlargement, stress incontinence, or pelvic organ prolapse, which may coexist with or mimic the symptoms of diabetic cystopathy.

Diabetic Bladder Dysfunction: Overlapping Symptoms and Lack of Validated Diagnostic Questionnaire

The diagnosis of overactive bladder (OAB) based on symptom scores has helped in classifying the degree of diabetic bladder dysfunction. A survey of 3,962 women demonstrated that OAB affects 21 % of diabetic women, compared to only 13 % of nondiabetic women (Lawrence et al. 2007). Using the OAB symptom score, Liu et al. (2011) demonstrated a high prevalence (23 %) of OAB in 1,359 type 2 diabetic patients. However, the prevalence of UAB – the opposite syndrome to the OAB – in DM population remains poorly understood due to a lack of validated diagnostic questionnaires. The clinical symptoms of UAB are poorly distinguishable from the obstructive lower urinary tract symptoms, e.g., weak stream, intermittency, hesitancy, and straining to void. Therefore, the diagnosis of UAB is challenging from the clinical symptoms only. The epidemiology study regarding DU in DM population is based on urodynamic study with variable diagnosis criteria (Table 11.1), and objective cutoffs for detrusor underactivity (DU) have not been standardized.

Epidemiology: DM Patients with or Without Urinary Symptoms

Kaplan et al. (1995) retrospectively analyzed the urodynamic findings of 115 male and 68 female diabetics with persistent voiding symptoms. Impaired detrusor contractility was defined by poorly sustained or weak detrusor contractions (<30 cmH_2O) and a catheterized urine flow rate of less than 12 ml/s. The results indicate that mean bladder capacity was 485 ± 89 ml with a mean first sensation of filling of 298 ± 67 ml. Of the 182 patients, 100 (55 %) had detrusor hyperreflexia, 42 (23 %) had impaired detrusor contractility, 20 (11 %) had indeterminate findings, 19 (10 %) had detrusor areflexia, and 1 (1 %) was normal. Surprisingly, the standard diabetic cystopathy is far less than detrusor overactivity. However, sacral cord signs correlated with either impaired detrusor contractility in 50 % or detrusor areflexia in 24 % of patients with diabetic cystopathy. These data suggest that classical diabetic cystopathy is not the most common urodynamic finding in patients with DM and voiding dysfunction, and in fact these patients may present with concomitant lesions, such as benign prostatic hyperplasia, and stress incontinence and make variable pathophysiological findings. The authors concluded that urodynamic studies in diagnosing voiding dysfunction in diabetics before initiation of therapy is important.

Impaired detrusor contractility may lead to incomplete bladder emptying and urinary retention. Yu et al. (2004) conducted a prospective study to compare voiding function between 176 female type 2 diabetic patients and 162 age-matched nondiabetic women, none of whom had ever sought treatment for voiding dysfunction.

Table 11.1 Prevalence of diabetic bladder dysfunction

	Patients	UAB criteria	UAB %	Predictors
Kaplan et al. (1995)	115 M, 68 F, between 48 and 93 years old, with voiding symptoms	Impaired detrusor contractility: poorly sustained or weak detrusor contractions (<30 cmH_2O) and a catheterized urine flow rate of less than 12 ml/s	23 % impaired detrusor contractility 10 % had detrusor areflexia	Sacral cord signs – impaired detrusor contractility in 21 (50 %) or detrusor areflexia in 10 (24 %)
Yu et al. (2004)	176 F; mean 62 years, all without voiding symptoms	Voiding difficulty was defined as a maximal flow rate (*Q*max) of <12 ml/s or a PVR of ≥100 ml on two or more determinations	22 % voiding difficulty; 14 % of the patients had high PVR levels ≥100 ml	DM ≥20 years and two or more episodes of UTI in the preceding year
Yamaguchi et al. (2007)	58 M, 26 F, mean 60.8 years, with LUTS	Schafer's nomogram: weak and very weak detrusor contractility or acontractile detrusor, taken as detrusor underactivity	23 % decreased bladder sensation (first sensation ≥300 ml), 6 % increased bladder capacity ≥600 ml), detrusor underactivity 48 %	
Kebapcı et al. (2007)	27 M, mean 58 years 27 F, mean 62 years; with LUTS	Diabetic cystopathy – impaired bladder sensation, volume at first desire to void > 150 ml, increased PVR ≥ 100 ml, increased capacity ≥500 ml, decreased contractility, a flat trace on cystometry	M – 50 % F – 44 %	DM at least 8–9 years
Lee et al. (2009)	86 F, mean 67 years; who had not sought treatment for DBD	Schafer and ICS nomograms	35 % detrusor underactivity	Impaired bladder sensation on Aδ and C fiber bladder afferent pathways

(continued)

Table 11.1 (continued)

	Patients	UAB criteria	UAB %	Predictors
Bansal et al. (2011)	52 M, mean 61 years, with LUTS	Delayed first sensation of >250 ml, increased capacity > 600 ml, DUA, detrusor contractility index >100, high PVR of more than one third of capacity	Delayed first sensation 21 %, increased capacity 25 %, DUA 79 %, high PVR 65 %	81 % had autonomic dysfunction; 58 % had peripheral neuropathy; high correlated with DU in conjunction with high PVR, but not DU alone
Lin et al. (2012)	181 F	Detrusor hyperactivity with insufficient contractility and detrusor underactivity with poor voiding efficiency		Age and recurrent UTI
He et al. (2014)	1,640 F, mean 53 years; 93 % with LUTS	International Urogynecological Association/International Continence Society (IUA/ICS) Standardization of Terminology Reports	48 % impaired detrusor contractility; 8 % detrusor areflexia	

Diabetic patients were 5 times as likely to have unrecognized voiding difficulty, defined a maximal flow rate <12 ml/s or a post-void residual (PVR) urine volume ≥100 ml. Notably, 22 % had voiding difficulty and 14 % had high PVR levels ≥100 ml. Duration of diabetes of ≥20 years appeared to be an independent predictor.

Fifty-four diabetic patients, half men and half women, with lower urinary tract symptoms were involved in an urodynamic investigation by Kebapcı et al. (2007). Bladder dysfunction was present in 74 % of men characterized by impaired bladder sensation – volume at first desire to void > 150 ml, increased PVR ≥ 100 ml, increased bladder capacity ≥500 ml, and decreased bladder contractility on urodynamics. Bladder dysfunction was noted in 59 % of diabetic women including UAB in 44 %, detrusor overactivity 31 %, urge incontinence 13 %, and stress urinary incontinence 12 %. Prolongation of QTc on electrocardiogram, abnormal esophageal transit and gastric emptying times, microalbuminuria, and diabetic retinopathy were associated with an increased risk of PVR ≥ 100 ml. The authors also found that PVR ≥ 100 ml was associated with 21 and 4 times increased risk of recurrent UTI in men and in women, respectively. The establishment of UAB 8 years after the diagnosis of type 2 DM may be an important prognosticator for future serious diabetic bladder dysfunction.

Lee et al. (2009) studied urodynamic characteristics and bladder sensory function by intravesical current perception threshold testing at frequencies of 5 and 250 Hz in 86 diabetic women who had not sought treatment for diabetic bladder dysfunction. Among them, 30 (35 %) were classified as having detrusor underactivity, 12 (14 %)

presented signs of detrusor overactivity, 11 (13 %) were referred to as having bladder outlet obstruction, and 33 (38 %) showed normal detrusor function. The detrusor underactivity group showed impaired emptying function and decreased sensation on cystometry and an increase in current perception threshold values associated with a decrease in bladder voiding efficiency on 5 and 250 Hz current perception threshold testing. The results support that impaired bladder sensation of Aδ and C fiber bladder afferent pathways may play a key role in diabetic bladder dysfunction.

Bansal et al. (2011) evaluated urodynamic study and sympathetic skin responses, motor and sensory nerve-conduction velocity studies in 52 diabetic men with lower urinary tract symptoms, and mean duration of DM of 11 years. Delayed first sensation of >250 ml was seen in 21 %, increased capacity of>600 ml was noted in 25 %, and high PVR of more than one third of capacity in 65 %. Other abnormalities, such as detrusor overactivity (36 %), bladder outlet obstruction (29 %), and decreased compliance (33 %), were also common. Only 8 % of patients had normal bladder function on urodynamic evaluation. A large majority (81 %) had electrophysiologic evidence of autonomic dysfunction. The authors reported that electrophysiologic evidence of peripheral neuropathy was seen in 58 % of patients with diabetic bladder dysfunction. UAB with an elevated PVR highly correlates with neurologic abnormalities.

He et al. (2014) reported in 918 diabetic patients with impaired detrusor contractility ($n=787$) or detrusor areflexia ($n=131$) that the mean first sensation of filling was 238 ml, with a mean maximum cystometric capacity of 624 ml, mean maximum flow rate of 9.6 ml/s, mean detrusor pressure at maximum flow rate of 32 cmH_2O, and mean PVR of 323 ml. Thirty-eight of 131 patients with detrusor areflexia had impaired renal function and bilateral hydronephrosis.

In a prospective study of 181 women with type 2 DM and lower urinary tract dysfunction, Lin et al. (2012) demonstrated that the duration of DM relative to the urodynamic diagnoses of these women was longer in those with detrusor hyperactivity with impaired contractility and with poor voiding efficiency. Regression analysis indicated that age and recurrent urinary tract infections were the two independent factors associated with developing voiding dysfunction.

Pathophysiology

Diabetes is associated with a systemic inflammation, neuropathy, vascular complications, and metabolic syndrome, all of which have been linked to DM cystopathy (Yoshimura et al. 2005). The biology of DM cystopathy is multifactorial and can be a result of an alteration or aberrant function of the detrusor smooth muscle cell, the innervation or the neuronal component, or urothelium. Watanabe and Miyagawa (1999) suggested that there are three primary causes of UAB in diabetics:

1. Overdistention due to deficient bladder sensation and polyuria
2. Fibrosis due to chronic cystitis
3. Motor disturbance due to autonomic neuropathy

Table 11.2 Neurologic diseases that may cause underactive bladder

Causes of neurogenic underactive bladder
Central nervous system diseases
Neurologic disorders: (a) Acute cerebrovascular accidents (b) Multiple sclerosis (MS) (c) Parkinson's disease
Injury to the spinal cord and cauda equina (a) Herniated disk (b) Cauda equina syndrome
Peripheral neuropathy
Infectious neurologic problems (a) AIDS (b) Neurosyphilis (tabes dorsalis) (c) Herpes zoster and herpes simplex (d) Guillain–Barré syndrome
After pelvic surgery and radiation therapy (a) Pelvic surgery (b) Pelvic and sacral fractures (c) Lesions of the pudendal nerve

Modified from Miyazato et al. (2013)

Diabetic neuropathy is characterized by demyelinization, axonal degeneration, fiber loss, and defect in bladder Aδ and C afferent fibers. Diabetic cystopathy-affected specimens have shown focal axonal degeneration and decreased bladder wall cholinergic nerve fibers (Van Poppel et al. 1988). Furthermore, many associations have been linked between bladder dysfunction and peripheral nerve system dysfunction in diabetes, e.g., somatic pain sensation, motor and sensory nerve conduction velocities in the limbs, and sympathetic skin responses (sweating) (Yamaguchi et al. 2007).

The cause of diabetic neuropathy is multifocal, including altered metabolism of glucose and hyperglycemic activation of the polyol pathway causing direct neuronal damage. Ischemia, superoxide-induced free-radical formation, impaired axonal transport, and metabolic derangement of the Schwann cell result in segmental demyelination and impairment of nerve conduction (Yoshimura et al. 2005; Lee et al. 2009). Neuronal dysfunction may reflect a deficiency of axonal transport of nerve growth factor that may induce diabetic neuropathy (Sasaki et al. 2003).

Other Neurological Diseases Causing UAB

UAB can be observed in many neurologic conditions, such as disturbed central nervous system function, peripheral neuropathy, and impaired bladder neurotransmission (Table 11.2), and this has been discussed in the recent comprehensive reviews (Miyazato et al. 2013; Andersson 2014).

Central Nervous System Diseases

Acute Cerebrovascular Accidents (CVA)

Brittain et al. (2000) reported a high prevalence (34 %) of urinary symptoms among community-dwelling stroke survivors. These symptoms have considerable impact on the lives of stroke survivors. Although urinary incontinence is the most common sequela of CVA, urinary retention may be the first event to occur in the acute phase of CVA. Poststroke urinary retention has been reported in 29 % of stroke patients within 72 h of admission (Kong and Young 2000). The exact mechanism is not clear but has been termed "cerebral shock" Retention may not necessarily be the outcome of the neurologic lesion itself, but rather from the impaired consciousness, immobility, and incompetence to express the need to void, with resulting overdistention of the bladder and failure to void.

Han et al. (2010) compared the urodynamic parameters in ischemic and hemorrhagic stroke patients with bladder dysfunction. They found that 71 % of ischemic stroke patients had detrusor overactivity and 29 % had detrusor underactivity, but 65 % of hemorrhagic stroke patients had underactive detrusor and 35 % had overactive detrusor. A recent study investigated the urodynamic patterns of poststroke urinary incontinence in 106 patients affected by ischemic stroke. The result showed normal studies in 15 %, detrusor overactivity in 56 %, detrusor overactivity with impaired contractility in 14 %, and detrusor underactivity in 15 % (Pizzi et al. 2014).

Parkinson's Disease

Parkinson's disease (PD) is a disorder of basal ganglia and usually caused by insufficient formation and action of dopamine. It is clinically characterized by muscle rigidity, tremor, and a slow physical movement. Lower urinary tract symptoms are estimated to occur in 65 % of patients with PD (Sakakibara et al. 2014). Storage symptoms are the most common including nocturia. Voiding symptoms can also occur in the patients with PD. UAB has been reported in up to 16 % of patients with PD. A greater percent of patients with PD have delay in initiating urination, prolongation/poor stream, and straining.

The most common finding in urodynamic studies of patients with PD is detrusor overactivity (67 %) (Sakakibara et al. 2014). Uchiyama et al. (2011) found that detrusor underactivity (50 %), impaired urethral relaxation such as detrusor–sphincter dyssynergia (8 %), and bladder outlet obstruction (16 %) were present in the voiding phase of untreated PD patients, respectively.

Multiple Sclerosis

Multiple sclerosis (MS) is a complex, autoimmune relapsing–remitting disorder of the CNS causing a wide spectrum of neurologic manifestation. The prevalence of lower urinary tract dysfunction in patients with MS has been reported to be between

50 and 90 % (Litwiller et al. 1999). Urinary urgency, frequency, and urgency incontinence are the most common symptoms (de Sèze et al. 2007). Voiding symptoms are also common in this population, occurring in 34–79 % of patients (de Sèze et al. 2007). In a recent study, Amarenco et al. (2013b) investigated 65 patients suffering from MS with urological dysfunction, and they found that 45 (69 %) patients suffered from OAB, 48 (73 %) from voiding dysfunction, and 14 (21 %) from urinary retention.

Urodynamic evaluation has an important role in determining proper bladder management in MS patients. The most common urodynamic finding is detrusor hyperreflexia in 62 % of these patients, followed by detrusor–sphincter dyssynergia in 25 % and hypocontractility in 20 % (Litwiller et al. 1999). A recent urodynamic investigation demonstrated detrusor overactivity in 70 % of cases and detrusor underactivity in 6 % of cases (Amarenco et al. 2014).

Underactive detrusor can be one of the main manifestations of MS-related bladder dysfunction, and the main cause of UAB in MS is often due to detrusor–sphincter dyssynergia (DSD) (Amarenco et al. 2014). It resulted from neurological lesions between the brainstem (pontine micturition center) and the sacral spinal cord (sacral micturition center) which may occur in MS patients. This incoordination between detrusor smooth muscle and external urethral sphincter and/or bladder neck induces an obstruction, which results in excessive bladder pressures during voiding and residual volume.

Few guidelines are currently available for the urological management of MS. Amarenco and colleagues (2013a) have designed a First-Line Urological Evaluation in Multiple Sclerosis (FLUE-MS) algorithm (Fig. 11.1) for neurologists and general practitioners, enabling identification of "red flags," timely patient referral to specialists, and appropriate first-line therapy.

Injury to the Spinal Cord and Cauda Equina

Any injury to the spinal cord including those caused by trauma, degenerative, developmental, vascular, infectious, and idiopathic injury may cause voiding dysfunction. Rabadi and Aston (2014) investigated 161 veterans with spinal cord injury (SCI); symptoms of neurogenic bladder was present in 133 (83 %). Veterans with NGB also had more severe spinal injury and more frequent UTI. Typically, SCI above the S1 level (suprasacral SCI) does not interrupt the integrity of parasympathetic (S2 through S4) and somatic nerves (S1 through S4). Only cortical inhibition of micturition reflex and detrusor–sphincter coordination regulated by the pontine micturition center are disturbed. Injury at the S2–S4 level (sacral SCI) can result in impairment of detrusor contractility and pudendal nerve dysfunction.

It is generally agreed that urodynamic study should be conducted to provide a precise diagnosis for each patient with SCI. According to the urodynamic manifestation, Dong et al. (2006) divided the patients with neurogenic bladder dysfunction caused by intervertebral disk hernia into three groups: the group of detrusor

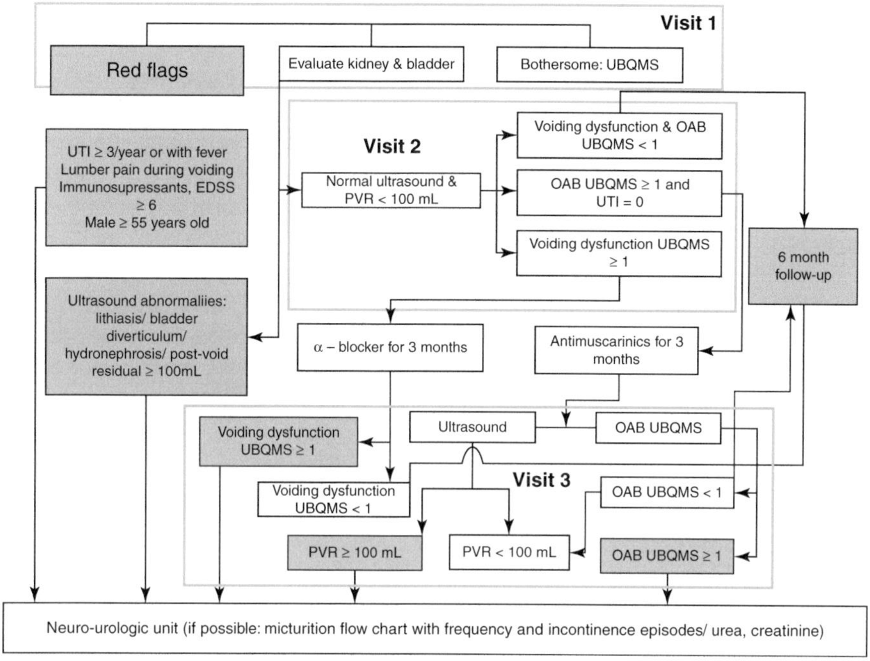

Fig. 11.1 Urological evaluation in MS (FLUE-MS) algorithm (Modified from Amarenco et al. (2013a)). *UBQMS* Urinary Bothersome Questionnaire in Multiple Sclerosis, *EDSS* Expanded Disability Status Scale

hyperreflexia without dyssynergia (10 %), the group of detrusor hyperreflexia with dyssynergia (43 %), and the group of DA (47 %). Hellstrom et al. (1986) evaluated bladder function urodynamically in 17 patients previously operated for the cauda equina syndrome caused by a prolapsed lumbar intervertebral disk and found that 36 % of patients had detrusor underactivity.

Peripheral Neuropathy

Infectious Neurologic Problems

AIDS

Both the central and peripheral nervous system is affected in 30–40 % of AIDS patients. Voiding disturbances may be related to recurrent or chronic UTI; central nervous system disturbances including encephalitis, cerebral toxoplasmosis, and HIV-related dementia; or peripheral neurologic deficits. Central and peripheral neurologic causes account for approximately 61 % of voiding dysfunction seen in AIDS-affected patients (Lebovitch and Mydlo 2008).

Neurosyphilis (Tabes Dorsalis)

Syphilis is a sexually transmitted disease caused by the spirochete *Treponema pallidum*. Tabes dorsalis is a demyelinating atrophy of the dorsal spinal cord that affects the posterior column, resulting in impaired bladder sensation, impaired detrusor contractility, sequential bladder overdistention, and eventual detrusor decompensation if left untreated. Voiding dysfunction secondary to neurosyphilis in current times is a very rare finding in the developed world, but may still be endemic in some underdeveloped countries. Urodynamic studies often demonstrate UAB with reduced or absent bladder sensation and increased bladder capacity. Suprasacral and sacral cord lesions may disturb the innervation of detrusor, leading to reduced bladder compliance, detrusor overactivity with detrusor–sphincter dyssynergia, or detrusor underactivity with high residual urine volume (Hattori et al. 1990).

Herpes Zoster and Herpes Simplex

Herpes zoster (HZ) is an acute viral infection caused by the varicella–zoster virus (VZV). It is usually a localized painful mononeuropathy associated with a vesicular eruption limited to the dermatome innervated by the nerve from a single spinal or cranial sensory ganglion. The rate of occurrence of urinary retention as a complication of herpes zoster is thought to be 4 % (Broseta et al. 1993). Chen et al. (2002) reviewed 423 patients infected by HZ and found that 17 (4 %) patients had real voiding dysfunction. Among them, the dermatomes of involvement were 14 (82 %) in the sacral area, 2 in the lumbar (12 %), and 1 in the thoracic (6 %). Four (24 %) of the 17 patients were classified as having neuritis-associated voiding dysfunction. They are clinically manifested with urinary retention and a reduced or absent filling sensation. Urodynamic studies were performed on 3 patients, and all revealed an UAB.

Guillain–Barré Syndrome

Guillain–Barré syndrome is an immune-mediated neuropathy affecting both small and large myelinated axons, causing acute progressive weakness. The syndrome is characterized by rapidly progressive signs of motor weakness and paresthesia progressing from the lower to upper extremities. The voiding dysfunction and related urodynamic studies are infrequently reported in Guillain–Barré syndrome (GBS). Sixty-five GBS patients were evaluated urodynamically by Sakakibara et al. (2009) and the result showed that 28 % of the patients had urinary dysfunction, including urinary retention in 9 %.

Pelvic Surgery

Pelvic nerve damage and bladder resection are the most common causes of postoperative voiding dysfunction after extirpative pelvic surgery. Both the storage and micturition functions of the bladder can be affected by the damage of pelvic surgery, and it may also unmask underlying voiding dysfunction such as bladder outlet obstruction. Symptoms of postoperative voiding dysfunction include frank urinary retention, decreased force of stream, urinary strain, hesitancy, intermittency, sense of residual, frequency, urgency, incontinence, and nocturia (Wagner and Russo 2000). Voiding dysfunction can also occur after abdominoperineal resection and hysterectomy.

Voiding dysfunction seen after pelvic surgery for rectal cancer may be caused by the damage to the sacral nerves that also innervate the urinary bladder. In addition, posterior tilting of the bladder that may occur after abdominoperineal resection could also cause difficulty in bladder emptying. The diagnosis of neurogenic bladder can be confirmed with a denervation supersensitivity test (Havenga et al. 2000). The most common urodynamic findings after abdominoperineal resection include detrusor underactivity with impaired sensation, increased capacity, and compliance with concomitant incompetence of the bladder neck, suggesting a combined injury to both parasympathetic and sympathetic innervation.

Similar to the pelvic surgery with APR for rectal cancer, the performance of radical hysterectomy has long been associated with the development of postoperative bladder dysfunction (Gilbaz et al. 2013). Patients after radical hysterectomy can suffer from voiding dysfunction caused by parasympathetic denervation.

Tseng et al. (2012) compared the feasibility and complications between nerve-sparing radical hysterectomy and conventional radical hysterectomy. A modified nerve-sparing radical hysterectomy was performed in 15 patients and none of them required intermittent catheterization. All 12 patients who underwent radical hysterectomy needed self-catheterization after discharge.

Management of DM and Neurogenic UAB

Generally, treatment of UAB caused by DM or neurologic diseases should be determined by the urodynamic findings. Current medical treatment for UAB includes the use of muscarinic receptor agonists, such as bethanechol, to stimulate detrusor muscarinic receptors or choline esterase inhibitors, like distigmine, to reduce the degradation of acetylcholine. α-Adrenergic blockers are also used to reduce urethral outlet resistance. However, available evidence shows that only limited beneficial effects can be obtained in preventing or treating UAB by oral medicine (Miyazato et al. 2013; Andersson 2014).

UAB may respond to physiotherapy in the form of maneuvers to facilitate detrusor activity. Activation of stretch receptors in the bladder wall can trigger a detrusor contraction, and so pressing or tapping over the bladder may initiate a detrusor contraction. However, suprapubic tapping and straining are risky maneuvers and should not be used in patients with increased intravesical pressure or vesicoureteral reflux.

For the DM or neurogenic UAB patients with urinary retention, clean intermittent catheterization is preferable to a chronic indwelling catheter. The most frequently used strategy for bladder rehabilitation is CIC (Hagen and Rekand 2014). Castel-Lacanal et al. (2013) prospectively evaluated the impact of clean intermittent catheterization on the quality of life of patients affected by MS and found that intermittent catheterization is well accepted and reduces the impact of urinary dysfunction on their quality of life. Clean intermittent catheterization should be continued until the return of bladder contractility. A period of at least 6 months should pass before considering any definitive surgical intervention in the patient with sphincteric incontinence or poor compliance, as the natural history of peripheral nerve injury suggests that function may return over time. However, the DM UAB is an end stage of bladder complication and is irreversible.

Neuromodulation and intravesical electrical stimulation has been reported to be potentially beneficial in selected patients. According to previous animal studies, to induce micturition, the perineal afferents must activate the parasympathetic excitatory inputs to the bladder but must also suppress the urethral sympathetic and sphincter somatic guarding reflexes. A suppression of guarding reflexes by sacral nerve stimulation (SNS), a urologic technique that has proved safe and minimally invasive, contributes to enhancement of voiding in patients with urinary retention (Miyazato et al. 2013). Pudendal afferent signaling serves as a common crossroad in the neurologic wiring of the lower urinary tract. Pudendal afferent inputs turn on voiding reflexes by suppressing the guarding reflex pathways, and pudendal afferent inputs to the sacral spinal cord also can turn off supraspinally mediated voiding reflex by blocking ascending sensory inputs (Leng and Chancellor 2005).

Conclusion

UAB can result from a variety of neurologic diseases, including central nervous system disorder and peripheral neuropathy. Pelvic surgery and trauma can also cause UAB. Diabetic patients with urinary tract symptoms, large bladder capacity, elevated residual urine volume, and urinary tract infections should undergo urodynamic evaluation for the detection of detrusor underactivity. However, due to the asymptomatic characteristic at the incipient stage of diabetic UAB, early diagnosis is still an unmet medical need. A reliable UAB questionnaire may help to identify the real prevalence of UAB in DM or neuropathic patients. Careful urodynamic evaluation is essential to determine the etiology of LUT symptoms and to screen for any urologic risk factors. Effective pharmacologic therapy for neurogenic UAB is still lacking and represents an important unmet medical need.

References

Allgot B, Gan D, King H et al (2003) Diabetes atlas: executive summary, 2nd edn. International Diabetes Federation, Brussels

Amarenco G, Chartier-Kastler E, Denys P, Jean JL, de Sèze M, Lubetzski C (2013a) First-line urological evaluation in multiple sclerosis: validation of a specific decision-making algorithm. Mult Scler J 19:1931–1937

Amarenco G, Raibaut P, Hubeaux K, Jousse M, Sheikh IS, Lapeyre E (2013b) Autonomic nervous system alteration in multiple sclerosis patients with urinary symptoms. Clinical, urodynamic and cardiovascular study. Prog Urol 23:1505

Amarenco G, de Sèze M, Ruffion A, Sheikh Ismael S (2014) Clinical and urodynamic evaluations of urinary disorders in multiple sclerosis. Ann Phys Rehabil Med 57:277–287

Andersson KE (2014) The many faces of impaired bladder emptying. Curr Opin Urol 24:363–369

Bansal R, Agarwal MM, Modi M, Mandal AK, Singh SK (2011) Urodynamic profile of diabetic patients with lower urinary tract symptoms: association of diabetic cystopathy with autonomic and peripheral neuropathy. Urology 77:699–705

Brittain K, Perry S, Peet S, Shaw C, Dallosso H, Assassa R, Williams K, Jagger C, Potter J, Castleden C (2000) Prevalence and impact of urinary symptoms among community-dwelling stroke survivors. Stroke 31:886–891

Broseta E, Osca JM, Morera J, Martinez-Agullo E, Jimenez-Cruz JF (1993) Urological manifestations of herpes zoster. Eur Urol 24:244–247

Castel-Lacanal E, Game X, De Boissezon X, Guillotreau J, Braley-Berthoumieux E, Terracol C, Gasq D, Labrunee M, Viala F, Rischmann P, Clanet M and Marque P (2013) Impact of intermittent catheterization on the quality of life of multiple sclerosis patients. World J Urol 31:1445–1450

Chancellor MB, Blaivas JG (1995) Chapter 14. Diabetic neurogenic bladder. In: Chancellor MB, Blaivas JG (eds) Practical neuro-urology: genitourinary complications in neurologic disease. Butterworth Heinemann, Stoneham, pp 149–154

Chang CH, Shau WY, Jiang YD et al (2010) Type 2 diabetes prevalence and incidence among adults in Taiwan during 1999–2004: a national health insurance data set study. Diabet Med 27:636–643

Chen PH, Hsueh HF, Hong CZ (2002) Herpes zoster-associated voiding dysfunction: a retrospective study and literature review. Arch Phys Med Rehabil 83:1624–1628

Daneshgari F, Liu G, Birder L, Hanna-Mitchell AT, Chacko S (2009) Diabetic bladder dysfunction: current translational knowledge. J Urol 182:S18–S26

de Sèze M, Ruffion A, Denys P, Joseph P-A, Perrouin-Verbe B & group IFN-Ues (2007) The neurogenic bladder in multiple sclerosis: review of the literature and proposal of management guidelines. Mult Scler 13:915–928

Dong D, Xu Z, Shi B, Chen J, Jiang X, Wang H (2006) Urodynamic study in the neurogenic bladder dysfunction caused by intervertebral disk hernia. Neurourol Urodyn 25:446–450

Frimodt-Moller C (1980) Diabetic cystopathy: epidemiology and related disorders. Ann Intern Med 92:318–321

Gilbaz E, Gungor Ugurlucan F, Aslay I, Yalcin O (2013) The effects of simple and radical hysterectomy and radiotherapy on lower urinary tract symptoms and urodynamics. Eur J Gynaecol Oncol 34:248–253

Guariguata L, Whiting DR, Hambleton I et al (2014) Global estimates of diabetes prevalence for 2013 and projections for 2035. Diabetes Res Clin Pract 103:137–149

Hagen EM, Rekand T (2014) Management of bladder dysfunction and satisfaction of life after spinal cord injury in Norway. J Spinal Cord Med 37:310–316

Han K-S, Heo SH, Lee S-J, Jeon SH, Yoo KH (2010) Comparison of urodynamics between ischemic and hemorrhagic stroke patients; Can we suggest the category of urinary dysfunction in patients with cerebrovascular accident according to type of stroke? NeurourolUrodyn 29:387–390

Hattori T, Yasuda K, Kita K, Hirayama K (1990) Disorders of micturition in tabes dorsalis. Br J Urol 65:497–499

Havenga K, Maas CP, DeRuiter MC, Welvaart K, Trimbos JB (2000) Avoiding long-term disturbance to bladder and sexual function in pelvic surgery, particularly with rectal cancer. Semin Surg Oncol 18:235–243

He CX, Yuan ZY, Yan SB, Wu CW, Huang YC, He W et al (2014) Clinical and urodynamic evaluation of women referred with diabetes mellitus. Int Urogynecol J 25:979–983

Hellstrom P, Kortelainen P, Kontturi M (1986) Late urodynamic findings after surgery for cauda equina syndrome caused by a prolapsed lumbar intervertebral disk. J Urol 135:308–312

Kaplan SA, Te AE, Blaivas JG (1995) Urodynamic findings in patients with diabetic cystopathy. J Urol 153:342–344

Kebapci N, Yenilmez A, Efe B, Entok E, Demirustu C (2007) Bladder dysfunction in type 2 diabetic patients. Neurourol Urodyn 26:814–819

Kong KH, Young S (2000) Incidence and outcome of poststroke urinary retention: a prospective study. Arch Phys Med Rehabil 81:1464–1467

Lawrence JM, Lukacz ES, Liu IL et al (2007) Pelvic floor disorders, diabetes, and obesity in women: findings from the Kaiser Permanente Continence Associated Risk Epidemiology Study. Diabetes Care 30:2536–2541

Lebovitch S, Mydlo JH (2008) HIV-AIDS: urologic considerations. Urol Clin North Am 35:59–68

Lee WC, Wu HP, Tai TY, Yu HJ, Chiang PH (2009) Investigation of urodynamic characteristics and bladder sensory function in the early stages of diabetic bladder dysfunction in women with type 2 diabetes. J Urol 181:198–203

Leng WW, Chancellor MB (2005) How sacral nerve stimulation neuromodulation works. Urol Clin North Am 32:11–18

Lin TL, Chen GD, Chen YC, Huang CN, Ng SC (2012) Aging and recurrent urinary tract infections are associated with bladder dysfunction in type 2 diabetes. Taiwan J Obstet Gynecol 51:381–386

Litwiller SE, Frohman EM, Zimmern PE (1999) Multiple sclerosis and the urologist. J Urol 161:743–757

Liu RT, Chung MS, Lee WC, Chang SW, Huang ST, Yang KD, Chancellor MB, Chuang YC (2011) Prevalence of overactive bladder (OAB) and associated risk factors in 1,359 patients with type 2 diabetes. Urology 78:1040–1045

Miyazato M, Yoshimura N, Chancellor MB (2013) The other bladder syndrome: underactive bladder. Rev Urol 15:11–22

Pizzi A, Falsini C, Martini M, Rossetti MA, Verdesca S, Tosto A (2014) Urinary incontinence after ischemic stroke: clinical and urodynamic studies. NeurourolUrodyn 33:420–425

Rabadi MH, Aston C (2014) Complications and urologic risks of neurogenic bladder in veterans with traumatic spinal cord injury. Spinal Cord. doi:10.1038/sc.2014.205. PMID: 25403501

Sakakibara R, Uchiyama T, Kuwabara S, Mori M, Ito T, Yamamoto T, Awa Y, Yamaguchi C, Yuki N, Vernino S, Kishi M, Shirai K (2009) Prevalence and mechanism of bladder dysfunction in Guillain-Barre Syndrome. NeurourolUrodyn 28:432–437

Sakakibara R, Tateno F, Nagao T, Yamamoto T, Uchiyama T, Yamanishi T, Yano M, Kishi M, Tsuyusaki Y, Aiba Y (2014) Bladder function of patients with Parkinson's disease. Int J Urol 21:638–646

Sasaki K, Yoshimura N, Chancellor MB (2003) Implications of diabetes mellitus in urology. Urol Clin North Am 30:1–12

Tseng CJ, Shen HP, Lin YH, Lee CY, Wei-Cheng Chiu W (2012) A prospective study of nerve-sparing radical hysterectomy for uterine cervical carcinoma in Taiwan. Taiwan J Obstet Gynecol 51:55–59

Uchiyama T, Sakakibara R, Yamamoto T, Ito T, Yamaguchi C, Awa Y, Yanagisawa M, Higuchi Y, Sato Y, Ichikawa T, Yamanishi T, Hattori T, Kuwabara S (2011) Urinary dysfunction in early and untreated Parkinson's disease. J Neurol Neurosurg Psychiatry 82:1382–1386

Van Poppel H, Stessens R, van Damme B et al (1988) Diabetic cystopathy: neuropathological examination of urinary bladder biopsies. Eur Urol 15:128–131

Wagner JR, Russo P (2000) Urologic complications of major pelvic surgery. Semin Surg Oncol 18:216–228

Watanabe T, Miyagawa I (1999) Characteristics of detrusor contractility during micturition in diabetics. Neurourol Urodyn 18:163–171

Yamaguchi C, Sakakibara R, Uchiyama T et al (2007) Overactive bladder in diabetes: a peripheral or central mechanism? Neurourol Urodyn 26:807–813

Yoshimura N, Chancellor MB, Andersson KE et al (2005) Recent advances in understanding the biology of diabetes-associated bladder complications and novel therapy. BJU Int 95:733–738

Yu HJ, Lee WC, Liu SP, Tai TY, Wu HP, Chen J (2004) Unrecognized voiding difficulty in female type 2 diabetic patients in the diabetes clinic: a prospective case-control study. Diabetes Care 27:988–989

Chapter 12
Geriatric Urology and Underactive Bladder

Marcus A. Austenfeld and Tomas L. Griebling

Introduction

According to the most recent published data from the United States Department of Health and Human Services, as of 2012, there were 43.1 million people aged 65 years or older, which represents 14 % of the total US population (U.S. Department of Health and Human Services 2013). The number of Americans who will reach 65 years of age in the next two decades increased by 24 % between 2002 and 2012. As a population, these patients are not only growing in number but are also experiencing increased overall longevity. Between 1980 and 2012, there was a 93 % increase in the number of people over 100 years of age living in the USA. This is a worldwide phenomenon, and similar increases are occurring in most developed countries. As the worldwide population lives longer and expects higher quality of life during those later years, attention must be turned to common geriatric health issues such as voiding dysfunction. This is a rapidly expanding portion of our population but one that is at great risk for possible neglect and mismanagement. Too often both clinicians and lay people attribute significant changes in urinary function to simply "growing older." Because of this, older adults may suffer unnecessarily from manageable clinical conditions that can substantially diminish functional status and quality of life and can potentially hasten institutionalization or even death. It has been estimated that 30 % of older adults admitted to nursing homes are placed in long-term care at least in part due to urinary incontinence (Nordling 2002).

M.A. Austenfeld, MD
Department of Urology, School of Medicine, The University of Kansas,
Kansas City, KS, USA

T.L. Griebling, MD, MPH (✉)
Department of Urology, School of Medicine, The Landon Center on Aging,
The University of Kansas, 3901 Rainbow Boulevard, Kansas City, KS 66160, USA
e-mail: tgriebling@kumc.edu

M.B. Chancellor, A.C. Diokno (eds.), *The Underactive Bladder*,
DOI 10.1007/978-3-319-23687-2_12

Detrusor underactivity is an important component that can contribute to lower urinary tract dysfunction in the geriatric population. The prevalence of underactive bladder (UAB) is estimated to be between 40 and 48 % in men and 12–38 % in women over 65 years of age (Abarbanel and Marcus 2007; Jeong et al. 2012; Resnick et al. 1989). Although there is a spectrum of clinical impact associated with detrusor underactivity, clinicians need to be able to differentiate between normal aging processes that affect the bladder, non-pathological changes in voiding habits, and bothersome or pathological changes in bladder function. Changes associated with other comorbid conditions and outcomes related to treatment interventions also need to be identified. Geriatric patients are more likely to underreport their symptoms compared to younger people and are at greater risk of living with silent urinary retention (Shah and Badlani 2002). Although a patient who voids infrequently and has rare urinary incontinence may be more convenient for caregivers, he or she is at increased risk for urinary tract infection (UTI), upper urinary tract deterioration, and development of worsening lower urinary tract symptoms.

Etiology of UAB in Older Adults

The causes of detrusor underactivity as a result of the typical aging process remain controversial. The bladder should remain adequately elastic and contractile despite a patient's age, and urinary incontinence should not be considered either an inevitable or normal part of aging (Elbadawi et al. 1997). Although several animal models have been developed to evaluate detrusor underactivity, the true relationship between microscopic and cellular changes to clinically significant bladder behavior is unclear, and the association between aging and detrusor underactivity is likely multifactorial.

Electron microscopy studies have demonstrated a number of changes that occur in the bladder with aging. These include widening of interstitial spaces between muscle cells and decreased numbers of intracellular receptor vesicles known as "caveolae" in aged detrusor muscle fibers, leading to the "dense band" pattern of muscle structure dedifferentiation (Elbadawi et al. 1993; Taylor and Kuchel 2006). This is thought to lead to an overall decrease in the maximum contractile power of the bladder (Griebling et al. 2014). Bladder innervation also changes with advancing age. The number of neurons in the bladder wall declines, and the ability to sense volume tends to decrease (Gilpin et al. 1986; Hotta et al. 1995). Over time, the smooth muscle to collagen ratio tends to decrease, and this may in part lead to reduced bladder contractility and changes in bladder compliance and maximum capacity.

Long-standing partial bladder outlet obstruction may also play a role in subsequent bladder decompensation. This has been characterized as a two-stage process. In the first phase, the bladder remains stable in both size and contractility despite partial obstruction. However, over time, the bladder decompensates and contractility tends to decline, leading either to a thin-walled fibrotic bladder with increased capacity and poor contractility or a thick-walled, low capacity, and poorly contractile bladder (Gosling et al. 2000). Bladder ischemia has also been postulated as a potential causative factor for underactive bladder in both animal models and in humans (Nomiya et al. 2012). Studies utilizing pelvic ultrasound have shown associations between decreased arterial flow to the bladder and detrusor dysfunction (Pinggera et al. 2008). Chronic overdistension of the bladder has also been postulated to cause temporary bladder ischemia which could lead to eventual detrusor dysfunction and UAB (Wada et al. 2012).

Diabetes mellitus, one of the most common comorbid conditions seen in older adults, may also play a role as a contributing factor to bladder dysfunction in geriatric patients. Patients with long-standing and poorly controlled diabetes may be at particular risk for developing what has been termed "diabetic cystopathy" (Yuan et al. 2015). This may be due to both neurogenic and myogenic factors. Sensation of bladder filling may change in some diabetic patients over time, and this can lead to prolonged intervoiding intervals. With time, bladder ischemia may contribute to this process and lead to subsequent bladder dysfunction. It is hypothesized that improved blood glucose control and better bladder hygiene with regular voiding habits may help to prevent these types of problems with advancing age in diabetic patients (Gomez et al. 2011).

Although the specific etiology of detrusor underactivity can be obscure, the geriatric patient with lower urinary tract symptoms is prone to a variety of medical comorbidities that merit additional investigation. Table 12.1 summarizes some of the more common comorbid conditions associated with urinary retention and incomplete bladder emptying in older adults. The most common etiologies of urinary retention in elderly men include bladder outlet obstruction from benign prostatic hyperplasia or urethral stricture. Outlet obstruction is quite uncommon in elderly women, who tend to be more prone to urinary incontinence. However, severe pelvic organ prolapse can lead to anatomic obstruction and difficulty voiding. Some of these patients describe having to use a finger in the vagina to reduce the prolapse in order to void spontaneously. Older adults often have problems with mobility that may limit physical transfers, which can lead to an increased risk of falls as patients rush to the toilet or predispose to skin breakdown and decubitus ulcers due to skin irritation from urinary leakage.

What Is "Normal" Geriatric Voiding?

Development of nocturia is a common change in voiding patterns that occur with advancing age. This can lead to negative outcomes on sleep quality and other aspects of quality of life. As age increases, the circadian rhythm of urine production shifts, and there is a greater volume of total urine production at night compared to during the day (Miller 2000). Nakamura and colleagues demonstrated a significant increase in urinary frequency between midnight and 6 am in elderly patients (Nakamura et al. 1996). A cohort study of 935 otherwise healthy men demonstrated that those

Table 12.1 Comorbid conditions in older adults that may predispose to urinary retention and incomplete bladder emptying

Comorbid condition	Direct and indirect effects
Benign prostatic hyperplasia (BPH)	Bladder outlet obstruction
Cognitive impairment (delirium, dementia)	Decreased sensation of filling
	Reduced awareness of need to void
Diabetes mellitus	Decreased sensation of filling
	Reduced awareness of need to void
	Diminished bladder contractility
Mobility impairment	Decreased ability to reach toilet facilities
	Increased bladder overdistension
Multiple sclerosis	Alterations in contractility
Parkinson's disease	Alterations in contractility
	Decreased ability to reach toilet facilities
Pelvic organ prolapse	Bladder outlet obstruction
Spinal cord injury	Alterations in contractility
	Decreased ability to reach toilet facilities
Spinal stenosis	Alterations in contractility
	Decreased ability to reach toilet facilities
Stroke	Decreased sensation of bladder filling
	Reduced awareness of need to void
	Alterations in contractility
	Decreased ability to reach toilet facilities
Urethral stricture	Bladder outlet obstruction

over 63 years of age had an average voided volume of 200 mL and had around 6 voids each day with an average of one each night (Huang Foen Chung and van Mastrigt 2009). This was in contrast to the comparison group of younger men, aged 38–62 years, who typically voided larger volumes and had between 5.5 and 6.0 voids daily, with 0–1 voids each night. Every participant had International Prostate Symptom Scores less than 10, suggesting mild lower urinary tract symptoms and a minimal contribution from prostatic hyperplasia. Clinical judgment must play a role in defining urinary frequency and bothersome nocturia for each patient, as confounding factors such as medications and regional variations in diet and activity preclude gross generalization of urinary habits in all older people.

Clinical Evaluation

Although it may seem obvious that a thorough history and physical examination is necessary in delineating the etiology of a geriatric patient's urinary dysfunction, these patients often require patience and coaching from their providers. Many receive clinical care from others or may have memory issues, comorbidities, or polypharmacy which could mask symptoms. The use of directed questions and prompting may be necessary. Visser and colleagues found that 64 % of women aged 55 years or older with urinary incontinence had not discussed their symptoms with their primary care provider (Visser et al. 2012). Urinary retention in the older patients is frequently multifactorial. Detrusor underactivity can be the result of chronic medical conditions such as Parkinson's disease, stroke, spinal cord trauma, or poorly controlled diabetes with subsequent neurogenic or myogenic dysfunction (Kebapci et al. 2007; Thorne and Geraci 2009).

Symptoms associated with urinary retention include weakened urinary stream, urinary tract infection, inability to urinate, or worsened constipation (Tan et al. 2001). Patients with complaints of recurrent urinary tract infections should be evaluated for the possibility of underlying urinary retention and incomplete bladder emptying. A voiding diary can be a useful adjunct measure, especially if the patient or caregivers can perform measurement of urine output and clean intermittent catheterization to measure postvoid volumes. More structured urodynamic evaluation may be useful to provide objective measures of bladder function in select patients. This can be particularly helpful in guiding treatment decisions, especially if prior treatments have been unsuccessful.

Elevated postvoid residual volumes can be measured either by catheterization or bladder ultrasound. In the geriatric population, intermittent catheterization can be invasive and uncomfortable, with the potential risk of introducing bacteria into the bladder. Ultrasound technology offers the benefit of being noninvasive and has been shown to be reasonably accurate and with reproducible results in the hands of trained staff (Ouslander et al. 1994; Borrie et al. 2001). However, the device is somewhat expensive and not every clinical setting will have access to this equipment. Currently, there is no clear consensus on what constitutes an abnormal PVR, particularly among geriatric patients. Volumes between 50 and 300 mL have all been used to define retention, and practitioners need to use these volumes as guidelines rather than absolute targets. In most settings, a volume of 100–150 mL may be a reasonable compromise.

Detrusor Hyperactivity with Impaired Contractility (DHIC)

The condition known as DHIC, or detrusor hyperactivity with impaired contractility, was first characterized by Resnick and Yalla in 1987 in a series of women with both urge urinary incontinence and elevated postvoid residual volumes associated with poor bladder contractility (Resnick and Yalla 1987). Pharmacological management of urinary urgency and urgency incontinence is usually contraindicated in patients with elevated postvoid residual volumes. This can make treatment of the condition more challenging and may also require the use of clean intermittent catheterization to regularly empty the bladder. Although bladder outlet obstruction has been shown in animal models to contribute to detrusor underactivity, men with DHIC or even pure detrusor underactivity may have their symptoms incorrectly attributed to purely BPH alone and undergo unnecessary surgical procedures to relieve obstruction. Thomas and colleagues demonstrated that men who underwent transurethral resection of the prostate with underlying detrusor underactivity experienced no significant symptomatic or urodynamic changes, compared to men with bladder outlet obstruction alone (Thomas et al. 2004). Because of this, urodynamic studies may be particularly useful to differentiate between these types of patients.

In a population of 181 men and women aged 70 years or older with LUTS, Abarbanel et al. found that 48 % of the men had impaired detrusor contractility, and of them, 67 % had associated detrusor hyperactivity (Abarbanel and Marcus 2007). Only 10 % had isolated bladder outlet obstruction, and 45 % had pure detrusor hyperactivity. Among the women in this study, impaired contractility was seen in 12 %, and half of these patients also had detrusor hyperactivity. Overall, only 32 % had pure detrusor overactivity. Regardless of gender, history of urinary retention or presence of indwelling catheter predicted those with detrusor underactivity. Because treatment of urgency urinary incontinence will paradoxically worsen the symptoms of patients with DHIC, older adults presenting with these symptoms should be carefully evaluated for underlying detrusor underactivity prior to initiation of pharmacologic or other therapy.

Medications and Urinary Retention in Older Adults

Approximately 80 % of people aged 65 years and older take an average of 2.9 prescription medications daily (American Geriatrics Society 2012 Beers Criteria Update Expert Panel 2012). In the geriatric population, critical attention must be paid to the potential adverse effects of medications, including drug-drug interactions, some of which may cause voiding dysfunction. Geriatric patients experience alterations in both pharmacokinetics and pharmacodynamics due to physiological alterations associated with the normal aging process. Absorption of medications may be slower, drug distribution may be altered by decreased lean muscle mass and increased adipose tissue, and both renal and hepatic metabolism may be diminished with advancing age (Willlams 2002). In order to help guide practitioners through these risks, the American Geriatrics Society recently published the fourth updated version of the Beers Criteria (American Geriatrics Society 2012 Beers Criteria Update Expert Panel 2012). These evidence-based recommendations can be useful in helping to avoid potentially inappropriate medications in this more vulnerable older population.

Medications with anticholinergic effects must be used with great caution due to potential worsening of urinary retention and constipation. One study of 738,004 men aged 20–84 years who were prescribed anticholinergic medications for lower urinary tract symptoms found a relative risk of acute urinary retention of 8.3 (95 %) within the first 30 days of therapy, although the relative risk decreased to 2.0 (95 %) with longer duration of use (Martin-Merino et al. 2009). Older patients are also more sensitive to the risk of dry mouth and xerostomia which can influence swallowing function and increase the risk of gingivitis and other tooth and gum disease. Other potential side effects of these medications include increased confusion and delirium and potential orthostatic hypotension. Glaucoma is common in older adults, and the anticholinergic medications are contraindicated in patients with a history of narrow angle, sometimes called closed angle glaucoma.

Opiate analgesics tend to increase external urethral sphincter tone and decrease the sensation of bladder fullness. They can also decrease overall mobility and increase risk for delirium in some older adults. The risk of urinary retention associated with these medications appears to be higher with the longer-acting pain medication (Darrah et al. 2009). Similarly, general anesthetics promote smooth muscle relaxation and can contribute to postoperative urinary retention. The risk is even higher in those patients treated with epidural pain management, with retention rates up to 23 % in some studies (Darrah et al. 2009).

Other types of medications commonly used by older adults which can worsen urinary retention include antiarrhythmics, antidepressants, antiepileptics, benzodiazepines, muscle relaxants, and neuroleptics used in the treatment of Parkinson's disease and other neurologic conditions (Miller 2000). Alpha-1 antagonists, particularly the nonselective agents, commonly prescribed to elderly men for the treatment of benign prostatic hyperplasia can induce or worsen orthostatic hypotension. These agents may be useful for the treatment of voiding dysfunction due to outlet obstruction but should be monitored closely.

Treatment of Acute Urinary Retention

Older adults are at greater risk of developing acute urinary retention. Jacobsen et al. demonstrated that a 60-year-old man has an approximately 23 % risk of developing an episode of acute urinary retention in the next 5 years of life (Jacobsen et al. 1997). Although this can be the acute result of exacerbation of other underlying comorbidity such as BPH or neurologic disorders, patients with detrusor underactivity may transition to acute urinary retention as well. This is best managed by immediate catheterization with bladder decompression.

Ongoing management may require addition of pharmacotherapies or treatment with clean intermittent catheterization if the patient remains unable to void adequately. Indwelling catheterization can be considered but is generally avoided for long-term management if possible due to risks of other complications including urinary tract infection, catheter colonization, bladder stones, or urothelial malignancy. Careful monitoring is needed to assess the effects of therapy and to identify any complications early, so appropriate treatment can be instituted.

Conservative Management of Incomplete Bladder Emptying

The impact of detrusor underactivity on older patients can range from minimal to severe. As previously discussed, an elevated PVR alone should be handled with prudence and taken in context of an overall clinical evaluation. Many patients respond well to conservative measures such as scheduled toileting, prompted voiding, or other treatments, particularly with the assistance of caregivers when needed. Double voiding, defined as urinating again after a brief delay from the initial void, can help to better empty the bladder in some patients. Bothersome nocturia may be improved by decreasing fluid intake several hours before retiring to bed. Patients with dependent edema in the lower extremities or an element of congestive heart failure may benefit from reclining with their legs elevated for a time before going to bed for the night. Timing of diuretic use is important, and these medications should be taken in the morning or early afternoon rather than closer to bedtime. Pelvic floor physical therapy and biofeedback training can be helpful in promoting urge suppression and may help with muscle relaxation during the voiding effort.

Urinary Catheterization in Older Adults

For those patients who fail voiding trials and have symptomatic urinary retention, clean intermittent catheterization is often the preferred method of management. Providers may have some hesitation about considering this treatment for older adults. There may be concern about the ability of an older adult to perform CIC on their own due to changes in cognition or hand dexterity. Assistance from caregivers may be needed in some cases. Clean intermittent catheterization has routinely been demonstrated to be safe and effective in older adults, with success rates reported between 82 and 95 % in patients over 65 years of age (Bennett and Diokno 1984; Parsons et al. 2012). Pilloni and colleagues demonstrated that in 21 patients over 70 years old with urinary retention who were started on a CIC schedule, 57 % could catheterize themselves independently (including one patient who was blind), 33 % were catheterized successfully by their partners, and 10 % by nurses or health-care aides (Pilloni et al. 2005). Overall, 86 % of patients in this study reported significant improvements in quality of life. Due to cost concerns, a clean rather than sterile technique is generally appropriate. One study looking at residents of a Veteran's Affairs nursing home and average age of 72 years found no significant differences between clean and sterile catheterization techniques regarding time to first urinary tract infection, or number of treatment episodes, and demonstrated an annual cost savings of $1460 per patient (Duffy et al. 1995).

About 5 % of nursing home residents have a chronic indwelling catheter, but nursing home residents who are catheterized for more than 76 % of their days in facilities are more than three times more likely to die within a year (Kunin et al. 1992; Rogers et al. 2008). The use of a chronic indwelling catheter is associated with increased risks of catheter colonization, urinary tract infection, limitations in mobility, urethral irritation and bladder spasms, bladder sediment and stone formation, urethritis, prostatitis, and epididymitis. Tension on the catheter or the balloon at the bladder neck can lead to urethral or bladder neck erosion and urinary incontinence. Repair and reconstruction of these types of injuries can be complex, particularly in elderly patients. Suprapubic catheter placement can obviate some of these risks for traumatic hypospadias or urethral or bladder neck erosion. However, rates of infection do not seem to be substantially different compared to urethral Foley catheters, and the placement does require a minor surgical procedure (Tenke et al. 2014). Chronic catheterization is also associated with an increased risk of bladder malignancy, particularly squamous cell carcinoma. Annual surveillance with cystoscopy is typically recommended in patients managed with either urethral or suprapubic catheters. Indwelling catheters are a useful short-term solution, but long-term catheterization must be a decision that is weighed carefully by physicians, patients, and their loved ones, with frequent reevaluation of catheter duration, benefit, and constant observation for potential side effects.

Sacral Neuromodulation and Older Adults

Sacral neuromodulation may be an effective intervention for some elderly patients with underactive bladder. This is clinically indicated in some patients with nonobstructive urinary retention and incomplete bladder emptying. The therapy offers several potential benefits including avoidance of medications which could be associated with polypharmacy or drug-drug interactions in geriatric patients. It may also be useful in those who either cannot perform or have not responded to other forms of behavioral therapy. Placement does require two short outpatient surgical procedures. One challenge in this particular population is that patients need to be actively engaged in changing device settings in response to their bladder symptoms. The programming device can be daunting for some patients who may be less technologically adept or in those with impaired cognition or hand dexterity. Other patients with other neurological conditions who need regular magnetic resonance imaging (MRI) examinations may not be good candidates for neuromodulation. Although some patients can undergo brain MRI with special imaging methods, body MRI is usually contraindicated in those with an implanted neurostimulator. Although these considerations must be taken into account when making decisions about this therapy, age alone should not be the sole factor against this therapy in older adults.

White et al. looked at a single center experience for sacral nerve stimulator placement in female patients 70 years or older with refractory overactive bladder and found that at a mean follow-up of 4 years, 65 % of geriatric patients had a functional generator with over 50 % improvement in symptoms (White et al. 2009). No significant difference in reprogramming requirements was appreciated between older patients and younger patients, although older patients tended to opt for device removal when perceived as ineffective. Although these data are promising, research on sacral neuromodulation in elderly patients is more limited than in younger adults, particularly for the indication of urinary retention. However, for appropriately screened candidates, sacral neuromodulation may be a viable treatment option.

Conclusions

Underactive bladder is a relatively common condition among older adults, although it should not be considered either a normal or inevitable part of the aging process. A wide variety of comorbidities and other factors appear to be associated with development of UAB in this population, and the etiology is likely multifactorial. Clinical evaluation is vital to understanding the potential causes of underactive bladder for a given patient and helps to guide selection of therapy. Treatment should be goal oriented and focus on specific needs of patients and their caregivers. Special consideration may be needed in geriatric patients with regard to interaction with underlying comorbidities and need for caregiver support, particularly for catheterization protocols. Whenever possible, clean intermittent catheterization is preferred as a treatment compared to indwelling catheterization. Ongoing follow-up is important to determine adequacy of treatment and to help identify and prevent complications. Successful treatment of underactive bladder may help to improve overall health and quality of life for older adults.

References

Abarbanel J, Marcus EL (2007) Impaired detrusor contractility in community-dwelling elderly presenting with lower urinary tract symptoms. Urology 69:436–440. 2007/03/27 edn. doi:10.1016/j.urology.2006.11.019

American Geriatrics Society 2012 Beers Criteria Update Expert Panel (2012) American Geriatrics Society updated Beers Criteria for potentially inappropriate medication use in older adults. J Am Geriatr Soc 60:616–631. 2012/03/02 edn. doi:10.1111/j.1532-5415.2012.03923.x

AoA U.S. Department of Health and Human Services A Profile of Older Americans (2013) http://www.aoaaclgov/Aging_Statistics/Profile/2013/docs/2013_Profilepdf. Accessed 2 Feb 2015

Bennett CJ, Diokno AC (1984) Clean intermittent self-catheterization in the elderly. Urology 24:43–45. 1984/07/01 edn

Borrie MJ, Campbell K, Arcese ZA, Bray J, Hart P, Labate T, Hesch P (2001) Urinary retention in patients in a geriatric rehabilitation unit: prevalence, risk factors, and validity of bladder scan evaluation. Rehabil Nurs (Off J Assoc Rehabil Nurs) 26:187–191. 2002/05/31 edn

Darrah DM, Griebling TL, Silverstein JH (2009) Postoperative urinary retention. Anesthesiol Clin 27:465–484. 2009/10/15 edn. doi:10.1016/j.anclin.2009.07.010

Duffy LM, Cleary J, Ahern S, Kuskowski MA, West M, Wheeler L, Mortimer JA (1995) Clean intermittent catheterization: safe, cost-effective bladder management for male residents of VA nursing homes. J Am Geriatr Soc 43:865–870. 1995/08/01 edn

Elbadawi A, Yalla SV, Resnick NM (1993) Structural basis of geriatric voiding dysfunction. IV. Bladder outlet obstruction. J Urol 150:1681–1695. 1993/11/01 edn

Elbadawi A, Hailemariam S, Yalla SV, Resnick NM(1997) Structural basis of geriatric voiding dysfunction. VII. Prospective ultrastructural/urodynamic evaluation of its natural evolution. J Urol 157:1814–1822. 1997/05/01 edn

Gilpin SA, Gilpin CJ, Dixon JS, Gosling JA, Kirby RS (1986) The effect of age on the autonomic innervation of the urinary bladder. Br J Urol 58:378–381. 1986/08/01 edn

Gomez CS, Kanagarajah P, Gousse AE (2011) Bladder dysfunction in patients with diabetes. Curr Urol Rep 12:419–426. 2011/09/07 edn. doi:10.1007/s11934-011-0214-0

Gosling JA, Kung LS, Dixon JS, Horan P, Whitbeck C, Levin RM (2000) Correlation between the structure and function of the rabbit urinary bladder following partial outlet obstruction. J Urol 163:1349–1356. 2000/03/29 edn

Griebling TL, DuBeau CE, Kuchel G, Wilde MH, Lajiness M, Tomoe H, Diokno A, Vereecke A, Chancellor MB (2014) Defining and advancing education and conservative therapies of underactive bladder. Int Urol Nephrol 46(Suppl 1):S29–S34. 2014/09/23 edn. doi:10.1007/s11255-014-0799-6

Hotta H, Morrison JF, Sato A, Uchida S (1995) The effects of aging on the rat bladder and its innervation. Jpn J Physiol 45:823–836.,1995/01/01 edn

Huang Foen Chung JW, van Mastrigt R (2009) Age and volume dependent normal frequency volume charts for healthy males. J Urol 182:210–214. 2009/05/19 edn. doi:10.1016/j.juro.2009.02.113

Jacobsen SJ, Jacobson DJ, Girman CJ, Roberts RO, Rhodes T, Guess HA, Lieber MM (1997) Natural history of prostatism: risk factors for acute urinary retention. J Urol 158:481–487. 1997/08/01 edn

Jeong SJ, Kim HJ, Lee YJ, Lee JK, Lee BK, Choo YM, Oh JJ, Lee SC, Jeong CW, Yoon CY, Hong SK, Byun SS, Lee SE (2012) Prevalence and clinical features of detrusor underactivity among elderly with lower urinary tract symptoms: a comparison between men and women. Korean J Urol 53:342–348. 2012/06/07 edn. doi:10.4111/kju.2012.53.5.342

Kebapci N, Yenilmez A, Efe B, Entok E, Demirustu C (2007) Bladder dysfunction in type 2 diabetic patients. Neurourol Urodyn 26:814–819. 2007/04/25 edn. doi:10.1002/nau.20422

Kunin CM, Douthitt S, Dancing J, Anderson J, Moeschberger M (1992) The association between the use of urinary catheters and morbidity and mortality among elderly patients in nursing homes. Am J Epidemiol 135:291–301. 1992/02/01 edn

Martin-Merino E, Garcia-Rodriguez LA, Masso-Gonzalez EL, Roehrborn CG (2009) Do oral antimuscarinic drugs carry an increased risk of acute urinary retention? J Urol 182:1442–1448. 2009/08/18 edn. doi:10.1016/j.juro.2009.06.051

Miller M (2000) Nocturnal polyuria in older people: pathophysiology and clinical implications. J Am Geriatr Soc 48:1321–1329. 2000/10/19 edn

Nakamura S, Kobayashi Y, Tozuka K, Tokue A, Kimura A, Hamada C (1996) Circadian changes in urine volume and frequency in elderly men. J Urol 156:1275–1279. 1996/10/01 edn

Nomiya M, Sagawa K, Yazaki J, Takahashi N, Kushida N, Haga N, Aikawa K, Matsui T, Oka M, Fukui T, Andersson KE, Yamaguchi O (2012) Increased bladder activity is associated with elevated oxidative stress markers and proinflammatory cytokines in a rat model of atherosclerosis-induced chronic bladder ischemia. Neurourol Urodyn 31:185–189. 2011/09/29 edn. doi:10.1002/nau.21191

Nordling J (2002) The aging bladder–a significant but underestimated role in the development of lower urinary tract symptoms. Exp Gerontol 37:991–999. 2002/09/06 edn

Ouslander JG, Simmons S, Tuico E, Nigam JG, Fingold S, Bates-Jensen B, Schnelle JF (1994) Use of a portable ultrasound device to measure post-void residual volume among incontinent nursing home residents. J Am Geriatr Soc 42:1189–1192. 1994/11/01 edn

Parsons BA, Narshi A, Drake MJ (2012) Success rates for learning intermittent self-catheterisation according to age and gender. Int Urol Nephrol 44:1127–1131. 2012/02/22 edn. doi:10.1007/s11255-012-0136-x

Pilloni S, Krhut J, Mair D, Madersbacher H, Kessler TM (2005) Intermittent catheterisation in older people: a valuable alternative to an indwelling catheter? Age Ageing 34:57–60.,2004/11/13 edn. doi:10.1093/ageing/afh233

Pinggera GM, Mitterberger M, Steiner E, Pallwein L, Frauscher F, Aigner F, Bartsch G, Strasser H (2008) Association of lower urinary tract symptoms and chronic ischaemia of the lower urinary tract in elderly women and men: assessment using colour Doppler ultrasonography. BJU Int 102:470–474. 2008/05/15 edn. doi:10.1111/j.1464-410X.2008.07587.x

Resnick NM, Yalla SV (1987) Detrusor hyperactivity with impaired contractile function. An unrecognized but common cause of incontinence in elderly patients. JAMA 257:3076–3081. 1987/06/12 edn

Resnick NM, Yalla SV, Laurino E (1989) The pathophysiology of urinary incontinence among institutionalized elderly persons. N Engl J Med 320:1–7. 1989/01/05 edn. doi:10.1056/nejm198901053200101

Rogers MA, Mody L, Kaufman SR, Fries BE, McMahon LF Jr, Saint S (2008) Use of urinary collection devices in skilled nursing facilities in five states. J Am Geriatr Soc 56:854–861. 2008/05/06 edn. doi:10.1111/j.1532-5415.2008.01675.x

Shah D, Badlani G (2002) Treatment of overactive bladder and incontinence in the elderly. Rev Urol 4(Suppl 4):S38–S43. 2006/09/21 edn

Tan TL, Lieu PK, Ding YY (2001) Urinary retention in hospitalised older women. Ann Acad Med Singapore 30:588–592. 2002/01/31 edn

Taylor JA 3rd, Kuchel GA (2006) Detrusor underactivity: clinical features and pathogenesis of an underdiagnosed geriatric condition. J Am Geriatr Soc 54:1920–1932. 2007/01/03 edn. doi:10.1111/j.1532-5415.2006.00917.x

Tenke P, Koves B, Johansen TE (2014) An update on prevention and treatment of catheter-associated urinary tract infections. Curr Opin Infect Dis 27:102–107. 2013/12/19 edn. doi:10.1097/qco.0000000000000031

Thomas AW, Cannon A, Bartlett E, Ellis-Jones J, Abrams P (2004) The natural history of lower urinary tract dysfunction in men: the influence of detrusor underactivity on the outcome after transurethral resection of the prostate with a minimum 10-year urodynamic follow-up. BJU Int 93:745–750. 2004/03/31 edn. doi:10.1111/j.1464-410X.2003.04719.x

Thorne MB, Geraci SA (2009) Acute urinary retention in elderly men. Am J Med 122:815–819. 2009/08/25 edn. doi:10.1016/j.amjmed.2009.05.009

Visser E, de Bock GH, Kollen BJ, Meijerink M, Berger MY, Dekker JH (2012) Systematic screening for urinary incontinence in older women: who could benefit from it? Scand J Prim Health Care 30:21–28. 2012/02/14 edn. doi:10.3109/02813432.2011.628244

Wada N, Watanabe M, Kita M, Matsumoto S, Kakizaki H (2012) Analysis of bladder vascular resistance before and after prostatic surgery in patients with lower urinary tract symptoms suggestive of benign prostatic obstruction. Neurourol Urodyn 31:659–663. 2012/04/11 edn. doi:10.1002/nau.21201

White WM, Mobley JD 3rd, Doggweiler R, Dobmeyer-Dittrich C, Klein FA (2009) Sacral nerve stimulation for refractory overactive bladder in the elderly population. J Urol 182:1449–1452. 2009/08/18 edn. doi:10.1016/j.juro.2009.06.049

Willlams CM (2002) Using medications appropriately in older adults. Am Fam Physician 66:1917–1924. 2002/12/10 edn

Yuan Z, Tang Z, He C, Tang W (2015) Diabetic cystopathy: a review. J Diabetes 7:442–447. 2015/01/27 edn. doi:10.1111/1753-0407.12272

Chapter 13
Underactive Bladder in Children

Israel Franco

Introduction

Underactive bladder and detrusor underactivity are not typically something that is on the top of the diagnostic differential in pediatric urology. In some instances, it is rarely mentioned in textbooks. Unfortunately, it does occur and is extremely difficult to manage in children. The term underactive bladder (UAB) is described in the International Children's Continence Society standardization document of 2014 as a clinical term that is "reserved for children who need to raise intra-abdominal pressure to initiate, maintain or complete voiding i.e. straining. The children may have low voiding frequency in the setting of adequate hydration but may also have frequency due to incomplete emptying with prompt refilling of the bladder. These children often produce an interrupted uroflow pattern and are usually found to have *detrusor underactivity* (DUA) if examined with invasive urodynamics. Flow patterns may be plateau-shaped; pressure flow studies will distinguish it from bladder outlet obstruction" (Austin et al. 2014). What is clear from this statement is that there are no well-defined criteria to identify UAB and DUA. There are no sets of uroflow parameters or urodynamic criteria, as the statement clearly does not allude to. There is a lack of consensus about the etiology of this condition in the adult literature as well as in the pediatric literature. With such a paucity of information on a problem that is so difficult to treat, we seem to be ignoring the elephant in the room.

I. Franco, MD
Section of Pediatric Urology, New York Medical College,
International Children's Continence Society,
Maria Fareri Children's Hospital, Valhalla, NY 10595, USA
e-mail: isifranco@gmail.com

M.B. Chancellor, A.C. Diokno (eds.), *The Underactive Bladder*,
DOI 10.1007/978-3-319-23687-2_13

DUA is a urodynamic diagnosis for all intents and purposes, and making the diagnosis in the pediatric population is difficult when as a rule, we tend to shy away from invasive testing in children. We are left with various proxy studies to help determine if the child has DUA. But even if they do have DUA, we are limited in what we can offer. Therefore, most parents will be hesitant to allow their child to have an invasive procedure such as urodynamics, especially, if there is no treatment available.

Epidemiology

Firlit et al. described one of the earliest descriptions of DUA utilizing pressure flow studies in 1977 (Firlit et al. 1977). They described what is the most common pattern seen in pediatric urology, the hyperactive external sphincter with detrusor hypotonia in 2/34 (6 %) of patients. More recently, Glassberg and his group have described a rate of 5–9 % of what they call detrusor underutilization (Glassberg et al. 2010; Van Batavia et al. 2011, 2014). Hoebeke in a 1000 patients saw an incidence of 4 % of children with expanded bladder capacities and hypocontractility (Hoebeke et al. 2001). LUTS is a major problem in children where it has its major effect in children between 3 and 14 years of age. The main symptom in children with LUTS is OAB, but in some cases, it is impossible to distinguish OAB symptoms from DUA symptoms since some of the symptoms overlap like hesitancy, weak stream, urgency, elevated post void residual (PVR) and intermittency, and straining to void. Recurrent UTIs in girls with OAB and external sphincter dyssynergia (EDSD) are indistinguishable from the girl with DUA, not until a more detailed evaluation is performed can the two be distinguished.

Bladder outlet obstruction due to bladder neck dysfunction or obstructive anatomic abnormalities like posterior urethral valves (PUV) and prune belly syndrome (PBS) are also causes of DUA. The most common cause of an anatomically related bladder underactivity that is not due to spinal dysraphisms and or spinal cord injury is PUV. The prevalence of boys with severe PUV is going down with the advent of increased in utero intervention and pregnancy terminations. Other anatomical causes leading to DUA in children are imperforate anus, bladder exstrophy, and cloacal anomalies. Other neurologic disorders such as Wolfram syndrome and multiple system atrophy account for a small portion of the cases of DUA.

Regardless of the cause, elevated PVR is a hallmark of DUA in children. Unlike in the adult population where chronic retention is classified as a PVR ≥300 ml or a palpable or percussable non-tender bladder, in children there is no definition for chronic retention of this magnitude, and PVR ≥20 ml is now considered abnormal (Chang et al. 2013). We are left with no set criteria to define where an elevated PVR is considered chronic or markedly abnormal. From our own experience, the child with DUA represents a small fraction of the children that we see with LUTS but make up a large proportion of the repeat visits in our clinic population.

Causes

Posterior Urethral Valves

Outlet obstruction in the adult male accounts for the majority of the cases of DUA. Playing on the same mechanisms of hypertrophy and changes in collagen, obstructive processes such as PUV can lead to DUA. In a systematic review of the literature in 2011 by Hennus et al. (2012) of studies of boys treated by endoscopic ablation of valves, they found that a hypocontractile bladder was seen in 35 % of patients (0–73 %), reported in eight studies. PVR was found in 31 % (0–56 %). In these three studies, bladder hypocontractility increased during follow-up, ranging from 0–27 % to 21–71 %. The percentage of patients with PVR increased from 4 to 29 % during 4.5 years follow-up and 0 to 43 % during 12.5 years after endoscopic valve ablation. This is disconcerting, since it indicates that whatever the process, there seems to be a progressive element in posterior urethral valve patients. This is in stark contrast to anterior urethral valve patients who when treated for their valves will have gradual resolution of hypercontractility, and no one develops hypocontractility (Kajbafzadeh et al. 2007). It is unclear if there are neurologic and neuroreceptor elements involved with the PUV patients since the bladder wall hypertrophy occurs during development, while anterior urethral valves are felt to occur postnatally due to a fold or a urethral diverticulum in the urethra and are identified around the time of toilet training. This later onset may be associated with reversibility and reduced risk for DUA.

Bladder Exstrophy

DUA has been reported in bladder exstrophy patients undergoing complete primary repair, which was popularized by Mitchell. We also know that patients that have classic repairs are also known to have DUA as well. In this group, the patients with multiple closures of the bladder are at more risk than those closed in one stage. Mesrobian (2014) reviewed the results of the complete primary repair and found that all 6 patients undergoing the procedure had an underactive bladder. He attributes this to the iatrogenic damage done to the pelvic plexus which lies adjacent to the urethral plate (Figs. 13.1 and 13.2) by the extensive mobilization of the bladder neck and bladder to tuck it into the pelvis as the primary cause of the damage. Aside from this study, there are numerous patients that have undergone exstrophy closures that have underactive bladders and are incapable of generating significant pressures.

Prune Belly Syndrome

In PBS, the bladder is thick walled and there is a large urachal remnant that gives it an hourglass appearance (Fig. 13.3). Histologically, the bladder demonstrates an altered connective tissue to smooth muscle ratio. There is smooth muscle

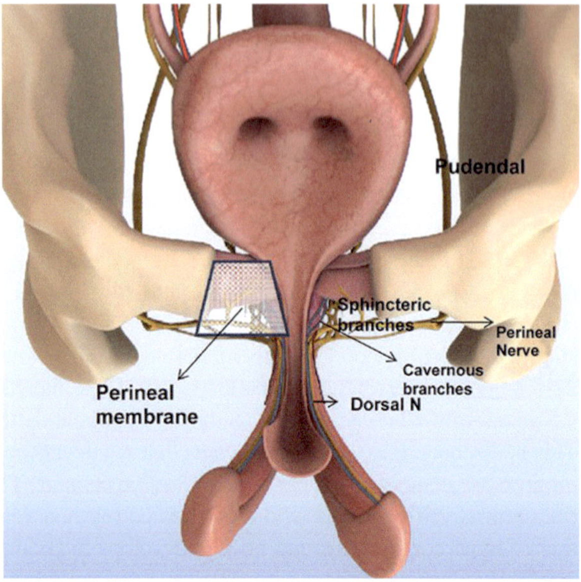

Fig. 13.1 Surgeon's view of bladder exstrophy during complete primary repair of bladder exstrophy; the pelvic diaphragm separates the pelvic sphincter mechanism from the bulbospongiosus, superficial transverse perineal muscle, and associated neurovascular structures that pierce it from (With permission from Mesrobian (2014))

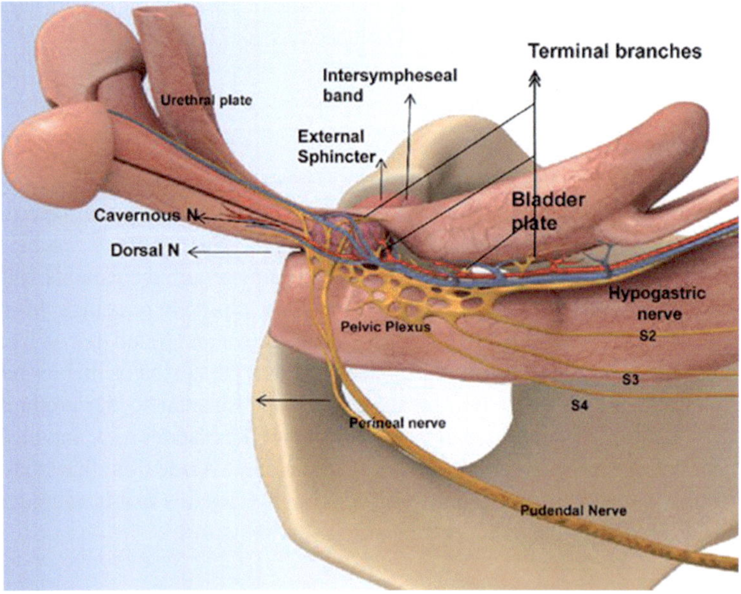

Fig. 13.2 Sagittal illustration of left pelvic plexus and its terminal branches; note relationship to bladder plate, prostatic urethra, and corpora cavernosa. The pelvic diaphragm is not shown (With permission from Mesrobian (2014))

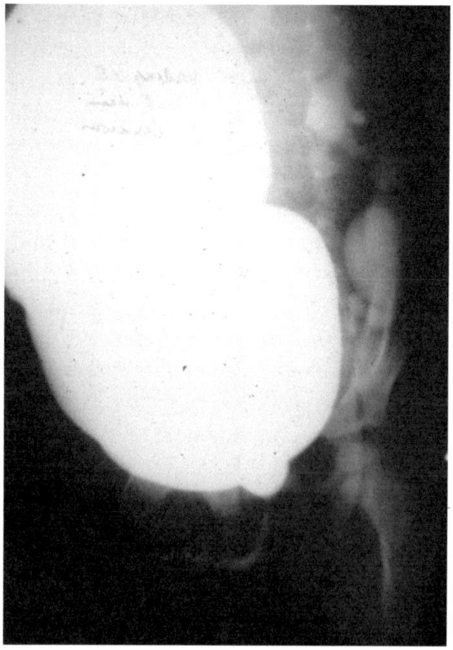

Fig. 13.3 Prune belly syndrome bladder with classic hourglass appearance and open bladder neck

hypertrophy, but the majority of the bladder thickness is due to fibrocytes and collagen. There is no abnormality in the distribution of ganglion cells. Classically, these bladders store urine well, and the urodynamic curve is shifted to the right with a range of voiding pressures noted. In less severe cases, there may be normal bladder pressures, and on the other end of the spectrum, there can be complete DUA.

There is no medical treatment for the DUA in PBS, and surgical intervention for the megacystis involves reduction cystoplasty, which was thought to lead to improved bladder emptying. Initially, it does lead to some improvements, but there appears to be no benefit between those that have undergone reduction cystoplasties and those that have not (Bukowski and Perlmutter 1994). Given these findings, reduction cystoplasty has fallen out of favor in these children. Most are relegated to emptying either by abdominal straining or intermittent catheterization when DUA is present.

Imperforate Anus and Cloacal Anomalies

In imperforate anus and cloacal anomalies, it was thought for many years that DUA was a result of surgical intervention and that it did not exist prior to surgical repair. After the posterior sagittal approach was popularized, preoperative testing was instituted since it was felt that the approach would not lead to the development of a neurogenic bladder. Much to the astonishment of investigators, it was found that the males with high imperforate anus have a high rate of neurogenic detrusor abnormalities that approaches 80 % preoperatively, and postoperatively, that number could be higher depending on the procedure performed.

In the case of the cloacal anomalies, some patients have detrusor underactivity prior to repair, and others seem to develop it after surgical correction (Camanni et al. 2009; Matsui et al. 2009). In these two studies, underactivity postoperatively was present in almost all patients who underwent total urogenital mobilization. This does not appear to be as prevalent in patients undergoing partial urogenital mobilization. We see a corollary with adults who undergo pelvic surgical dissection for an abdominal perineal pull through or extensive dissection between the bladder and the uterus, and these bladders are affected by the damage to the pelvic plexus, which leads to iatrogenic underactivity. Unfortunately, many of these patients probably have abnormal development of the pelvic plexus or sacral nerve roots and/or spinal cord as seen in the classic Vater syndrome. If we add on the potential for injury from extensive mobilization of the bladder, we have a high rate of DUA in these patients with imperforate anus and cloacal anomalies.

Functional Issues

The scenario that is most commonly encountered is the child with DUA due to functional voiding problems. As previously mentioned, it makes up about 4–9 % of the children with lower urinary tract problems seen in large practices that care for these children. Many will present with urgency and urge incontinence. It is not unusual that they also present with recurrent urinary tract infections due to incomplete emptying and stasis. What is noteworthy is that some will have tower flows consistent with high Qmax and then not empty all the way leaving behind large residual urine. In this scenario, there may be a shortening of the effective contraction time of the void resulting in incomplete emptying. In some cases, we may see external sphincter dyssynergia along with evidence of bladder neck dysfunction or isolated bladder neck dysfunction. On VCUG and videourodynamics, we can see delay in opening of the bladder neck and then a narrow and contracted prostatic urethra and external sphincter in some of these children. In this scenario, there is a loss of energy during the contraction that cannot be recovered, and this leads to incomplete emptying and eventual muscle hypertrophy of the bladder. The detrusor contraction along with abdominal straining can lead to these tower curves and therefore give the impression of good voiding pressures even though DUA can exist.

The other pattern that is not unusual is the patient with the plateau flow curve and low Qmax, which is what we would think is most synonymous with these patients that have DUA. In this scenario, the detrusor is not contracting at its full potential and leading to the delay in emptying and usually incomplete emptying. It is also possible that the bladder neck fails to adequately open, along with some degree of detrusor hypocontractility in some patients. We have seen this scenario in some patients with associated autonomic dysfunction. Again there is very little data on these patients with DUA since they make up the minority of the patients that have urodynamics, and recently, there has been a move to refrain from doing urodynamics in children. Moving forward we may have even less data available to define this entity.

It is not uncommon that in cases where the bladder neck is involved, we have seen a large number of patients present with evidence of autonomic dysfunction complaining of dizziness on standing, and in a subgroup that was tested with tilt table testing, we saw clear evidence of autonomic dysfunction. This dysfunction can be affecting the micturition reflexes at Onuf's nucleus where serotonergic input is responsible for the relaxation of the sphincter. These pathways emanate from the frontal lobes in the anterior cingulate gyrus and the prefrontal cortex, and they are long uninterrupted serotonergic pathways. It is conceivable that in this subset of patients, there could be some form of autonomic dysregulation possibly due to frontal lobe dysfunction. We have some data that points to serotonin being involved in this process from a series of patients that had a history of OAB and elevated PVRs who responded to 5-HT4 agonists (Franco et al. 2010). In the vast majority of patients that exhibit the aforementioned patterns, we can improve emptying by reducing outlet resistance either by correcting the EDSD and/or the internal sphincter dyssynergia (IDSD). In some instances, correction of constipation is all that is necessary to obtain a complete resolution of symptoms.

Glassberg's group (Van Batavia et al. 2014) describes a subset that engages in voiding postponement volitionally but does not exhibit DUA as specifically described by the ICCS guidelines which includes straining to void, fractionated stream, or low detrusor pressure on urodynamics. They term them DUD (detrusor underutilization disorder). They claim that these patients do not have detrusor underactivity on urodynamics and the majority exhibited normal bell curve patterns. These patients responded well to conventional urotherapy measures. Therefore, we should be weary of the criteria of large bladder capacity and infrequent voiding as a primary definer of DUA in children.

Other Causes

A viral illness that can affect the motor tracts and lead to detrusor areflexia with an intact sensation is the poliomyelitis. However, certain group A and B Coxsackie viruses (especially A7), several echoviruses, and enterovirus type 71 may produce similar findings, and typically these will be temporary. West Nile virus infection can also cause an acute flaccid paralysis that is clinically indistinguishable from paralytic poliomyelitis due to polioviruses.

Lyme's disease can also present with micturition problems via two mechanisms. The first is direct invasion of the organism into the bladder, and the second is related to neuroborreliosis, leading to meningoencephalopathy, transverse myelitis, myeloradiculitis, and demyelinating lesions of the spinal cord. Micturition disorders can appear in diverse forms such as detrusor hyperreflexia, detrusor-sphincter dyssynergia, and detrusor areflexia (Chancellor et al. 1993). One out of four Lyme encephalomyelitis patients can present with urinary dysfunction (Ackermann et al. 1988).

Vitamin B12 deficiency causes posterior long tract disease by demyelination of the lateral and dorsal (posterior) spinal columns as well as peripheral nerves leading to loss of proprioception with signs of upper motor neuron disease such as Babinski's response. There is a loss of bladder sensation and increased residual urine due to detrusor areflexia. Sphincteric EMG is intact since the corticospinal tracts are not involved. Erectile function will also be affected. These findings will also be seen in neurosyphilis and vitamin E deficiency.

Wolfram syndrome is a syndrome that manifests with diabetes insipidus, diabetes mellitus, optic atrophy, neurosensory deafness, urinary tract dilatation, and bladder dysfunction which will usually result in death in the third to fourth decade of life. The causative gene (WFS1) which encodes the wolframin protein (in the endoplasmic reticulum) has been identified, and a number of loss-of-function mutations have been described. In a publication in 1998, 6 out of 14 patients (42 %) had atonic bladders, and in a more recent publication, 45 % had elevated post-void residual. In our own experience, bladder emptying can be improved in some by improving outlet resistance, but residuals persist due to DUA.

Weber et al. (2011) describe a homozygous loss-of-function mutation of muscarinic acetylcholine receptor M3 (CHRM3) (1q41-q44) in five brothers with a PBS-like syndrome. CHRM3 encodes the M3 subtype of muscarinic acetylcholine (ACh) receptors. This mutation leads to a megacystis and prune-like abdominal wall defects. Aside from the DUA in the bladder, all of the brothers exhibited dilated pupils that reacted poorly to light and dry mouth. The mother, father, and sister of the boys were all heterozygous for the mutation. Unfortunately, their bladder function was not tested so we do not know if the heterozygous state can lead to some degree of hypocontractility.

Another mutation has been identified in ACTA2, R179H, that causes a syndrome characterized by dysfunction of smooth muscle cells throughout the body, leading to aortic and cerebrovascular disease, fixed dilated pupils, hypotonic bladder, malrotation and hypoperistalsis of the gut, and pulmonary hypertension (Milewicz et al. 2010). The urinary and gastrointestinal problems found in these patients are similar to complications of megacystis-microcolon-intestinal hypoperistalsis syndrome (MMIHS), an autosomal recessive condition typically lethal shortly after birth. MMHIS is characterized by megacystis and hydronephrosis, microcolon/short bowel with malrotation, and hypoperistalsis. The underlying genetic defect has not been identified, but the overlap of MMIHS with the ACTA2 R179H phenotype suggests a defect of smooth muscle cell contractile function, possibly from recessive or de novo ACTA2 mutations. Interestingly, congenital mydriasis has been reported in a patient with MMIHS.

Medications

Certain medications may be capable of producing DUA. Drugs with known anticholinergic activities are at risk for producing DUA. Other drugs not commonly thought of as having negative effects on detrusor activity include nonsteroidal anti-inflammatories (Minami et al. 2007), and its mode of action is on the PGE2 receptors in the bladder. Ketorolac, which is used commonly for its ability to suppress bladder spasms in children who underwent reflux surgery, is an indicator of this groups potential for a relaxing effect on the detrusor.

We have seen children have a marked change in bladder emptying with the introduction of cetirizine, a histamine h1 receptor antagonists. The whole group of h1 receptor antagonists is capable of producing this effect and is something that the clinician needs to be aware of.

Medications that cause constipation can have an indirect effect on the detrusor via rectal dilation. It is known that rectal dilation can inhibit bladder contractions and impair bladder emptying (Godec 1980; Miyazato et al. 2005).

Evaluation

Uroflowmetry

The uroflow study is capable of giving the practitioner a clue as to the possible diagnosis of DUA, but it is not capable of making a definitive diagnosis. Uroflowmetry with perineal EMG adds more information which helps to better define what is occurring at the sphincter. Unfortunately, the majority of uroflows are done without EMG, and few except for a handful of centers (ours included) will do dual EMG of the perineum and abdominal muscles. Without both EMGs, it is hard to tell if abdominal straining is occurring. Firlit et al. (1977) described the use of dual EMG evaluation as a means of identifying abdominal straining and removing the guesswork if abdominal straining was present (Fig. 13.4).

Interpretation of isolated flow curves is only suggestive of possible DUA, and several patterns are considered to be synonymous with DUA. One is the interrupted flow pattern which the international children's continence society (ICCS) states in the terminology document, "Each peak represents abdominal muscle straining creating the main force for urine evacuation. In between each strain, the flow ceases." This is supposed to be indicative of DUA, but without some form of verification, it is not possible to confirm this. It is true that there could be straining but also complete cessation of voiding due to EDSD, or detrusor weakness could account for this as well (Fig. 13.5a, b).

With regard to plateau pattern, the ICCS terminology document describes that a plateau curve "may be seen with an underactive bladder during a long continuous abdominal strain." Again, unless abdominal EMG is done, we cannot confirm that

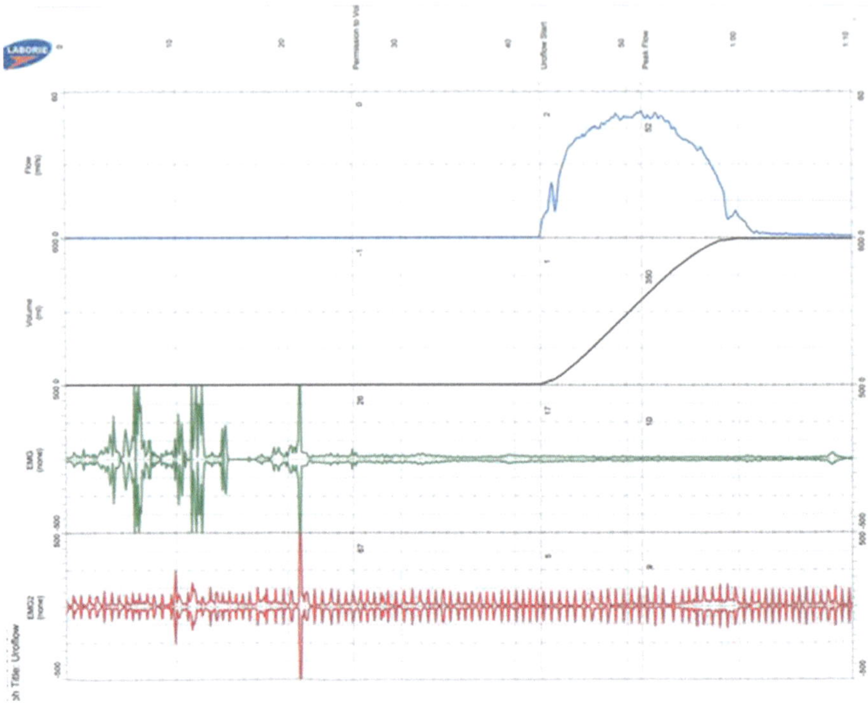

Fig. 13.4 A 14-year-old girl with a tower-type uroflow curve with a Qmax = 52 ml/s and Qavg = 17.1 ml/s on a voided volume of 600 ml and a PVR of 300 ml. There is no evidence of external sphincter dyssynergia in this case with only a minimal amount of abdominal straining at the end of urination. This is not a classic appearance of detrusor underactivity but has been confirmed by urodynamic testing. This patient benefited from alpha-blockers since there was evidence of bladder neck dysfunction based on a prolonged lag time and on voiding cystourethrogram

abdominal straining is occurring nor it is necessary to be present in someone that has DUA and that exhibits a plateau pattern (Fig. 13.6).

What is evident is that we are hampered by an inexact science, which is interpretation of uroflowmetry. Uroflowmetry is subjective and lacks objective criteria and set protocols for its performance. Societies need to go back and reevaluate the terminology and criteria being used to define DUA with regard to uroflowmetry.

Urodynamics

Urodynamic evaluation of the child with suspected DUA is typically not a common occurrence due to the reticence that most pediatric urologists have to perform invasive testing in children with intact sensation. But when we look at guideline documents such as the standardization document produced by the ICCS, we see that there are no specific guidelines set forth in the document. They talk of reduced

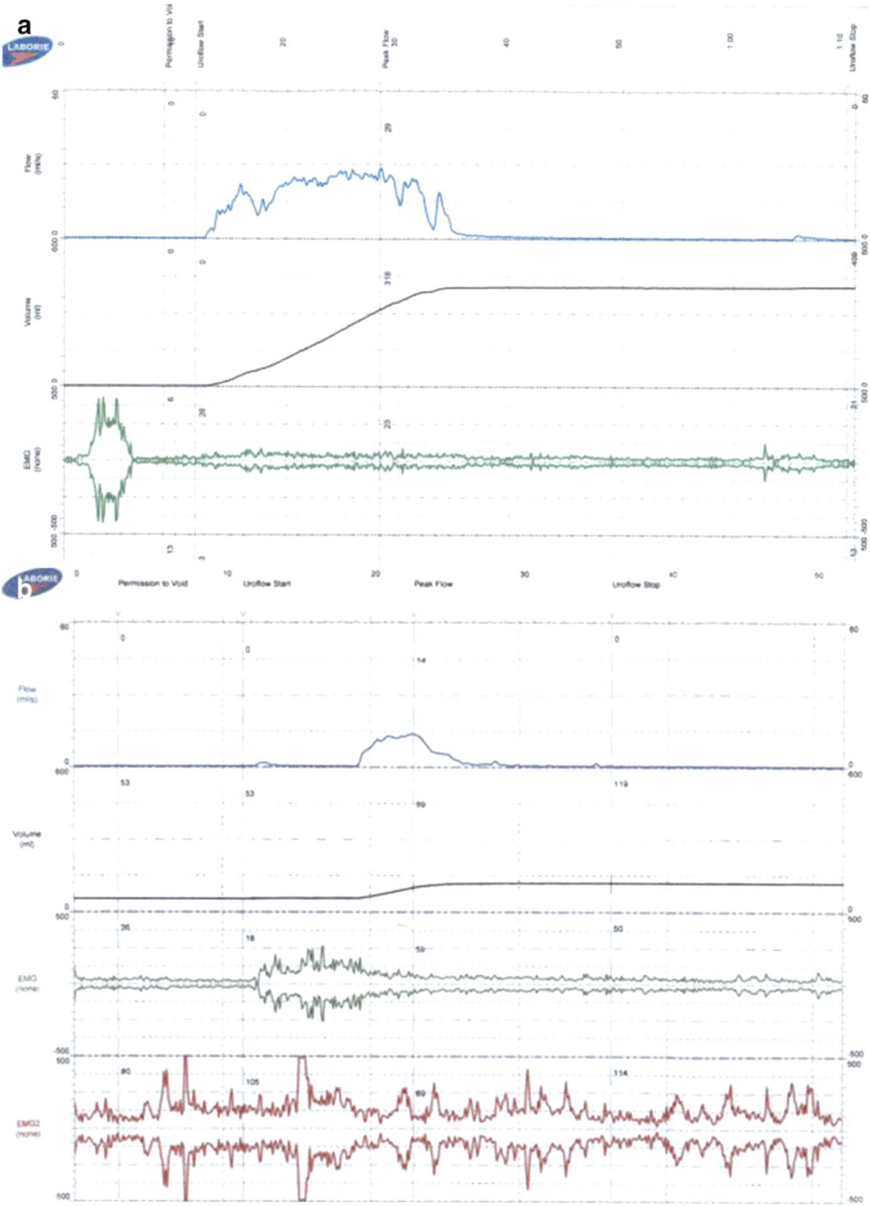

Fig. 13.5 (**a**) This is a 12-year-old boy with a stubby incomplete cord and detrusor underactivity confirmed on urodynamics. This is a staccato pattern with evidence of external sphincter activity. He voided 410 ml with a 214 ml PVR. Qmax = 28.6 ml/s and Qavg = 12.2 ml/s. Again simple observation of this study would not lead one to know that this patient has detrusor underactivity based on the present society recommendations. (**b**) A 12-year-old boy with Wolfram syndrome, OAB symptoms, and marked bladder underactivity with significant abdominal straining and EDSD at the start of urination that persists throughout the void. Qmax = 13.8 ml/s, Qavg = 5.0 ml/s, voided volume = 140 ml, and PVR = 140 ml

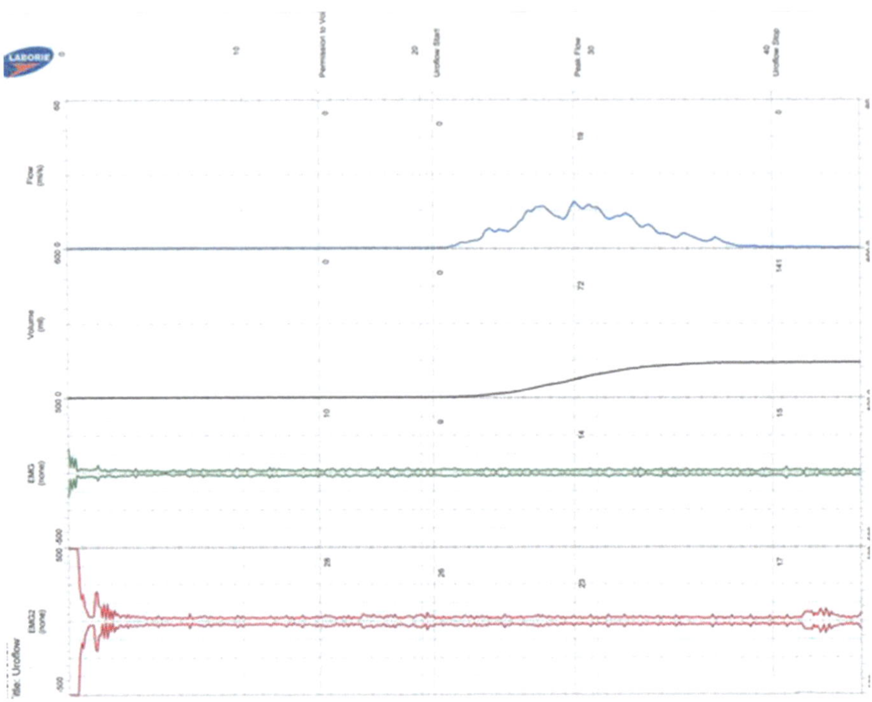

Fig. 13.6 A 14-year-old girl with known autonomic dysfunction (orthostatic hypotension, positive tilt test) and bladder neck dysfunction on VCUG, with DUA and no abdominal or perineal sphincter activity. Bladder emptying was markedly improved on alpha-blockers but still remains high. Plateau pattern with some staccato overtones. Qmax = 18.5 ml/s and Qavg = 7.6 ml/s. Voided volume = 140 ml and PVR = 214 ml

bladder sensation which is defined as "diminished awareness throughout bladder filling and absent bladder sensation" as no bladder sensation whatsoever. So what do we make of the children with DUA who have OAB. It is understood that children with DUA can have OAB and not all will have reduced sensation. This appears to be a carry-over from the lazy bladder descriptions of the past. A revision of the guidelines is in order with respect to sensation.

The ICCS document stresses that there are selective times when pressure flow studies are of clinical value in children in order to distinguish between two clinical conditions that will result in low flow on uroflowmetry – an underactive bladder versus bladder outlet obstruction (BOO). With the former, there is detrusor underactivity, whereas with BOO, the detrusor pressure is elevated. Unfortunately, we do not have a defined pressure to use as a baseline where scientists can go back and use as a reference point. Some studies use voiding pressures as low as 20 cmH_2O. The adult literature appears to suffer from such a lack of coordination as well with detrusor pressure at maximum flow rate ranging from 30 to 45 cmH_2O in men to a low of 10 cmH_2O in women. It may prove better to consider using the total power output of the bladder contraction than relying simply on the maximal or peak power. This is synonymous to an engine that can sustain a very short burst of horsepower versus a long sustained generation of power. Which is better? Obviously we need to find out more about this in the future to answer this question.

EMG activity should be measured during the urodynamic study since an intermittent and/or fluctuating flow rate may be due to intermittent contractions of the periurethral striated or levator ani muscles during voiding. This is especially necessary in patients that have urodynamics without video. The EMG will help delineate if the patient could benefit from interventions to correct the EDSD and improve bladder emptying in light of a weak detrusor.

Treatment

Eliminate Obstruction

Anatomic

The first step in the management of the patient with PUV or PBS is to eliminate the obstruction as early as possible. This involves in utero intervention. The damage is done to the kidneys early on in the developmental process, but we have seen some boys with PUV and PBS where in utero intervention with decompression of the bladder using vesico-amniotic stenting has resulted in better than expected bladder function, irrespective of upper tract function. Providing a similar effect is spontaneous in utero shunting either by a patent urachus in PBS patients or by spontaneous rupture of the bladder in PUV. The shunting process reduces the pressure in the bladder and mitigates the destructive effects of the ensuing collagen and elastin changes in the bladder. This in turn leads to a more compliant bladder that is less prone to DUA and can empty spontaneously.

Bladder Neck

Patients with known bladder neck dysfunction are best treated with alpha-blockers. Identifying the bladder neck dysfunction as early as possible is critical. Starting on the appropriate alpha-blocker is also important. In patients with OAB symptoms, we have found that the least selective alpha-blockers (i.e., terazosin and doxazosin) seem to help with OAB symptoms and provide relief of the obstruction of the bladder neck. In patients where OAB is not a concern, the more selective alpha-blockers seem to do a better job (tamsulosin and silodosin). In some cases, improving the emptying process will reduce the resistance at the bladder neck and the urethral sphincter complex allowing for a weakened detrusor to empty better and reduce the residual urine.

External Sphincter

In cases where the obstruction is at the external sphincter, the first-line treatment is elimination of constipation. This is the most common reason that results in EDSD in children. Sometimes, a simple matter such as eliminating rectal dilation can have a profound effect on EDSD. During bladder sonography pre-biofeedback, we will identify rectal dilation in excess of 4 cm, and invariably, these children will have a tight sphincter and have a difficult time relaxing the sphincter at the time of biofeedback. We know that the rectal dilation can have an inhibitory effect on the bladder contractility as previously described, and eliminating rectal dilation and bringing rectal diameter to less than 4 cm in children is a critical goal of our therapy to improve bladder emptying and reduce PVR in children. Aggressive use of cathartics and not just softeners is critical in the management of these children. We have seen that stool softeners by themselves generally have a poorer success rate in reducing rectal diameter than a combination of softeners and cathartics.

Second-line therapy is biofeedback training for EDSD. This has been found to be useful in appropriately selected children. As with all procedures when candidates are not adequately selected for the procedure, the overall efficacy can be reduced as recently documented in a meta-analysis of biofeedback in the literature. In more selected settings, it does work if the appropriate criteria for patient selection are used.

Third-line therapy would be the use of botulinum toxin A into the external sphincter in children both males and females. It represents a useful option for refractory patients that fail biofeedback. What we learned from our series of patients (Franco et al. 2007) in whom we injected with botulinum toxin A is that the refractory patients had a significant neuropsychiatric comorbidity and that if adequate management of that comorbidity was not provided, the vast majority of patients would revert back to having EDSD and require repeat injections.

Improving Detrusor Function

Improving the detrusor contractility is the Holy Grail in the management of DUA in children. We have found that in some cases, the use of serotonin agonists appears to work. In the past when tegaserod was available in the US market, we treated patients with the medication initially for severe constipation. We found that in some patients, the PVR was markedly reduced and OAB symptoms also were improved. We then started to use the medication on patients who had controlled constipation but had persistent elevated PVRs, and we found that the residuals went down as well. Once these patients came off the medication when the drug was taken off the market even if their constipation was controlled, we found that the residual urines trended back up again. In lieu of tegaserod, we had to use SSRIs and found that for some, they did continue to have benefits, while others had no significant benefit with the new drug. It is hard to convince parents to have their children take an SSRI when they have no symptoms of depression or anxiety, making routine use of this modality difficult.

Recently, we have begun to use prucalopride which is a selective, high-affinity serotonin (5-HT4) receptor agonist similar to tegaserod and have had success in selected cases in improving bladder emptying, but unfortunately, the drug is not available in the USA, and patients must procure it from Canada at their own cost. In one particular case, we had a young man with a 1200 ml PVR reduce his PVR down to 250 ml with the use of prucalopride.

Sacral Nerve Stimulation (SNS)

There is a paucity of data on DUA outcomes in children who have had SNS. There is only one large series of SNS in children at this time (Dwyer et al. 2014). This study and others appear to have good success with OAB symptoms, but the outcomes for patients with DUA are not as good as those with OAB. Even in Fowler's series of women with the syndrome, they reported that long term the average PVR was 75 ml in their group (Dasgupta et al. 2004). Our own experience with these patients is similar, in that we saw a prompt response to the elimination of OAB symptoms and urinary and fecal incontinence. But residual urine has remained high in these patients. There is a reduction in the number of UTIs that the patients have, and this may be a result of elimination of the OAB symptoms.

Reduction Cystoplasty

The use of reduction cystoplasty has fallen out of favor since the publication in 1994 showed that there was minimal value in patients with PBS in the long-term. The majority of these patients had an improvement initially, but eventually they regressed and bladder emptying did not seem to be any better than preop. With the introduction of catherizable stomas, which reduced the discomfort to sensate patients from CIC, there has been a virtual elimination of this procedure in pediatric urology.

Clean Intermittent Catheterization (CIC)

Intermittent catherization is the mainstay of management of the patient with neurogenic bladder, and advances in stoma techniques have made the procedure easier to create and more reliable. Abdominal catherizable stomas have allowed for the acceptance of CIC in sensate male patients who traditionally would shun CIC due to discomfort. It has become routine practice to consider placement of a catherizable stoma in patients with PBS and PUV when it is clear that they have DUA. The ability to empty these bladders regularly allows for improved continence rates and a reduction in hydronephrosis. These stomas allow for overnight catheter placement in patients that have diabetes insipidus which is commonly seen in patients with severe renal impairment. Overnight drainage has resulted in improved bladder function in some patients by reducing the inherent overstretching of the bladder that occurs at night in these patients. In a similar scenario, we have some PUV bladders rebound and show improved contractility and emptying after placing the patient on CIC for 1–2 years, enough so that the patients were able to stop performing CIC altogether. In these cases, aggressive decompression of the bladder especially early in life can give remarkable outcomes indicating that there is some pliability in the system and that function can be recovered if the detrusor is put to rest and allowed to remodel.

Conclusion

At the present time, the state of affairs for children with underactive bladder is dismal. We have no truly effective surgical techniques; stimulation techniques appear to address the OAB symptoms well but do not address the detrusor underactivity issue well enough. Medication research is lacking in the field, the one medication that we found that appeared to be effective in some children is not FDA approved, and the likelihood that it would be approved is minimal. At this time, the best we can do for these patients is to improve bladder emptying by reducing outlet resistance, by either improving bladder neck function or eliminating sphincter dyssynergia. We can only make sure that these children avoid certain medications that will aggravate their conditions and keep their rectal diameters to a minimal size to prevent bouts of retention. In all we suffer from a lack of research and options in this field, learning more about detrusor underactivity and underactive bladder needs to become a priority in pediatric urology.

References

Ackermann R, Rehse-Kupper B, Gollmer E, Schmidt R (1988) Chronic neurologic manifestations of erythema migrans borreliosis. Ann N Y Acad Sci 539:16–23

Austin PF, Bauer SB, Bower W, Chase J, Franco I, Hoebeke P, Rittig S, Vande Walle J, von Gontard A, Wright A, Yang SS, Neveus T (2014) The standardization of terminology of lower urinary tract function in children and adolescents: update report from the Standardization Committee of the International Children's Continence Society. J Urol 191:1863–1865

Bukowski TP, Perlmutter AD (1994) Reduction cystoplasty in the prune belly syndrome: a long-term followup. J Urol 152:2113–2116

Camanni D, Zaccara A, Capitanucci ML, Mosiello G, Iacobelli BD, De Gennaro M (2009) Bladder after total urogenital mobilization for congenital adrenal hyperplasia and cloaca–does it behave the same? J Urol 182:1892–1897

Chancellor MB, McGinnis DE, Shenot PJ, Kiilholma P, Hirsch IH (1993) Urinary dysfunction in Lyme disease. J Urol 149:26–30

Chang SJ, Chiang IN, Hsieh CH, Lin CD, Yang SS (2013) Age- and gender-specific nomograms for single and dual post-void residual urine in healthy children. Neurourol Urodyn 32: 1014–1018

Dasgupta R, Wiseman OJ, Kitchen N, Fowler CJ (2004) Long-term results of sacral neuromodulation for women with urinary retention. BJU Int 94:335–337

Dwyer ME, Vandersteen DR, Hollatz P, Reinberg YE (2014) Sacral neuromodulation for the dysfunctional elimination syndrome: a 10-year single-center experience with 105 consecutive children. Urology 84:911–917

Firlit CF, Smey P, King LR (1977) Micturition urodynamic flow studies in children. Trans Am Assoc Genitourin Surg 69:8–11

Franco I, Landau-Dyer L, Isom-Batz G, Collett T, Reda EF (2007) The use of botulinum toxin A injection for the management of external sphincter dyssynergia in neurologically normal children. J Urol 178(4 Pt 2):1775–1779; discussion 1779–1780

Franco I, Cagliostro S, Collett-Gardere T, Kearins M, Zelkovic P, Dyer L, Reda E (2010) Treatment of lower urinary tract symptoms in children with constipation using tegaserod therapy. Urotoday Int J 3:5784–5792

Glassberg KI, Combs AJ, Horowitz M (2010) Nonneurogenic voiding disorders in children and adolescents: clinical and videourodynamic findings in 4 specific conditions. J Urol 184: 2123–2127

Godec CJ (1980) Detrusor hyperreflexia inhibited by anal dilatation. Urology 15:321–324

Hennus PM, van der Heijden GJ, Bosch JL, de Jong TP, de Kort LM (2012) A systematic review on renal and bladder dysfunction after endoscopic treatment of infravesical obstruction in boys. PLoS One 7:e44663

Hoebeke P, Van Laecke E, Van Camp C, Raes A, Van De Walle J (2001) One thousand videourodynamic studies in children with non-neurogenic bladder sphincter dysfunction. BJU Int 87:575–580

Kajbafzadeh AM, Payabvash S, Karimian G (2007) Urodynamic changes in patients with anterior urethral valves: before and after endoscopic valve ablation. J Pediatr Urol 3:295–300

Matsui F, Shimada K, Matsumoto F, Obara T, Kubota A (2009) Bladder function after total urogenital mobilization for persistent cloaca. J Urol 182:2455–2459

Mesrobian HG (2014) Complete primary repair of bladder exstrophy is associated with detrusor underactivity type of neurogenic bladder. Urology 83:1139–1144

Milewicz DM, Ostergaard JR, Ala-Kokko LM et al (2010) De novo ACTA2 mutation causes a novel syndrome of multisystemic smooth muscle dysfunction. Am J Med Genet A 152A: 2437–2443

Minami H, Matsutani R, Mizokami A, Namiki M (2007) Case of acute urinary retention as a result of non-steroidal anti-inflammatory drugs. Int J Urol 14:368–369

Miyazato M, Sugaya K, Nishijima S, Morozumi M, Ohyama C, Ogawa Y (2005) Rectal distention inhibits the spinal micturition reflex via glycinergic or GABAergic mechanisms in rats with spinal cord injury. Urol Int 74:160–165

Van Batavia JP, Combs AJ, Hyun G, Bayer A, Medina-Kreppein D, Schlussel RN, Glassberg KI (2011) Simplifying the diagnosis of 4 common voiding conditions using uroflow/electromyography, electromyography lag time and voiding history. J Urol 186(4 Suppl):1721–1726

Van Batavia JP, Fast AM, Combs AJ, Glassberg KI (2014) The bladder of willful infrequent voiders: underactive or underutilized? J Pediatr Urol 10:517–521

Weber S, Thiele H, Mir S et al (2011) Muscarinic acetylcholine receptor M3 mutation causes urinary bladder disease and a prune-belly-like syndrome. Am J Hum Genet 89:668–674

Chapter 14
Public Health and Advocacy for UAB

David D. Chancellor and Hikaru Tomoe

Introduction

Patients with UAB are unable to completely empty their bladder and have a diminished sense of when their bladder is full. UAB can impact a patient in a variety of ways (Fig. 14.1). UAB can lead to increased residual urine and urinary tract infections. Urine left behind in the bladder over the long-term can lead to kidney damage or bladder stones. The clinical symptoms of UAB can lead to psychological ones as well. Loss of bladder control may negatively affect a patient's ability to sleep or work. When confronted with the symptoms of a debilitating and poorly understood condition such as UAB, it is easy for social isolation to set in. Overall, while the exact UAB symptoms usually vary from one person to another, they are almost always associated with impaired quality of life.

The loss of voluntary bladder control from UAB can enact a physical, mental, and economic cost to the patient. The physical and psychological impact which UAB exerts should not be understated. When UAB affects a patient, its burden can reverberate through to caregivers, family members, and, eventually, the community as a whole. As a result, UAB is a public health focus that should concern us all.

D.D. Chancellor, BS (✉)
Executive Director, Underactive Bladder Foundation, Pittsburgh, PA, USA
e-mail: David@underactivebladder.org

H. Tomoe, MD, PhD
Department of Urology and Pelvic Reconstructive Surgery,
Tokyo Women's Medical University, Tokyo, Japan
e-mail: Tomoeur@dnh.twmu.ac.jp

M.B. Chancellor, A.C. Diokno (eds.), *The Underactive Bladder*,
DOI 10.1007/978-3-319-23687-2_14

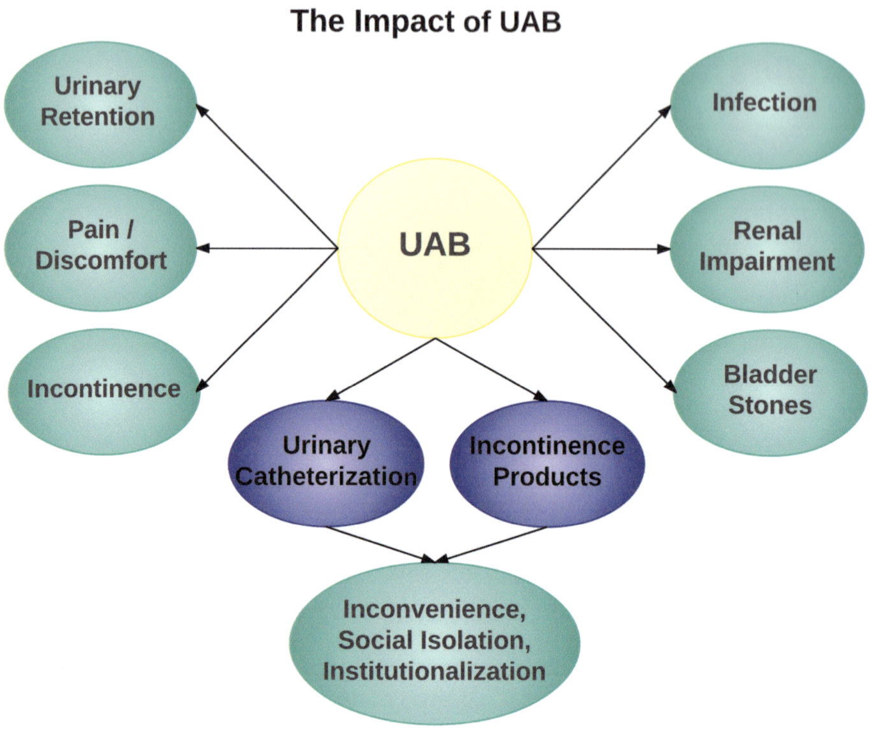

Fig. 14.1 Underactive bladder (UAB) may affect an individual in a variety of ways. Some of the potential impacts of UAB include urinary retention, pain/discomfort, incontinence, urinary tract infections (infection), renal impairment, and bladder stones. Additionally, the use of products to manage the condition such as urinary catheters or diapers can have an isolating effect on a patient

Epidemiology and Current Management of UAB

The precise epidemiology of UAB is uncertain; however, the condition is prevalent with no regard to gender. UAB can be present at any age. Recent research suggests that UAB is more prevalent than previously thought, perhaps because the incidence of the condition increases with age. Although little is known about the underlying causes of UAB, the decline of both bladder and urethral function is associated with aging. With an aging population across the developed world, it is clear that UAB is a growing issue.

There is no cure for UAB. Available pharmacotherapy is currently lacking. A class of drugs called cholinergic agonists is the most commonly used drugs for the condition. These products are too often marginally effective, ineffective and are associated with systemic side effects.

Chronic clean intermittent catheterization (CIC) is the most relied upon treatment for UAB. CIC enables many UAB patients to manage the condition and endure. Without CIC, UAB would be more strongly associated with mortality.

Although CIC remains the mainstay of UAB treatment for the foreseeable future, it does have issues.

Many patients are unable to perform CIC. Patients using CIC on a daily basis experience discomfort, stigma, and inconvenience. Additionally, chronic CIC is associated with complications including urinary tract infections and bleeding. This is troublesome as a single episode of a urinary tract infection can be costly to the patient and health system.

Unfortunately, with existing catheter technology, the only way to reduce the risk of CIC-related complications is to reduce the duration and frequency of CIC. Portable bladder scanners which accurately measure bladder volume are widely available, are inexpensive, and may help in this regard. These scanners can be used effectively to reduce the number of CICs which can decrease the risk of infections. Additionally, to combat complications of CIC, healthcare providers need to be aware of the current guidelines which help ensure patient safety. We still need alternative strategies and new tools to improve the management of UAB.

UAB is a significant reason for nursing home placement of the elderly. Patients who are unable to catheterize themselves are too often forced to enter a nursing home. Nursing homes are costly and can be detrimental to the long-term health of a patient. As populations age, the number of people and associated costs of UAB will continue to escalate. If we can find a way to better treat the condition, it would allow for substantial medical savings while allowing countless individuals to remain independent. In the era of ever rising healthcare costs, this is an issue we cannot afford to ignore.

Increasing UAB Awareness

Although UAB affects many people, it has received a disproportionately low level of attention. Despite a growing interest in the medical community, UAB's public profile remains limited. There are serious issues standing in the way of understanding UAB that result in the condition being overlooked and misdiagnosed too often.

Compared to other bladder conditions, UAB has received substantially less attention in academic and public circles. Comparatively, there is limited research in the scientific literature regarding the diagnosis, epidemiology, and treatment of UAB. This may be due to a lack of research stemming from confusion over terminology, definition, and diagnosis. Indeed, the medical community is still exploring the optimal name for the condition. We are in the early stage of rectifying this deficit in understanding.

As with many bladder dysfunction issues, there is a stigma attached to UAB. UAB patients often suffer silently, because they often appear healthy. This contributes to the relative obscurity of UAB. Support services can make a difference to patients coping with UAB, and more of these services still need to become available.

The gap in understanding UAB has perpetuated a lack of awareness of the condition. Public awareness and familiarity with UAB and other associated clinical urinary terms (detrusor underactivity, atonic bladder, lazy bladder, etc.) remain low. UAB remains an underappreciated entity by the medical community and industry.

Patient Advocacy

The negative impact of UAB is not a problem of one, rather UAB affects us all. The best way to combat the issue is by working together as a community. Patient advocacy is increasingly relied on to tackle the most difficult public health problems. Patient advocacy is one of the most effective tools available to fight for a cure.

The medical community requires better organization related to UAB. All organizations, be it for profit, nonprofit, or government, can do their part to seek out patients and let their voice be heard. We need organizations to reach out and advocate for UAB, with the Underactive Bladder Foundation being one example.

The *Underactive Bladder Foundation* (Pittsburgh, PA) is a volunteer-run charity dedicated to supporting efforts in UAB education, advocacy, and research. For additional details and contact information about the Underactive Bladder Foundation, see the foundation's website at www.underactivebladder.org or twitter feed @UABFoundation.

Please contact the Underactive Bladder Foundation to help improve awareness and find new and effective treatments for UAB.

There are a number of other aging- and urology-focused organizations as well. New groups are encouraged to form. Industry and government may contribute by sponsoring these efforts. As a community, we must do more to stress that UAB is an issue worth discussing and that UAB is not a normal part of aging. Efforts to support dissemination of research and publication continue to be important in overcoming the paucity of information on UAB

The future is highly encouraging. In recent years, well-known nonprofits and foundations have begun to feature UAB on a more frequent basis. The healthcare industry has begun to develop new technology and approaches for this indication. Finally, the National Institutes of Health has also begun to target UAB, notably with the creation of the first federally funded grant opportunities for aging UAB, starting with PA-15-049. There is good reason to be hopeful.

Beginning in 2014, the CURE-UAB series of meetings have sought to identify gaps in the collective understanding in order to prioritize future efforts in UAB. During these meetings, delegates identified critical research priorities including establishment of definition, development of effective animal research models, and establishment of clinical guidelines for diagnosis and treatment of UAB. Meeting workshops aimed at reviewing current knowledge and identifying research opportunities for UAB in older adults.

The first meeting was held in Bethesda, MD, in February 2014. The outcomes of that workshop are summarized in a September 2014 special issue of International Urology and Nephrology, Volume 46, Supplement 1, pages 1–46, with broad conclusions that further progress is needed on consensus disease definition, clinical guidelines, therapeutic directions, and suitable animal models to allow accurate testing of potential therapeutic candidates for UAB. Additional enduring material and videos and slides from CURE-UAB talks are also available (http://www.underactivebladder.org/index.php/for-professionals/videos-and-webcasts).

CURE-UAB is a series of meetings. At the time of this book, the next meeting will occur in December 2015 in Denver, CO (Fig. 14.2).

Conclusion

Medical problems can have social solutions. We need to continue to advocate for funding specifically earmarked for research on UAB diagnosis, epidemiology, and treatment. These efforts should extend beyond targeting lawmakers. As a

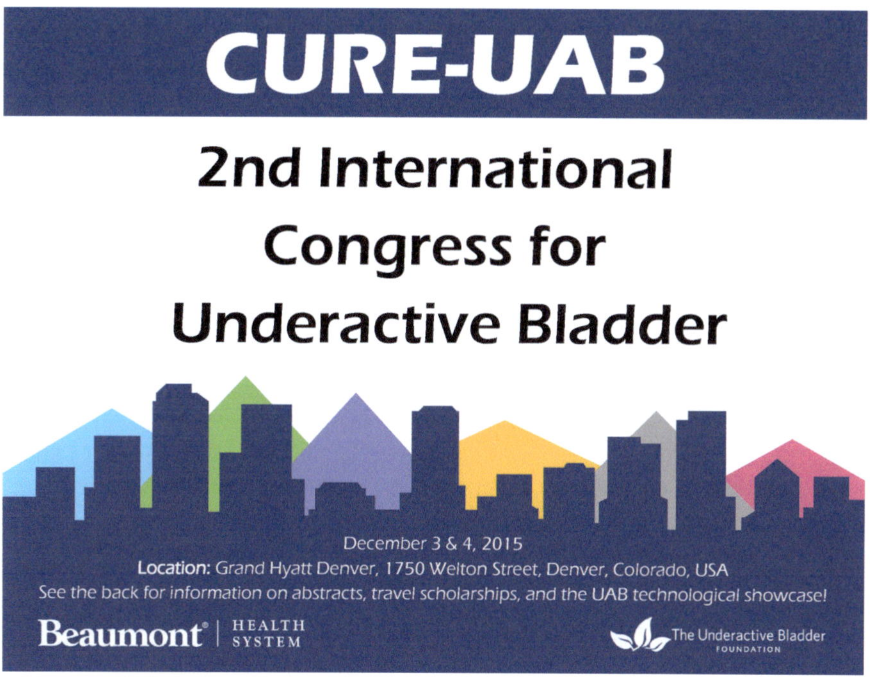

Fig. 14.2 Second international CURE-UAB congress

Dear Colleague,

We are pleased to invite you to attend the 2nd International Congress for Underactive Bladder (CURE-UAB). This 1.5 day program will feature the cutting edge research, clinical care, and technological advancements for underactive bladder.

The event will feature presentations from a world renowned faculty, panel discussions, work groups, and poster sessions. This international gathering will appeal to basic researchers, nurses, clinicians, academicians, industry representatives, and other stakeholders from the fields of urology, geriatrics, gynecology, neurology, and general medicine.

CURE-UAB provides an unparalleled platform for learning, participating, networking, collaborating, and discussing the emerging field of underactive bladder.

I hope to that you will join us in Denver to make the 2nd International Congress for Underactive Bladder a success.

Sincerely,

Michael B. Chancellor, MD
Chair, 2nd International Congress for Underactive Bladder

Abstracts
We will be accepting abstracts for poster presentation at CURE-UAB. The deadline for abstract submission is October 2, 2015. Please use the contact information below for more information and guidelines.

Travel Scholarships
A limited number of travel scholarships will be available to individuals who have submitted an abstract for poster presentation. Please use the contact information below for more information.

UAB Technological Showcase
The latest technology will be showcased to demonstrate clinical advancements in UAB management.

Results of the 1st CURE-UAB
- Special Edition of International Urology and Nephrology: http://link.springer.com/journal/11255/46/1/suppl/page/1
- Enduring Material: http://underactivebladder.org/index.php/for-professionals/videos-and-webcasts

Contact Information
Please contact Andrew Vereecke with questions or requests for information regarding CURE-UAB, abstracts, or scholarships: andrew.vereecke@beaumont.edu ▪ +1 248 551-3483

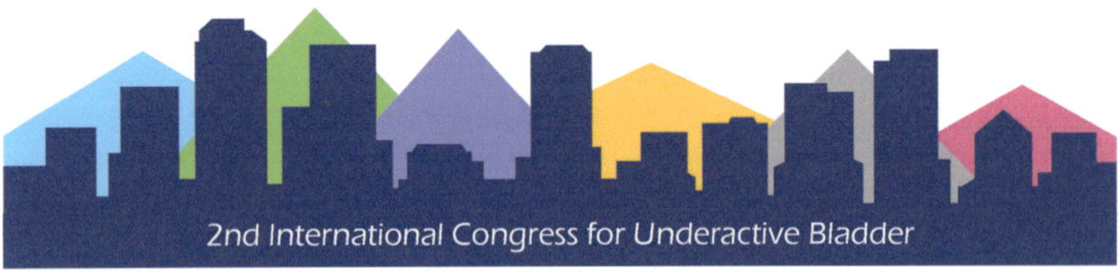

Fig. 14.2 (continued)

community, advocacy can be also focused on motivating the private sector and pharmaceutical industry to support UAB outreach as well.

As a community, we would be well served to acknowledge the significant UAB public health concerns and plot a course for effective disease advocacy and scientific exploration of the problems to reduce the societal and patient burden of UAB once and for all. By reading this book, you are far more educated than the majority of caretakers and the public, many of whom are still unfamiliar with the condition.

In spite of the tremendous progress that has already taken place, there are still many that misunderstand, misdiagnose, and do not acknowledge UAB. Today, it may still take years for a patient to be properly diagnosed and begin a management course. In time the advocacy efforts we initiate today will yield the desired results. Over the long-term, we can effectively combat the public health effects of UAB to bring the condition out into the open for discussion. Only by speaking openly about UAB and working together can we improve the welfare of UAB patients.

Appendix 1: Guide to Underactive Bladder Care (What Your Patients Should Know)

Symptoms of UAB

Each person has a different set of symptoms. Typically no two people have the same symptoms or order of their symptoms. Symptoms of UAB can include:

- *Decreased sensation that the bladder is full*
- *Small amount of urine during voiding*
- *Straining with urination:* The feeling that you have to bear down to empty your bladder
- *Double voiding*: Returning to the bathroom to urinate several minutes after voiding
- *Weak urinary stream:* Urine dribbles out
- *Urinary retention:* This is when you are unable to empty your bladder fully. Some people can only produce a "dribble" of urine. Others strain to push out urine, can't completely empty their bladder, or can't urinate at all.
- *Urinary* Incontinence*:* Urine leakage that you can't control. You may leak just a few drops of urine. Sometimes you may gush a large amount of urine. Sometimes urine will leak while you sleep.
- *Frequency:* Going to the bathroom many times during the day or night. (You may produce only small amounts of urine.) The number of times someone urinates is different from person to person. Many experts agree that going to the bathroom more than eight times in 24 hours is "frequent urination". Some people purposely urinate frequently to manage symptoms such as incontinence.
- *Recurrent (repeated) urinary tract infections* (UTI): When an infection occurs more than 2 times in 6 months or greater than 3 times in one year, this may be the first symptom of UAB. It can become a chronic illness caused by harmful bacteria, viruses or yeast growing in the urinary tract.

M.B. Chancellor, A.C. Diokno (eds.), *The Underactive Bladder*,
DOI 10.1007/978-3-319-23687-2

Treatments

Prescription medication Current treatments are limited due to the lack of consensus on the definition and the lack of research related to UAB. Presently there are three prescription medications used: Bethanechol (Urecholine, Duvoid) stimulates the nerves of the bladder to squeeze more effectively. Dosage is 10–15 mg taken three to four times daily. Side effects may limit effectiveness. Side effects include dizziness and lightheadedness, nausea, vomiting, abdominal cramps and pain, diarrhea, increased saliva, increased urination, sweating, flushing, watery eyes, and headache.

Nerve stimulation This therapy works by stimulating the sacral nerves, located near the tailbone, with mild electrical pulses. If this therapy works for you and you are able to urinate with less effort, you may want to consider having the device placed into your body. This device once implanted through a surgical procedure sends pulses of electricity to the nerves around your bladder (Chap. 8). This treatment has some success, yet it doesn't work in every case nor does it always relieve all symptoms. Because you can test it before it is implanted, many people agree to test this device.

InFlow device Women with UAB who require catheterization, either intermittently or continuously, now have an option for emptying their bladder. The FDA recently approved the InFlow device for use in the United States. The InFlow is a valve-pump device made of silicone and inserted into the urethra. At any time the woman needs to void, one can sit on a toilet, hold a remote control over the lower pelvic area, and press a button. This magnetically activates the miniature internal pump within the device, which results in the bladder emptying at a normal flow rate. When the button is released, the valve is engaged, blocking further urine flow (Chap. 10). The device must be changed every 29 days initially by a health-care provider. Family or significant other can perform future device changes. Clinical studies illustrate the effectiveness of the product as well as increasing the quality of life of the participants.

Reflex voiding double or triggered reflex voiding. Triggered reflex voiding consists of various stimulation techniques, which include squeezing the glans penis or scrotal skin, pulling the pubic hair, tapping the suprapubic area, stroking the skin of the thigh or sole of the foot, and digital rectal stimulation. If you cannot find your trigger zone, speak to a health-care professional.

Use of pads for incontinence To absorb urine leakage many people will wear incontinence pads or adult diapers. With limited incontinence treatments, these products allow many people to work, remain social, and sleep without interruption. Yet these absorbent products may result in leakage onto clothing or sheets, create skin issues such as rashes and breakdown of skin, cause infections, and can be expensive over time. Pads and diapers must be properly fitted and changed frequently to avoid these complications. There are many types of products on the market today, and many improvements in absorption and skin issues have been addressed by the manufacturers over time. As the number of baby boomers continues to rise, a larger number of consumers of such products have resulted. Should you decide to use such products, please be aware of the following:

- Disposable pads or guards
- Briefs (diapers)
- Washable underwear that is designed for use with incontinent pads
- Swimwear pads
- Incontinent pads for the bed washable or disposable
- Mattress pads

Proper fit Fit may be more important than absorbency. In order to limit leakage onto clothing, products should be properly fitted. As there are many types of products, you may want to request samples from a manufacturer or medical product supplier. You should be able to receive several types of products to try. A search on the internet using the following words "incontinence product samples" will provide you with a number of choices. By using a medical supplier, you may have the opportunity to speak with a knowledgeable representative who can provide you with more information than you would receive in the grocery store or pharmacy.

Style More absorbent products may be larger and impact your ability to wear them with regular or tight-fitting clothes. Many people choose an elastic waist brief because they can fit just like underwear making toileting a bit easier as opposed to using pads.

Costs Investigate as to whether insurance will cover the products you need. Medical suppliers know what products may be covered and with what types of insurance or health savings account programs.

Skin Care Issues

Using diapers and other products can make skin problems worse. Although they may keep bedding and clothing cleaner, these products allow urine or stool to be in constant contact with the skin. Over time, the skin breaks down. Special care must be taken to keep the skin clean and dry. This can be done by:

- Cleaning and drying the area right away after urinating or having a bowel movement
- Cleaning the skin with mild, dilute soap and water then rinsing well and gently patting dry

Use soap-free skin cleansers that do not cause dryness or irritation. Follow the product's instructions. Some products do not require rinsing. Moisturizing creams can help keep the skin moist. Avoid products that contain alcohol, which may irritate the skin. If you are receiving radiation therapy, ask your health-care provider if it is OK to use any creams or lotions.

Consider using a skin sealant or moisture barrier. Creams or ointments that contain zinc oxide, lanolin, or petrolatum form a protective barrier on the skin. Some skin care products, often in the form of a spray or a towelette, create a clear, protective film over the skin. A doctor or nurse can recommend barrier creams to help protect the skin.

Even if these products are used, the skin must still be cleaned after each episode of incontinence. Reapply the cream or ointment after cleaning and drying the skin. Incontinence problems can cause a yeast infection on the skin. This is an itchy, red, pimple-like rash. The skin may feel raw. Products are available to treat a yeast infection:

- If the skin is moist most of the time, use a powder with antifungal medication, such as nystatin. Do NOT use baby powder.
- A moisture barrier or skin sealant may be applied over the powder.
- If severe skin irritation develops, see the health-care provider.

Catheterization

Intermittent self-catheterizations to drain the bladder This is the preferred method of bladder emptying over long-term indwelling catheterization. A small plastic tube covered with lubrication is placed in the urethra to drain the bladder. If you agree to perform this, it is important to recognize that this procedure may need to be performed several times daily. Draining all the urine from the bladder allows the bladder to deflate several times daily, and this may also limit bacteria from multiplying in the bladder. Once the urine is removed, the single-use tube is then removed, and the tube should be discarded. If you cannot catheterize yourself, you may want to ask a significant other to assist you. It may be a difficult procedure (especially for women) to perform as the urethra is not as visible as it is in men. There are many types of catheters on the market, and patient preference should occur; however, insurance companies may limit the type and number that you receive.

Indwelling urethral catheter A tube is placed into the bladder through the urethra, and this catheter is held in place in the bladder by a small balloon that contains saline. The end is attached to a drainage bag that comes in many sizes. The tube needs to be changed on a monthly basis and drainage bags need to be more frequently. Complications include damage to the urethra, infection, blockages in the tube, sepsis, decreased self-esteem, impact on sexual function, odor, and daily management. Urethral catheters are not preferred for long-term use.

Suprapubic catheter Inserting a urethral catheter surgically through the abdomen into the bladder can limit the complications that occur with an indwelling urethral catheter. The same drainage systems are used as with urethral catheters. Drainage devices may be changed during the day depending on the size needed for collection, clothing choice, or activity.

External catheter for men Using a sheath and external collection device is an option for men who are incontinent; however, this is not preferred as the bladder may not fully empty. Infection, skin breakdown, lack of a good fit, urine leakage, constriction of the penis, and equipment malfunctions can occur. These treatments are unfortunately not cures. They can slow the process of bladder dysfunction and help limit the damage of UAB on the kidneys.

Catheterization can be the source of recurrent infection. The following strategies may limit infection:

- Drink sufficient amounts of water throughout the day.
- Review your diet for protein intake and make sure that you are ingesting adequate amounts. Protein is an important nutrient required for the building, maintenance, and repair of tissues in the body. The recommended daily allowance for protein for men is 56 g daily and for women is 46 g daily.
- Consider the use of cranberry supplements as research documents decreased rates of infection.
- Catheterize according to schedule determined by your health-care team.
- Use sufficient lubrication on the catheter with each catheterization.
- Clean catheter drainage bags between use.
- Proper hygiene to perineal area.
- Ensure use of lubrication to the vagina during intercourse.
- Women should void immediately upon intercourse.
- Women may want to consider vaginal estrogen.

Managing UAB Symptoms

Although medication alone may not provide adequate management of symptoms, there are other ways to help you manage your symptoms. These can include managing your diet, timed voiding, exercising, and physical therapy. All of these behavioral strategies require both time and effort. Considering that your symptoms may not have appeared overnight, they cannot go away in one day. However, with time and patience, you may find success.

Diet Diet can have a profound effect on your voiding patterns. Some symptoms may be able to be managed just by altering your diet. You may want to complete a voiding diary and monitor your fluid intake to see if you are able to find any relationship between your intake and urination or incontinence patterns. Certain foods may impact bladder function, and you may want to monitor food intake as well.

Daily fluid consumption There are many people who believe that to stay healthy you must drink at least eight glasses of water per day. Drinking that much fluid may result in urinary urgency and incontinence. Sipping on fluids all day (this is common in people who have dry mouth complaints) may also worsen symptoms. While drinking fluid over a longer period of time may reduce the frequency of voids, larger fluid volumes over a short period of time may create a need to urinate one to two hours after a large fluid intake. Since dry mouth complaints from medication or high blood glucose can create the thirst urge, the use of a moisturizing product for your mouth such as hard candy or gum such as the assortment of products by Biotene can limit dry mouth. Sugar-free products can reduce the risk of dental cavities, high glucoses, or undesirable weight gain. As fluid intake is also important in managing constipation, it is important to drink enough fluids compared to too little fluids during the day. Concentrated urine can increase the risk of recurrent infections.

Fluid intake at bedtime If you do not drink for several hours (at least 3 h) before bedtime, you may wake up fewer times at night to urinate. If your legs become swollen during the day, you may want to recline in bed or a chair with your legs elevated above your heart for several hours in the late afternoon or evening. This will help return fluids into your system and may decrease the number of times that you urinate or the amount of incontinence you experience during the night. These tactics may also help in cases where fluid retention occurs.

Caffeine Caffeine is a powerful substance that may impact bladder function. Drinking sodas, coffee, and tea can result in urgency, frequency, and/or incontinence. If you choose to limit products with caffeine to see if that can improve your symptoms, do so slowly over a period of several weeks, as strong headaches may result during the withdrawal period. Caffeine impacts bladder symptoms in overactive bladder; however, the effects of caffeine on UAB are not known at this time. Only you will be able to determine if there is improvement in your symptoms should you attempt to limit caffeine.

Alcohol Alcohol has also been shown to impact the bladder, triggering symptoms of incontinence. It may impair your level of conscience and impact your ability to toilet. In addition, it acts as a diuretic and may induce greater bladder filling up with urine and frequency of urination or incontinence.

Daily Activities

Timed voiding If you find that you are not maintaining continence and constantly rushing when you feel it's time to urinate, then urinating every two to three hours is a method that you might find effective. This timed voiding strategy can work well if you are able to remember to do this. Remember, you must REMIND yourself to use the toilet when following a pattern of timed voiding. You can do this by leaving clues at your desk, setting your watch, using the timer of your smartphone, or asking others to help you with this timed activity.

Management of bowel movements Constipation may impact bladder function, and adjusting your diet to include more fiber may be helpful. Fiber supplements can be beneficial. As fiber is not significantly digested, it binds water within the intestine, therefore softening stools especially if they are hard. Laxative may be required especially when abdominal bloating occurs. Impairments in both rectal and anal sensations, as well as impaired motor function of pelvic floor muscles and the anal sphincter, may cause bowel incontinence. Impaired mobility can cause bowel incontinence due to not having sufficient time to find a commode. As bowel incontinence can increase the risk of urinary infection and skin breakdown, this can be managed by working with your medical team and monitoring your symptoms and diet. As UAB and bowel symptoms may be related, working to have regular bowel movements may improve your bothersome urinary symptoms.

Pelvic Floor and Kegel Exercises

Kegel exercises can help make the muscles under the uterus, bladder, and bowel (large intestine) stronger. They can help both men and women who have problems with urine leakage or bowel control. A pelvic floor muscle training exercise is like pretending that you have to urinate and then holding it. You relax and tighten the muscles that control urine flow. It's important to find the right muscles to tighten.

A physical therapist or continence expert with special training related to the pelvic floor can assist you with pelvic floor muscle training to assure you do it correctly. They may use biofeedback and electrical stimulation to help find the correct muscle group to work. Biofeedback is a method of positive reinforcement. Electrodes are placed on the abdomen and along the anal area. Some therapists place a sensor in the vagina in women or the anus in men to monitor the contraction of pelvic floor muscles. A monitor will display a graph showing which muscles are contracting and which are at rest. The therapist can help find the right muscles for performing pelvic floor muscle training exercises.

The information found in this appendix is provided as an information source only and is not to be used or relied on for any diagnostic or treatment purposes. It is not intended or implied to be a substitute for professional medical advice. Please consult your health-care provider before making any health-care decisions or for guidance about specific medical conditions.

Appendix 2: Resources to Underactive Bladder Care

Public education on UAB is necessary to increase awareness and promote improved care. It is our hope that this awareness will be the catalyst to generating public interest in this condition resulting in funding for UAB research and, ultimately, a cure for this life-altering condition. Public awareness campaigns will need to be developed to emphasize the importance of this condition and improve both public and professional recognition. A number of professional organizations will be key stakeholders in expanding knowledge, especially at the grass root level. This will help to stimulate research in the commercial, public, and private funding arenas both in countries around the world (Fig. 1).

There is a critical need for more effective treatment options beyond those currently available. Improved understanding and awareness will, in turn, lead to changes in health-care policy, which could have a substantial positive impact on care for those with underactive bladder.

Resources

The Underactive Bladder Foundation. www.underactivebladder.org
National Institute on Aging (NIA). www.nia.nih.gov
National Institute of Diabetes and Digestive and Kidney Diseases (NIDDK)

Fig. 1 The Underactive Bladder Foundation (http://www.underactivebladder.org/)

M.B. Chancellor, A.C. Diokno (eds.), *The Underactive Bladder*,
DOI 10.1007/978-3-319-23687-2

www.kidney.niddk.nih.gov
Urology Care Foundation. info@urologycarefoundation.org
Simon Foundation for Continence. www.simonfoundation.org
National Association for Continence (NAFC). www.nafc.org
Caregiver Action Network (CAN). www.caregiveraction.org
Health in Aging Foundation. www.healthinagingfoundation.org
National Multiple Sclerosis Society (NMSS). www.nmss.org
United Spinal Associations. www.unitedspinal.org
Men's Health Network. www.menshealthnetwork.org
Women's Health Foundation. www.womenshealthfoundation.org
HDIS, The largest supplier of urinary products. www.HDIS.com
Har-Kel Medical Supplies, 1800-257-1830. www.harkel.com
Printable Diary. http://www.niddk.nih.gov/health-information/health-topics/urologic-disease/daily-bladder-diary/Documents/diary_508.pdf
http://nihseniorhealth.gov/talkingwithyourdoctor/planningyourdoctorvisit/keeping_track_your_medicines.pdf

MIX
Papier aus verantwortungsvollen Quellen
Paper from responsible sources
FSC® C105338

If you have any concerns about our products,
you can contact us on
ProductSafety@springernature.com

In case Publisher is established outside the EU,
the EU authorized representative is:
Springer Nature Customer Service Center GmbH
Europaplatz 3, 69115 Heidelberg, Germany

Printed by Libri Plureos GmbH
in Hamburg, Germany